T0348636

Thyroid Cancer

Editor

MINGZHAO XING

ENDOCRINOLOGY AND METABOLISM CLINICS OF NORTH AMERICA

www.endo.theclinics.com

Consulting Editor
ADRIANA G. IOACHIMESCU

March 2019 • Volume 48 • Number 1

ELSEVIER

1600 John F. Kennedy Boulevard • Suite 1800 • Philadelphia, Pennsylvania, 19103-2899

http://www.theclinics.com

ENDOCRINOLOGY AND METABOLISM CLINICS OF NORTH AMERICA Volume 48, Number 1
March 2019 ISSN 0889-8529, ISBN 13: 978-0-323-61078-0

Editor: Stacy Eastman
Developmental Editor: Meredith Madeira

© **2019 Elsevier Inc. All rights reserved.**

This periodical and the individual contributions contained in it are protected under copyright by Elsevier, and the following terms and conditions apply to their use:

Photocopying
Single photocopies of single articles may be made for personal use as allowed by national copyright laws. Permission of the Publisher and payment of a fee is required for all other photocopying, including multiple or systematic copying, copying for advertising or promotional purposes, resale, and all forms of document delivery. Special rates are available for educational institutions that wish to make photocopies for non-profit educational classroom use. For information on how to seek permission visit www.elsevier.com/permissions or call: (+44) 1865 843830 (UK)/(+1) 215 239 3804 (USA).

Derivative Works
Subscribers may reproduce tables of contents or prepare lists of articles including abstracts for internal circulation within their institutions. Permission of the Publisher is required for resale or distribution outside the institution. Permission of the Publisher is required for all other derivative works, including compilations and translations (please consult www.elsevier.com/permissions).

Electronic Storage or Usage
Permission of the Publisher is required to store or use electronically any material contained in this periodical, including any article or part of an article (please consult www.elsevier.com/permissions). Except as outlined above, no part of this publication may be reproduced, stored in a retrieval system or transmitted in any form or by any means, electronic, mechanical, photocopying, recording or otherwise, without prior written permission of the Publisher.

Notice
No responsibility is assumed by the Publisher for any injury and/or damage to persons or property as a matter of products liability, negligence or otherwise, or from any use or operation of any methods, products, instructions or ideas contained in the material herein. Because of rapid advances in the medical sciences, in particular, independent verification of diagnoses and drug dosages should be made.

Although all advertising material is expected to conform to ethical (medical) standards, inclusion in this publication does not constitute a guarantee or endorsement of the quality or value of such product or of the claims made of it by its manufacturer.

Endocrinology and Metabolism Clinics of North America (ISSN 0889-8529) is published quarterly by Elsevier Inc., 360 Park Avenue South, New York, NY 10010-1710. Months of issue are March, June, September, and December. Periodicals postage paid at New York, NY and additional mailing offices. Subscription prices are USD 371.00 per year for US individuals, USD 761.00 per year for US institutions, USD 100.00 per year for US students and residents, USD 454.00 per year for Canadian individuals, USD 941.00 per year for Canadian institutions, USD 497.00 per year for international individuals, USD 941.00 per year for international institutions, and USD 245.00 per year for international and Canadian and foreign students/residents. To receive student/resident rate, orders must be accompanied by name of affiliated institution, date of term, and the signature of program/residency coordinator on institution letterhead. Orders will be billed at individual rate until proof of status is received. Foreign air speed delivery is included in all *Clinics* subscription prices. All prices are subject to change without notice. **POSTMASTER:** Send address changes to *Endocrinology and Metabolism Clinics of North America*, Elsevier Health Sciences Division, Subscription Customer Service, 3251 Riverport Lane, Maryland Heights, MO 63043. **Customer Service: Telephone: 1-800-654-2452** (U.S. and Canada); **1-314-447-8871** (outside U.S. and Canada). **Fax: 1-314-447-8029. E-mail: journalscustomerservice-usa@elsevier.com (for print support); journalsonlinesupport-usa@elsevier.com (for online support).**

Reprints. For copies of 100 or more, of articles in this publication, please contact the Commercial Rights Department, Elsevier Inc., 360 Park Avenue South, New York, NY 10010-1710; phone: +1-212-633-3874; fax: +1-212-633-3820; E-mail: reprints@elsevier.com.

Endocrinology and Metabolism Clinics of North America is covered in *MEDLINE/PubMed (Index Medicus), EMBASE/Excerpta Medica, Current Contents/Clinical Medicine, Current Contents/Life Sciences, Science Citation Index, ISI/BIOMED, BIOSIS,* and *Chemical Abstracts.*

Contributors

CONSULTING EDITOR

ADRIANA G. IOACHIMESCU, MD, PhD, FACE
Professor of Medicine (Endocrinology) and Neurosurgery, Emory University School of Medicine, Atlanta, Georgia, USA

EDITOR

MINGZHAO XING, MD, PhD
Dean, School of Medicine, Southern University of Science and Technology, Shenzhen, Guangdong, China; Professor of Medicine, Oncology, Pathology, and Cellular and Molecular Medicine, Department of Medicine, Division of Endocrinology, Diabetes, and Metabolism, Director, The Johns Hopkins Thyroid Tumor Center, Johns Hopkins School of Medicine, Baltimore, Maryland, USA

AUTHORS

EHAB S. ALAMEER, MD
Department of Surgery, Tulane University School of Medicine, New Orleans, Louisiana, USA

ANGKOON ANUWONG, MD, FRCST, FACS
Department of Surgery, Minimally Invasive and Endocrine Surgery Division, Police General Hospital, Bangkok, Thailand

SYLVIA L. ASA, MD, PhD
Professor, Department of Laboratory Medicine and Pathobiology, University of Toronto, Toronto, Ontario, Canada

SAAD AL AWWAD, MD
Department of Surgery, Tulane University School of Medicine, New Orleans, Louisiana, USA

KEITH C. BIBLE, MD, PhD
Division of Medical Oncology, Mayo Clinic, Rochester, Minnesota, USA

BERNADETTE BIONDI, MD
Associate Professor of Endocrinology, Department of Clinical Medicine and Surgery, University of Naples Federico II, Naples, Italy

JUAN P. BRITO, MD, MSc
Division of Diabetes, Endocrinology, Metabolism, and Nutrition, Department of Medicine, Knowledge and Evaluation Research Unit, Mayo Clinic, Rochester, Minnesota, USA

ASHISH V. CHINTAKUNTLAWAR, MBBS, PhD
Division of Medical Oncology, Mayo Clinic, Rochester, Minnesota, USA

DAVID S. COOPER, MD
Division of Endocrinology, Diabetes, and Metabolism, Johns Hopkins School of Medicine, Baltimore, Maryland, USA

ROSSELLA ELISEI, MD
Endocrine Unit, Department of Clinical and Experimental Medicine, University of Pisa, Pisa, Italy

AHMAD M. ELTELETY, MBBCh, MSc, MD-PhD, MRCS (ENT)
Clinical Fellow, Endocrine Head and Neck Surgery, Otolaryngology Department, Medical College of Georgia, Augusta University, Augusta, Georgia, USA; Lecturer, Otolaryngology Department, Faculty of Medicine, Cairo University, Cairo, Arab Republic of Egypt

ROBERT L. FOOTE, MD
Department of Radiation Oncology, Mayo Clinic, Rochester, Minnesota, USA

MEGHAN E. GARSTKA, MD, MS
Department of Surgery, Tulane University School of Medicine, New Orleans, Louisiana, USA

BRYAN R. HAUGEN, MD
Professor of Medicine and Pathology, Division of Endocrinology, Metabolism and Diabetes, University of Colorado School of Medicine, Aurora, Colorado, USA

IAN D. HAY, MD, PhD, FRCP
Division of Diabetes, Endocrinology, Metabolism, and Nutrition, Department of Medicine, Mayo Clinic, Rochester, Minnesota, USA

YASUHIRO ITO, MD, PhD
Department of Surgery, Kuma Hospital, Kobe, Japan

PORNPEERA JITPRATOOM, MD, FRCST
Department of Surgery, Minimally Invasive and Endocrine Surgery Division, Police General Hospital, Bangkok, Thailand

ISARIYA JONGEKKASIT, MD, FRCST
Department of Surgery, Minimally Invasive and Endocrine Surgery Division, Police General Hospital, Bangkok, Thailand

DIPTI KAMANI, MD
Department of Otolaryngology, Division of Thyroid and Parathyroid Endocrine Surgery, Massachusetts Eye and Ear Infirmary, Boston, Massachusetts, USA

EMAD KANDIL, MD, MBA
Professor, Department of Surgery, Tulane University School of Medicine, New Orleans, Louisiana, USA

JAN L. KASPERBAUER, MD
Division of Head and Neck Surgery, Mayo Clinic, Rochester, Minnesota, USA

PAUL W. LADENSON, MD
Professor of Medicine, Division of Endocrinology, Diabetes, and Metabolism, Johns Hopkins School of Medicine, Baltimore, Maryland, USA

CAROLYN MAXWELL, MD
Associate Professor of Medicine, Division of Endocrinology and Metabolism, Stony Brook University School of Medicine, Stony Brook, New York, USA

SARAH E. MAYSON, MD
Assistant Professor of Medicine, Division of Endocrinology, Metabolism and Diabetes, University of Colorado School of Medicine, Aurora, Colorado, USA

AKIRA MIYAUCHI, MD, PhD
Department of Surgery, Kuma Hospital, Kobe, Japan

CARMELO NUCERA, MD, PhD
Laboratory of Human Thyroid Cancers Preclinical and Translational Research, Division of Experimental Pathology, Department of Pathology, Cancer Research Institute (CRI), Cancer Center, Center for Vascular Biology Research (CVBR), Beth Israel Deaconess Medical Center, Harvard Medical School, Boston, Massachusetts, USA; Broad Institute of MIT and Harvard, Cambridge, Massachusetts, USA

GREGORY W. RANDOLPH, MD, FACS, FACE
Department of Otolaryngology, Division of Thyroid and Parathyroid Endocrine Surgery, Massachusetts Eye and Ear Infirmary, Boston, Massachusetts, USA

BENJAMIN R. ROMAN, MD, MSHP
Department of Surgery, Division of Head and Neck, Memorial Sloan Kettering Cancer Center, New York, New York, USA

PRASANNA SANTHANAM, MBBS, MD
Assistant Professor of Medicine, Division of Endocrinology, Diabetes, and Metabolism, Johns Hopkins School of Medicine, Baltimore, Maryland, USA

THANYAWAT SASANAKIETKUL, MD, FRCST
Department of Surgery, Minimally Invasive and Endocrine Surgery Division, Police General Hospital, Bangkok, Thailand

CAROLYN DACEY SEIB, MD, MAS
Clinical Instructor of General Surgery, University of California, San Francisco, San Francisco, California, USA

STEVEN I. SHERMAN, MD
Naguib Samaan Distinguished Professor and Department Chair, Department of Endocrine Neoplasia and Hormonal Disorders, The University of Texas MD Anderson Cancer Center, Houston, Texas, USA

JENNIFER A. SIPOS, MD
Professor of Medicine, Division of Endocrinology and Metabolism, The Ohio State University Wexner Medical Center, Columbus, Ohio, USA

JULIE ANN SOSA, MD, MA
Leon Goldman, MD Distinguished Professor of Surgery, Chair, Department of Surgery, Professor, Department of Medicine, University of California, San Francisco, San Francisco, California, USA

DAVID J. TERRIS, MD, FACS, FACE
Regents Professor of Otolaryngology and Endocrinology, Surgical Director, Otolaryngology Department, Augusta University, Thyroid and Parathyroid Center, Augusta, Georgia, USA

R. MICHAEL TUTTLE, MD
Endocrinology Service, Department of Medicine, Memorial Sloan Kettering Cancer Center, New York, New York, USA

FERNANDA VAISMAN, MD, PhD
Endocrinology Service, Instituto Nacional do Cancer, Universidade Federal do Rio de Janeiro, Rio de Janeiro, Rio de Janeiro, Brazil

VERONICA VALVO, PhD
Laboratory of Human Thyroid Cancers Preclinical and Translational Research, Division of Experimental Pathology, Department of Pathology, Cancer Research Institute (CRI), Cancer Center, Center for Vascular Biology Research (CVBR), Beth Israel Deaconess Medical Center, Harvard Medical School, Boston, Massachusetts, USA

DOUGLAS VAN NOSTRAND, MD, FACP, FACNP
Department of Nuclear Medicine, Nuclear Medicine Research, MedStar Health Research Institute and MedStar Washington Hospital Center, Washington, DC, USA

DAVID VIOLA, MD
Endocrine Unit, Department of Clinical and Experimental Medicine, University of Pisa, Pisa, Italy

LEONARD WARTOFSKY, MD, MACP
Thyroid Cancer Research Center, MedStar Health Research Institute, Washington, DC, USA

STEVEN P. WEITZMAN, MD
Associate Professor, Department of Endocrine Neoplasia and Hormonal Disorders, The University of Texas MD Anderson Cancer Center, Houston, Texas, USA

MINGZHAO XING, MD, PhD
Dean, School of Medicine, Southern University of Science and Technology, Shenzhen, Guangdong, China; Professor of Medicine, Oncology, Pathology, and Cellular and Molecular Medicine, Department of Medicine, Division of Endocrinology, Diabetes, and Metabolism, Director, The Johns Hopkins Thyroid Tumor Center, Johns Hopkins School of Medicine, Baltimore, Maryland, USA

DORINA YLLI, MD, PhD
Thyroid Cancer Research Center, MedStar Health Research Institute, Washington, DC, USA

Contents

Thyroid cancers of follicular cell derivation provide excellent phenotype-genotype correlations. Current morphologic classifications are complex and require simplification. Benign adenomas have follicular or papillary architecture and bland cytology. Well-differentiated thyroid carcinomas exhibit follicular architecture, expansile growth, and variable cytologic atypia and invasiveness; low-risk tumors have excellent prognosis after surgical resection whereas widely-invasive and angioinvasive tumors warrant total thyroidectomy and radioablation. Papillary carcinoma is less differentiated; indolent microcarcinomas can be managed by active surveillance, whereas clinical lesions with local or distant spread require therapy. Progression gives rise to poorly differentiated and anaplastic carcinomas that are less common but far more aggressive.

The incidence of thyroid cancer worldwide has increased significantly over the past 3 decades, due predominantly to an increase in papillary thyroid cancer. Although most of these cancers are small and localized, population-based studies have documented a significant increase in thyroid cancers of all sizes and stages, in addition to incidence-based mortality for papillary thyroid cancer. This suggests that the increasing incidence of thyroid cancer is due in large part to increasing surveillance and over-diagnosis, but that there also appears to be a true increase in new cases of thyroid cancer.

Thyroid cancer is the most common endocrine malignancy. Its incidence and mortality rates have increased for patients with advanced-stage papillary thyroid cancer. The characterization of the molecular pathways essential in thyroid cancer initiation and progression has made huge progress, underlining the role of intracellular signaling to promote clonal evolution, dedifferentiation, metastasis, and drug resistance. The discovery of genetic alterations that include mutations (BRAF, hTERT), translocations, deletions (eg, 9p), and copy-number gain (eg, 1q) has provided new biological insights with clinical applications. Understanding how molecular pathways interplay is one of the key strategies to develop new therapeutic treatments and improve prognosis.

Clinical Diagnostic Evaluation of Thyroid Nodules

Carolyn Maxwell and Jennifer A. Sipos

The presence of a thyroid nodule may be recognized by the patient or the clinician on palpation of the neck or it may be an incidental finding during an imaging study for some other indication. The method of detection is less important, however, than distinguishing benign lesions from more aggressive neoplasms. This article outlines the diagnostic algorithm for the evaluation of thyroid nodules including biochemical testing, imaging, and, when appropriate, fine-needle aspiration. In addition, the authors review the natural history of benign nodules, follow-up strategies, and indications for repeat aspiration.

Sarah E. Mayson and Bryan R. Haugen

The historical management approach for many patients with indeterminate thyroid nodule fine needle aspiration cytology is a diagnostic lobectomy or thyroidectomy. However, the majority of patients undergo surgery unnecessarily, because most are proven to have benign disease on histology. Molecular testing is a diagnostic tool that can be used to help guide the clinical management of thyroid nodules with indeterminate cytology results. Testing has evolved substantially over the last decade with significant advances in testing methodology and improvements in our understanding of the genetic basis of thyroid cancer.

Fernanda Vaisman and R. Michael Tuttle

Thyroid cancer management is rapidly evolving to a personalized management approach. Risk stratification systems are designed to assist in personalized management. Differentiating patients who may benefit from aggressive therapy and intense follow-up as opposed to those who can be successfully treated with minimalized initial management options and follow-up is crucial to the development of the right treatment plan for the right patient in order to optimize initial therapy and follow-up testing. This article aims to describe and discuss the risk stratification systems currently recommended for differentiated thyroid cancer.

Mingzhao Xing

Controversies exist on how to optimally manage thyroid cancer because the prognosis is often uncertain based on clinical backgrounds. This can now be helped with prognostic genetic markers in thyroid cancer, exemplified by *BRAF* V600E and *TERT* promoter mutations, which have been well characterized and widely appreciated. The genetic duet of *BRAF* V600E/*RAS* and *TERT* promoter mutations is a most robust prognostic genetic pattern for poor prognosis of differentiated thyroid cancer. The high negative predictive values of the prognostic genetic markers are equally valuable. The best prognostic value of genetic markers in thyroid cancer is achieved through a clinical risk level-based and genotype-individualized manner.

called a true scarless surgery; however, there is a scarcity of long-term studies about its safety and feasibility. Because thyroid cancer is a slow-growing lesion, with adequate follow-up and surveillance, TOETVA is a surgical procedure for the management of low-risk DTC without any difference of surgical and oncological outcome.

normally be required to maintain a euthyroid state. The basis of this therapy is the knowledge that TSH is a growth factor for thyroid cancer, so that lower serum TSH levels might be associated with decreased disease activity. However, clinical studies have not documented improved outcomes with TSH suppression, except in patients with the most advanced disease. Furthermore, there are a number of negative outcomes related to aggressive thyroid hormone therapy, including osteoporosis, fracture, and cardiovascular disease. Therefore, a graded approach to TSH suppression is recommended by the American Thyroid Association, based on initial risk and ongoing risk assessment.

Serum thyroglobulin monitoring along with anatomic and functional imaging play key roles in the surveillance of patients with differentiated thyroid cancer after initial treatment. Among patients with a disease stage justifying thyroid remnant ablation or with suspected metastatic disease, radioiodine whole-body scans are essential in the months after surgery. For patients with low to moderate-risk cancers, ultrasonography of the neck (with measurement of serum thyroglobulin on thyroid hormone replacement) are the best initial diagnostic modalities, and are often the only tests required. In individuals suspected of having distant metastases, CT, MRI, and 18F-FDG PET can make important contributions in localizing residual disease and monitoring its progression and responses to therapy, provided they are used in the appropriate setting.

Systemic therapy options have emerged for treatment of progressive, radioiodine-refractory differentiated thyroid carcinoma. Approved therapies that target tumor angiogenesis, lenvatinib and sorafenib, improve progression-free survival and, in an older subset, lenvatinib can prolong overall survival. Treatments based on targeting specific somatic genetic alterations are also available, which potentially also may prolong progression-free survival but are not yet approved for use by the Food and Drug Administration for this specific disease. More novel approaches that may benefit select patients include resensitization therapies that allow further radioiodine utilization and new immunotherapy concepts.

Anaplastic thyroid cancer (ATC) is a devastating and usually incurable diagnosis. Clinical and pathologic diagnosis is best assessed at a tertiary center with concentrated ATC expertise. Expeditious multidisciplinary management is recommended for optimal patient outcomes. Based on multiinstitutional and population-based studies, multimodal therapy that includes chemoradiotherapy with surgery (when feasible) is the preferred

ENDOCRINOLOGY AND METABOLISM CLINICS OF NORTH AMERICA

VISIT THE CLINICS ONLINE!
Access your subscription at:
www.theclinics.com

ENDOCRINOLOGY AND
METABOLISM CLINICS OF
NORTH AMERICA

FORTHCOMING ISSUES

June 2019
Transgender Medicine
Vin Tangpricha, Editor

September 2019
Pregnancy and Endocrine Disorders
Mark E. Molitch, Editor

December 2019
Endocrine Hypertension
Amir Hamrahian, Editor

RECENT ISSUES

December 2018
Hypoparathyroidism
Michael A. Levine, Editor

September 2019
Innovations in the Management of
Neuroendocrine Tumors
Ashley Grossman, Editor

June 2018

ISSUES OF RELATED INTEREST

Hematology/Oncology Clinics, December 2018 (Vol. 32, Issue 6)
Head and Neck Cancer
Available at: http://www.theclinics.com

VISIT THE CLINICS ONLINE!
Access your subscription at:
www.theclinics.com

Foreword
Thyroid Cancer

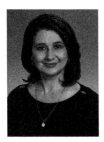

Adriana G. Ioachimescu, MD, PhD, FACE
Consulting Editor

The "Thyroid cancer" issue of the *Endocrinology and Metabolism Clinics of North America* offers a comprehensive update on a topic that underwent significant transformation in recent years. The guest editor is Mingzhao Xing, MD, PhD, Professor of Medicine, Oncology Pathology and Cellular and Molecular Medicine at Johns Hopkins University School of Medicine. Dr Xing is a distinguished researcher in the field of thyroid neoplasia whose work had an important impact on the development of molecular-based management of thyroid tumors. The authors have various backgrounds, making possible a multidisciplinary approach that contains pertinent information for endocrinologists, surgeons, pathologists, nuclear medicine specialists, oncologists, and basic scientists.

A large amount of scientific information has accumulated that facilitates risk stratification and individualized treatment plans for patients with thyroid cancer. The issue contains essential updates for medical professionals who treat this condition. For example, new information is presented regarding epidemiology, histological classification, and genetic and molecular markers used to establish the diagnosis and prognosis of thyroid nodules. The issue tackles all types of thyroid cancer, including papillary, anaplastic, and medullary. The clinical evaluation and management of patients with thyroid cancer are also thoroughly reviewed, including surgical options, radioiodine therapy, thyroid hormone suppression therapy, and new therapies for refractory cases. Last but not least, the active surveillance option of the low-risk papillary thyroid cancer patients is carefully appraised.

I hope you will find this issue of the *Endocrinology and Metabolism Clinics of North America* interesting to read and helpful in your practice. I thank Dr Xing for

Endocrinol Metab Clin N Am 48 (2019) xv–xvi
https://doi.org/10.1016/j.ecl.2018.12.002
0889-8529/19/© 2018 Published by Elsevier Inc.

guest-editing this ample issue and the authors for their excellent contributions. I would like to acknowledge the Elsevier editorial staff for their support.

Adriana G. Ioachimescu, MD, PhD, FACE
Emory University School of Medicine
1365 B Clifton Road, Northeast, B6209
Atlanta, GA 30322, USA

E-mail address:
aioachi@emory.edu

Preface

Entering an Era of Precision Management of Thyroid Cancer

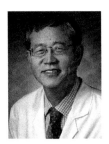

Mingzhao Xing, MD, PhD
Editor

Thyroid cancer is a common endocrine malignancy, which has seen a rapidly rising incidence and an unprecedentedly large number of accumulated living cases in recent years. The vast majority of patients with thyroid cancer have an excellent clinical prognosis. Yet, there are patients, albeit in a minority, who have poor clinical outcomes. The fate of thyroid cancer is thus not destined the same in all patients, imposing a constant challenge as to how the management of patients would be most appropriate. The classical philosophy of optimizing the management of thyroid cancer by maximizing the treatment benefits while minimizing the adverse treatment effects has evolved into today's concept of individualized precision management. It seems to have been challenging, however, to practice this apparently simple concept as until recently overtreatments of naturally low-risk cases of thyroid cancer and undertreatment of inherently aggressive cases had been common. This situation has changed today, driven by the principle of evidence-based medicine and the abundance of sound scientific and clinical data (evidence) that has occurred in recent years. Understanding of the molecular pathogenesis and mechanisms and clinical behaviors of thyroid cancer is now fundamentally better than ever, which underpins today's profoundly improved accuracy in achieving optimal management of thyroid cancer. This considerable progress has occurred virtually in all clinical aspects of thyroid cancer. These include, for example, modern histopathology classification, contemporary epidemiology, clinical and molecular diagnosis, dynamic clinical assessment, genetic-based risk stratification and management, optimal designing and performance of thyroidectomy, precise determining of neck lymph node dissection, cosmetically superior endoscopic surgical treatment, measured selection and administration of radioiodine therapy, stratified thyroid hormone suppression, cost-effective diagnostic strategy in posttreatment follow-up surveillance, extent-appropriate treatment of low-risk thyroid cancer, novel

Endocrinol Metab Clin N Am 48 (2019) xvii–xviii
https://doi.org/10.1016/j.ecl.2018.12.001
0889-8529/19/© 2018 Published by Elsevier Inc.

drug treatment of progressive differentiated thyroid cancer, and special management of anaplastic thyroid cancer and medullary thyroid cancer.

All of these areas have been comprehensively covered in the 19 articles in this issue of Elsevier's *Endocrinology and Metabolism Clinics of North America* dedicated to thyroid cancer. It is advisable that this series be read as a whole, so that it can be appreciated that all the clinical areas in the management of thyroid cancer are systemically connected while patients are managed individually. Specifically, patients with thyroid cancer are treated on a large multistep systemic management spectrum, within which specific steps are specially emphasized and precisely pursued for individual patients as the disease fits. With each of these steps, as extensively discussed in each corresponding article in this series, the principle of individualized precision management is applied.

We are now entering into an era of rapid progress and improvement in precision thyroid cancer medicine. I am honored to be invited by Elsevier as the Editor to assemble and edit this timely series dedicated to this topic. It is a great fortune to have this opportunity to work with such a distinguished panel of internationally outstanding scholarly experts in the thyroid cancer field who made this series possible. I am extremely grateful for their generous acceptance of the invitation to contribute a beautiful article in each of the important areas discussed above. I am certain that these contributions will prove to be extremely valuable references to the thyroid cancer field in the years to come. As always, science continues to progress, which constantly changes our concepts, and individual human opinion bias virtually always occurs. Therefore, readers are advised to exert their own judgment in reading, understanding, and accepting the contents in this series.

Mingzhao Xing, MD, PhD
School of Medicine
Southern University of Science and Technology
Shenzhen, Guangdong 518055, China

Department of Medicine
Johns Hopkins University School of Medicine
Baltimore, MD 21207, USA

E-mail address:
mxing1@sustc.edu.cn

The Current Histologic Classification of Thyroid Cancer

Sylvia L. Asa, MD, PhD*

KEYWORDS

- Thyroid cancer • Classification • Histomorphology • Cytology
- Genotype-phenotype correlations • Prognosis

KEY POINTS

- Genotype-phenotype correlations in differentiated thyroid tumors identify "RAS-like" follicular neoplasms or "BRAF-like" papillary carcinomas; the former are more differentiated in morphology and expression profiling.
- Follicular tumors can be benign when they lack nuclear atypia, low risk with cytologic atypia but no or minimal invasion, or aggressive invasive tumors with angioinvasion predicting distant metastasis.
- Benign tumors with papillary architecture and benign cytology account for functioning tumors that cause clinical or subclinical hyperthyroidism; they have unique mutations in the TSH receptor signaling pathway.
- Papillary carcinomas can be indolent microcarcinomas that can be subjected to active surveillance or invasive lesions that require clinical management; variants of these tumors, including hobnail, tall cell, and columnar variants, have additional genetic and/or epigenetic events accounting for aggressive behavior.
- Progression occurs in thyroid carcinomas with additional mutations, rearrangements, and/or copy number variations that give rise to poorly differentiated and anaplastic carcinomas.

INTRODUCTION

Thyroid cancer has a wide spectrum of morphologies and behaviors that include the most common and indolent tumors as well as the most aggressive and rapidly lethal malignancies. The importance of pathology in the identification, diagnosis, and

Disclosure Statement: Dr S.L. Asa is a member of the Medical Advisory Boards of Leica Biosystems Pathology Imaging and Ibex Medical Analytics. There is no conflict of interest with the material presented in this publication
Department of Laboratory Medicine and Pathobiology, University of Toronto, Elizabeth Street, Toronto, Ontario M5G 2C4, Canada
* Department of Pathology, University Health Network, 200 Elizabeth Street, 11th floor, Toronto, Ontario M5G 2C5, Canada.
E-mail addresses: sylvia.asa@utoronto.ca; Pathlady01@gmail.com

Endocrinol Metab Clin N Am 48 (2019) 1–22
https://doi.org/10.1016/j.ecl.2018.10.001
0889-8529/19/© 2018 Elsevier Inc. All rights reserved.

prognostication of thyroid cancer cannot be underestimated. The last decade has seen tremendous progress in understanding the molecular basis of thyroid cancer in a field where genotype-phenotype correlations have proven to be very tight. However, molecular studies have also shown that prognosis in this area is dependent on more than just genetic alterations. The importance of genetic and epigenetic alterations and adverse histopathologic features has emerged from multiple studies.

This review concentrates on the histologic features of tumors of thyroid follicular cell derivation. The reader is reminded that there are many other types of thyroid cancer, including medullary carcinomas that derive from parafollicular calcitonin-producing C cells, tumors that arise from parathyroids, thymus, and salivary gland structures that can be within or adjacent to the thyroid, as well as stromal malignancies, lymphoid tumors, and metastatic lesions. Discussion of all these entities is beyond the scope of this work.

In this review, the major classes of thyroid tumors of follicular cell derivation are discussed within the context of historical data, molecular correlates, and more recent information on the significance of the various components of histologic features, including architecture, growth pattern, cytology, and invasion patterns. The impact of these features on the determination of prognosis is reviewed. Advances in the understanding of the histologic types of thyroid cancer have impacted the role of cytology in screening and diagnosis, as well as the management of patients that now includes active surveillance, surgical resection that may be hemithyroidectomy or may require total thyroidectomy with or without lymph node dissection, radioactive iodine therapy or more aggressive oncologic approaches. The new risk stratifications that emerge from the revised classifications point to the need for clinicopathologic correlations, rational use of resources, and balanced management approaches that weigh patient compliance and the real and perceived risks of undertreatment and overtreatment.

MORPHOLOGIC CLASSIFICATIONS: A HISTORICAL PERSPECTIVE

The classification of thyroid cancers has undergone multiple alterations over the last century. At the time of publication of the first Armed Forces Institute of Pathology Fascicle on thyroid tumors, published in 1953, the classification of differentiated thyroid cancer was very simple (**Table 1**): there were benign and malignant tumors and they each came in 2 variants, papillary and follicular, that were distinguished based on architecture.[1,2] The classification of a lesion as malignant was dependent on identifying invasive behavior that could be infiltration of the tumor capsule, surrounding tissue and/or vessels. Interestingly, at that time, although most adenomas were follicular (**Fig. 1**), tumors classified as "papillary cystadenomas" were the second most common type of adenoma[3]; however, with reports of metastatic disease even in noninvasive papillary tumors, it soon became evident that almost any tumor with papillary architecture could metastasize. Thus, the existence of a truly benign papillary tumor

Table 1		
Classification of primary thyroid neoplasms of follicular cell derivation circa 1953		
Benign		Follicular adenoma
		Papillary cystadenoma
Malignant	Differentiated	Follicular carcinoma
		Papillary carcinoma
	Undifferentiated	Anaplastic carcinoma

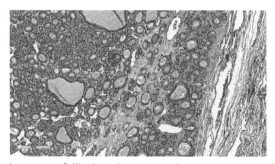

Fig. 1. Follicular adenoma. A follicular adenoma is a benign neoplasm of thyroid follicular cells. It is usually well delineated and noninvasive and is composed of follicles lined by bland epithelial cells that have monotonous nuclei that are round and dark (hematoxylin-eosin, magnification bar = 200 μm).

came into question,[4] and it was proposed that all papillary neoplasms should be classified as malignancies.[5,6] Sadly, the concept of a papillary adenoma was eliminated and has not been revived despite clear clinical and molecular data supporting its existence (**Fig. 2**) as the basis for functioning nodules.[2,7–11]

The classification based on architecture was complicated by the reality that many "papillary carcinomas" had prominent areas of follicular architecture.[12–14] Thus came the era of "mixed papillary and follicular" carcinomas, despite the fact that these tumors behaved in the same fashion as classical papillary carcinomas.

The real challenge in this field was precipitated by the recognition of the cytologic features of papillary carcinoma. The characteristic nuclear enlargement associated with clearing and peripheral margination of chromatin that provides a "ground-glass appearance" and irregular nuclear contours (**Fig. 3**) was recognized by Lindsay in 1960,[14] who reported the same nuclear alterations in tumors with follicular architecture that developed lymph node metastasis. This nuclear atypia became known as "Orphan Annie eye nuclei" because of their resemblance to the eyes of the cartoon character Little Orphan Annie, as appreciated by Nancy Warner.[15] Despite the fact that nuclear clearing may occasionally be seen as an artifact in thyroid,[16,17] nuclear atypia gained paramount importance and was reinforced by the 1977 paper by Chen and Rosai that popularized the term "follicular variant of papillary carcinoma."[18] Thus, variants of papillary carcinoma became the predominant type of thyroid cancer.

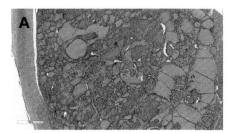
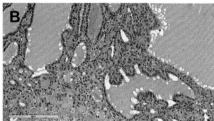

Fig. 2. Papillary adenoma. A benign tumor of follicular epithelium that is hyperactive is characterized by papillary architecture that is different from the disorganized papillae of papillary carcinoma. These tumors have true papillae, but they are organized within follicles and have a distinct centripetal orientation (A) (hematoxylin-eosin, magnification bar = 700 μm). The nuclei lining the papillae are crowded, but they remain round, relatively uniform, and basally oriented; there is striking scalloping of the colloid at the cell surface (B) (hematoxylin-eosin, magnification bar = 200 μm).

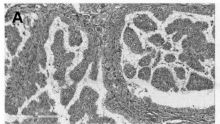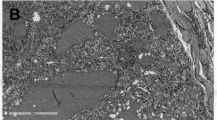

Fig. 3. Nuclear atypia in differentiated thyroid cancers. Papillary carcinoma is characterized by a constellation of nuclear features (*A*) (hematoxylin-eosin, magnification bar = 200 μm) that include enlargement, elongation, crowding, and overlapping, clearing of nucleoplasm with peripheral margination of chromatin, and irregular nuclear contours that can be seen as linear grooves or may be so florid as to cause intranuclear cytoplasmic pseudoinclusions; there are multiple micronucleoli. In follicular patterned tumors, the nuclear atypia is less florid; there is usually less crowding, overlap, and elongation, but the nuclei still have clearing with peripheral margination of chromatin and prominent, often multiple nucleoli and irregular shapes (*B*) (hematoxylin-eosin, magnification bar = 200 μm).

Poorly differentiated thyroid carcinomas were initially recognized in the 1980s as rare but aggressive forms of thyroid carcinoma that were not as undifferentiated or as rapidly lethal as anaplastic carcinoma[19,20] (**Table 2**).[21] The following decades also saw new variants of papillary carcinomas that behaved in a more aggressive way than conventional papillary thyroid carcinoma (PTCs); those included tall cell carcinomas,[22–25] the very rare columnar cell type,[26,27] and most recently, the hobnail cell variant.[28–30] Many of these arose within differentiated carcinomas, and some were associated with anaplastic dedifferentiation, paving the way for the concept of progressive dedifferentiation in thyroid carcinoma.[31]

By 2004, the World Health Organization (WHO) book on endocrine tumors[32] classified all tumors that displayed "distinctive nuclear features" as papillary carcinoma variants[32] (**Table 3**). Those nuclear features were elegantly portrayed in 3-dimensional reconstructions[33] and using stains for the nuclear membrane component emerin to highlight nuclear morphology.[34,35] Architecture became irrelevant, and because invasion was not required for papillary carcinoma, it no longer held importance for the diagnosis of malignancy. More and more follicular-patterned tumors were reclassified as papillary carcinoma, and the incidence of follicular carcinoma decreased.[36]

Table 2		
Classification of primary thyroid neoplasms of follicular cell derivation circa 1992		
Benign		Follicular adenoma • Conventional • Variants
Malignant	Differentiated	Follicular carcinoma Papillary carcinoma • Conventional • Variants
	Poorly differentiated	Insular carcinoma Others
	Undifferentiated	Anaplastic carcinoma

Adapted from Rosai J, Carcangiu ML, DeLellis RA. Tumors of the thyroid gland. atlas of tumor pathology, Third Series, Fascicle 5. Washington, DC: Armed Forces Institute of Pathology; 1992; with permission.

Table 3 Classification of primary thyroid neoplasms of follicular cell derivation circa 2004		
Benign		Follicular adenoma • Multiple variants Hyalinizing trabecular tumor
Malignant	Differentiated	Papillary carcinoma • Multiple variants Follicular carcinoma • Minimally invasive • Widely invasive
	Poorly differentiated	Poorly differentiated carcinoma
	Undifferentiated	Anaplastic carcinoma

Adapted from DeLellis RA, Lloyd RV, Heitz PU, et al. Pathology and genetics of tumours of endocrine organs. Lyon (France): IARC Press; 2004; with permission.

However, the threshold for the diagnosis of follicular variant papillary thyroid carcinoma (FVPTC) became one of the most controversial areas in pathology with significant intraobserver and interobserver variation.[37–40] In 2016, an entire study was dedicated to developing consensus for the recognition and grading of nuclear atypia.[41] Moreover, nuclear atypia of the same type is also seen in reactive settings, such as thyroiditis, where it may represent dysplasia[42] and is common at the site of previous biopsy.[43]

The classification of invasion has not generated as much controversy in the published literature. When extensive, it is not difficult to assess. However, microscopic invasion is much harder to evaluate because of several factors.[44] One important determinant of invasion is the degree of scrutiny; the more capsular tissue submitted and the more sections examined, the more likely one is to identify microscopic invasion. Another controversy is the amount of invasion required to classify a lesion as invasive: does it require full-thickness invasion or is infiltration into the capsule sufficient? Third, because the vast majority of patients now have preoperative biopsy, the distinction of true invasion from postbiopsy artifact can be difficult.[43]

When the diagnosis of malignancy in follicular neoplasms was entirely dependent on the identification of florid invasion, it appeared that papillary carcinomas were less aggressive because they manifested less vascular invasion and usually metastasized to locoregional lymph nodes, whereas invasive follicular carcinomas often involved blood vessels, metastasized hematogenously, and caused distant metastases. Thus began the belief that papillary carcinoma is the most indolent of all cancers, and that follicular carcinoma is more aggressive.

The advent of molecular tools to interrogate thyroid cancers provided the opportunity to understand the morphology of thyroid cancers based on genetic alterations and gene expression profiles, resulting in new ideas that challenge the concepts as they evolved over time.

THE IMPACT OF MOLECULAR GENETICS: GENOTYPE-PHENOTYPE CORRELATIONS

As far back as 1987, genetic alterations were identified in PTCs. The initial identification of the *RET/PTC* oncogene[45] provided evidence of chromosomal rearrangements resulting in fusion proteins that cause cell transformation. Ongoing studies added new information with rearrangements involving *TRK*[46] and *PAX8-PPARG*.[47,48] Association of thyroid cancer with previous head and neck radiation had been proven,[49–51] and the survivors of the nuclear bombs in Japan and the Chernobyl nuclear disaster provided evidence that radiation underlies these chromosomal alterations.[52–58] It soon became apparent, however, that the most common finding in sporadic papillary carcinoma was the BRAF^{V600E} activating mutation.[59–61] Thus, there were 2 pathways implicated in the development of papillary carcinomas, one based on point mutations in sporadic cancers and the other implicating radiation in gene rearrangements.[62–64]

The dominant molecular alterations identified in follicular-patterned lesions were mutations in the RAS family genes[64]; these mutations were found in tumors classified as follicular thyroid carcinomas (FTCs) and FVPTCs but also in benign follicular adenomas and even in dominant nodules of sporadic nodular goiter.[64–75] There was controversy around the importance of these RAS mutations as possibly predictive of aggressive behavior,[75] but the identification of these mutations in apparently benign lesions suggested that they are early events in thyroid follicular epithelial transformation and do not predict aggressive malignancy.

The significance of these genetic alterations was emphasized by the TCGA study of PTC.[76] This study classified tumors based on their genetic alterations and identified several novel mutations and rearrangements that are discussed in Veronica Valvo and Carmelo Nucera's article, "Coding Molecular Determinants of Thyroid Cancer Development and Progression," in this issue. A major finding is that tumors classified as PTCs fall into 2 distinct categories: "BRAF-like" tumors that exhibit either the BRAF^{V600E} mutation or several of the rearrangements, and "RAS-like" tumors that harbor RAS mutations. The BRAF-like tumors comprised classical variant PTCs with either diffuse or focal papillary architecture and usually infiltrative growth, whereas the RAS-like tumors were the well-delineated, expansile FVPTCs. Even tumors without these specific mutations or rearrangements fell into these categories in a manner that reflected their architecture. Additional insights were obtained from the expression profiling of these tumors. What became apparent was that follicular-patterned lesions are more differentiated than those with papillary architecture, a feature that should not come as a surprise to pathologists. The consistency of these findings and the similarity of FVPTCs to FTCs based on molecular profiling questions the validity of the separation of FVPTC from FTC. Indeed, a far simpler approach to this classification would be to recognize that nuclear atypia is a feature of any thyroid carcinoma, not just papillary carcinomas, and that differentiated thyroid cancers should be classified as follicular or papillary based on their architecture.[77] The natural sequelae of that proposition are that the categories of each tumor type will change, and that follicular carcinoma will increase in incidence dramatically, with a large number of low-risk cancers that may show no or only minimal invasion and only nuclear atypia.

This problem was brought to the fore by the move to reclassify noninvasive encapsulated FVPTC, which is known to be a low-risk cancer, to reduce overtreatment. This initiative, although admirable in its stated goal, resulted in a proposal to rebrand such tumors as Non-Invasive Follicular Thyroid neoplasm with Papillary-like nuclear features (NIFT-P),[41] an unfortunate name that maintains the confusion concerning the significance of nuclear atypia, and also created uncertainty when the entity was suddenly reclassified as "not cancer"[78] despite the fact that they can metastasize even when rigid criteria are applied.[79,80] The importance of not overtreating low-risk thyroid cancers is critical, but there are other ways of educating clinicians and developing guidelines for the management of low-risk disease.[81] The goal of reducing overdiagnosis is not likely to be addressed by this renaming, because the incidence of NIFT-P is not high, especially outside the United States.[79,80,82–84] Moreover, these lesions require surgery for diagnosis, and the real impact is on the use of radioactive iodine. Indeed, this reclassification does not impact the real cause of overdiagnosis that involves the early detection of microcarcinomas[85] that could be managed with active surveillance.[86]

The complexity of the current classification of thyroid cancer is seen in the 2017 WHO classification of endocrine tumors (**Table 4**).[87] The addition of multiple variants of borderline tumors, including NIFT-P and "Uncertain Malignant Potential" (UMP), provides pathologists with the opportunity to equivocate but does not offer firm guidelines on how to distinguish truly benign lesions from those that have a low but unequivocal possibility of metastatic behavior.[79,80,83]

MORPHOLOGIC PATTERNS OF THYROID CANCERS

Despite the many controversies and changes that have evolved over the past 70 years, it remains irrefutable that thyroid cancer manifests a spectrum of morphologies that correlates with clinical behavior.

Well-differentiated tumors have follicular architecture and resemble normal thyroid. They can be benign when they have no nuclear atypia (see **Fig. 1**) and no evidence of invasion into a capsule, if there is one, or into surrounding parenchyma if there is no capsule. They can be low-risk cancers when they exhibit nuclear atypia and/or minimal local invasion (**Fig. 4**). These neoplasms are diagnosed based on thorough histopathological examination[88] that can only be performed after surgical resection; the important learning for good clinical management is based on a willingness to perform hemithyroidectomy on low-risk patients (based on American Thyroid Association guidelines[81]) who have well-delineated, homogenous expansile masses on ultrasound or other imaging. High-risk follicular carcinomas are identified based on more aggressive invasion, including multifocal and gross invasion of the capsule and surrounding tissue, and/or vascular invasion (**Fig. 5**). However, even vascular invasion is the

Table 4
World Health Organization classification of primary thyroid neoplasms of follicular cell derivation 2017

Benign	Follicular adenoma	
Borderline/uncertain	Hyalinizing trabecular tumor	
	Other encapsulated follicular-patterned tumors	Follicular tumor of UMP
		Well-differentiated tumor of UMP
		NIFT-P
Malignant	PTC	Papillary carcinoma
		Follicular variant of PTC
		Encapsulated variant of PTC
		Papillary microcarcinoma
		Columnar cell variant of PTC
		Oncocytic variant of PTC
	FTC	FTC, minimally invasive
		FTC, encapsulated angioinvasive
		FTC, widely invasive
	Hürthle (oncocytic) cell tumors	Hürthle cell carcinoma
	Poorly differentiated thyroid carcinoma	
	Anaplastic thyroid carcinoma	

Adapted from Lloyd RV, Osamura RY, Kloppel G, et al. WHO classification of tumours of endocrine organs (4th edition). Lyon (France): IARC Press; 2017; with permission.

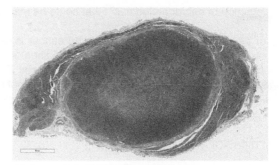

Fig. 4. Low-risk follicular carcinoma. These tumors are well delineated and may be completely encapsulated. There may be superficial invasion into the capsule but no widespread invasion and no angioinvasion (hematoxylin-eosin, magnification bar = 2 mm).

subject of controversy,[89,90] and the use of this feature to determine aggressive management requires the application of criteria that are meaningful to predict distant metastasis.[89]

Based on molecular profiling, papillary carcinoma should be considered a less well-differentiated carcinoma than follicular carcinoma. These BRAF-like tumors have at least focal if not diffuse papillary architecture and usually have florid nuclear atypia (**Fig. 6**). They are most often infiltrative but may have a well-delineated nidus or may be well-circumscribed expansile lesions or even have complete intracystic growth. Microcalcifications are common in this tumor type and are usually due to psammoma bodies that are the hallmark of classical PTC. This type of calcification is contrasted with the eggshell type of calcification that can be seen, usually at the periphery, in the capsule of any thyroid lesion. Previous studies showing that the *BRAF*^{V600E} mutation predicted worse prognosis actually are explained by the ability of this mutation to separate the classical variant PTCs from the FVPTCs[91]; however, among classical PTCs, those with the mutation are no more aggressive than those without when all other parameters, such as tumor size and patient demographics, are comparable.[92]

Most thyroid cancers with *RET/PTC* rearrangements are classical PTCs or their variants[76,93]; those with *RET/PTC3* tend to be solid variant or have solid areas.[94–96] *TRK* rearrangements tend to be more common in patients with a history of radiation and in the pediatric population.[46,50,55,58,97,98] In contrast, the *PAX8-PPARG* rearrangement, which was initially identified in follicular carcinomas,[47] is characteristically found in FVPTCs.[99] A unique form of PTC known as the diffuse sclerosing variant is a type of

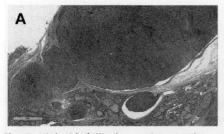
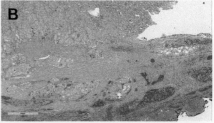

Fig. 5. High-risk follicular carcinoma. These tumors are widely invasive (*A*) (hematoxylin-eosin, magnification bar = 2 mm) and/or may exhibit invasion into vascular channels (*B*) (hematoxylin-eosin, magnification bar = 500 μm), providing evidence of the ability to give rise to distant metastases.

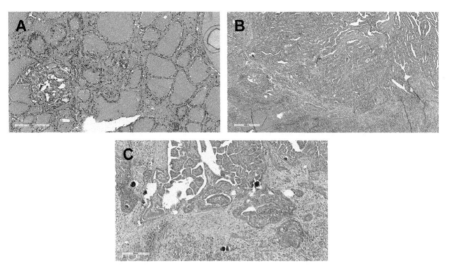

Fig. 6. Papillary carcinoma. Classical papillary carcinoma may be a small and indolent lesion that can be found incidentally as a microcarcinoma (*A*) (hematoxylin-eosin, magnification bar = 200 μm) or may be a large and infiltrative tumor. These lesions have complex papillary architecture (*B*) (hematoxylin-eosin, magnification bar = 400 μm) and may contain psammoma bodies (*C*) (hematoxylin-eosin, magnification bar = 200 μm), concentric whorls of calcification that have been considered to be degenerate tips of papillae but actually form in the cytoplasm of tumor cells that then rupture.

classical PTC that occurs usually in children and young adults. Many PTCs have stromal fibrosis and may be misdiagnosed as this variant; the true diffuse sclerosing PTC is a highly infiltrative lesion that causes thyroid enlargement but does not have a discrete central mass; it therefore may be difficult to visualize on imaging or even grossly.[100–103] While the tumor forms classical papillae, they are embedded within fibrous stroma and have a propensity to infiltrate through lymphatics, involving the entire gland and adjacent lymph nodes. Psammoma bodies are usually numerous and widespread. These lesions do not typically harbor the *BRAF*[V600E] mutation and have been reported to have gene rearrangements including *RET/PTC* and *ALK* fusions.[104–106]

Specific subtypes of papillary carcinoma are of prognostic significance, including the hobnail,[28–30] tall cell,[22–25] and columnar cell[26,27] variants (**Fig. 7**) that are thought to be more aggressive. The morphologic criteria defining these lesions are mainly cytologic: hobnail cells have apical nuclei within a surface bulge of the cell that resembles a hobnail; tall cells are defined as having a height-to-width ratio that exceeds 3:1, and columnar cells are elongated and spindle-shaped with stratified nuclei and vacuolation. There are also some architectural features that are characteristic of these tumors: tall cell PTCs have elongated "tram-track" follicles; columnar cell tumors are said to resemble endometrioid tumors, and hobnail cell tumors have large edomatous and/or fibrotic papillae. These tumors often harbor the *BRAF*[V600E] mutation and are BRAF-like lesions.[76] In addition, tall cell PTCs have epigenetic alterations that segregate them into a more aggressive subtype of PTC,[76] and they may have TERT promoter mutations that can explain more aggressive behavior.[107] Recent studies showed that hobnail cell tumors that do poorly have TERT and p53 mutations.[108,109] Poorly differentiated thyroid carcinomas (**Fig. 8**) exhibit loss of thyroid morphology and are instead composed of solid nests or trabeculae with individual tumor cell necrosis and high mitotic activity.[19,20,110,111] The solid nesting pattern resembles that

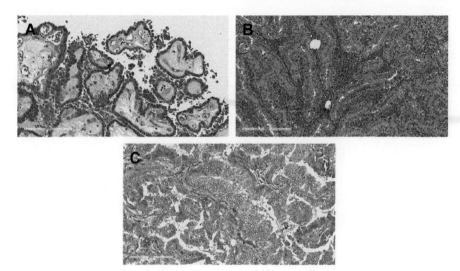

Fig. 7. Hobnail, tall cell, and columnar variants of papillary carcinoma. These variants of papillary carcinoma represent more aggressive tumors that have classical papillary architecture but are distinguished based on cytology and some unusual features. Hobnail cell tumors (A) have cells that exhibit surface extrusions resembling hobnails; they also usually have dilated edematous papillae. Tall cell tumors are composed of crowded elongated cells that have a height-to-width ratio that exceeds 3:1 (B); they also tend to form a tram-track appearance. Columnar cell tumors have significant crowding and overlap with stratified nuclei and cytoplasmic vacuolation (C) (hematoxylin-eosin, magnification bar = 200 μm).

of neuroendocrine tumors; therefore, they are also sometimes classified as "insular" carcinoma,[19] whereas the trabecular forms are more cribriform in appearance.

Anaplastic carcinomas are completely undifferentiated malignancies (**Fig. 9**) that have no features that confirm their origin in thyroid follicular epithelium; the evidence of their derivation is proven by identifying areas of differentiated and poorly differentiated thyroid carcinoma that is usually present when carefully investigated, proving that this entity arises by progressive dedifferentiation.[31] When not present, this is a diagnosis of exclusion, because they may resemble sarcomas or other lesions.

Variants of both types of differentiated thyroid cancer can be identified based on cytologic features, such as oncocytic change and clear cell change. Oncocytic and clear cell change are often associated, and although occasional tumors have clear cytoplasm due to accumulation of glycogen or lipid, most clear cell change is related to mitochondrial abnormalities. The concept that these are variants of conventional carcinomas is controversial. It is widely accepted that oncocytic change (**Fig. 10**) can be seen focally or diffusely in follicular adenomas, follicular carcinomas, and papillary carcinomas,[32] and indeed, mitochondrial DNA alterations as well as mutations in GRIM19 have been identified in such tumors associated with the usual driver alterations, including mutations and rearrangements.[112–118] It is also evident that poorly differentiated carcinoma can have extensive oncocytic change[119–121] explaining more aggressive oncocytic malignancies that have been called "Hürthle cell carcinoma" (which, incidentally, is a misnomer that should be avoided, since Karl Hürthle actually described C cells[122]). Recent studies have confirmed mitochondrial gene alterations as well as significant copy number changes in the more aggressive examples of these oncocytic poorly differentiated tumors.[123,124]

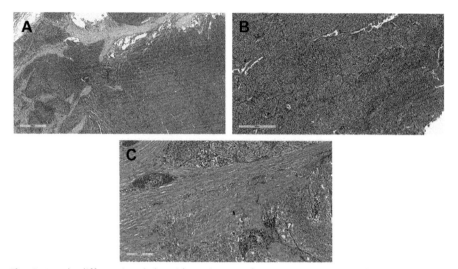

Fig. 8. Poorly differentiated thyroid carcinoma. These tumors are less differentiated than follicular or papillary carcinomas but not as undifferentiated as anaplastic carcinoma. They are usually composed of solid nests and sheets of cells that resemble neuroendocrine tumors, hence the terminology "insular" carcinoma. They are usually widely invasive (A) (hematoxylin-eosin, magnification bar = 700 μm), have individual tumor cells necrosis (B) (hematoxylin-eosin, magnification bar = 300 μm), and usually exhibit angioinvasion (C) (hematoxylin-eosin, magnification bar = 200 μm).

PROGNOSTIC FACTORS

A major clinical goal for those who manage patients with thyroid cancer is to identify morphologic and molecular features that provide the ability to identify tumors of any given type that will behave more aggressively than others.

In differentiated thyroid cancers, several biomarkers, molecular alterations, and epigenetic features, including microRNAs, have been proposed.[125] Morphologic features that predict progression are also important.[126] Clinical parameters, including age, gender, and risk factors, are also of critical relevance.[127]

It is generally accepted that size and rate of growth are important clinical parameters that distinguish a classical papillary microcarcinoma that can be subjected to

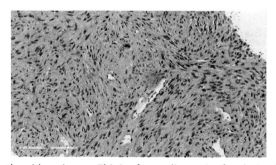

Fig. 9. Anaplastic thyroid carcinoma. This is often a diagnosis of exclusion because these tumors are composed of completely undifferentiated spindle and giant cells that lack biomarkers of thyroid differentiation; they have frequent and often atypical mitoses. The diagnosis is confirmed by the identification of differentiated elements within the lesion that prove progression from a thyroid carcinoma (hematoxylin-eosin, magnification bar = 200 μm).

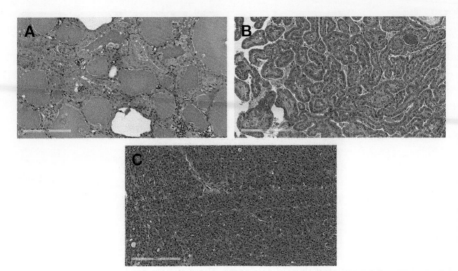

Fig. 10. Oncocytic tumors. Oncocytic change can be seen in any type of thyroid tumor, including follicular adenomas (not shown), follicular carcinoma or follicular variant papillary carcinoma (*A*), classical papillary carcinoma (*B*), and poorly differentiated carcinoma (*C*) (hematoxylin-eosin, magnification bar = 200 μm).

active surveillance from a large, infiltrative classical PTC that requires surgery.[86] Minimally invasive FTCs and encapsulated FVPTCs or NIFT-P lesions, and even low-risk classical PTCs in the clinically detectable range, can be considered adequately treated by surgical resection[41,128,129] without total thyroidectomy or lymph node dissection.[130,131] In contrast, PTCs with morphologic features, such as hobnail, tall, or columnar cell features, warrant more careful assessment to determine whether they have developed extrathyroidal extension or regional lymph node metastases. Carcinomas of either papillary or follicular type that show unequivocal angioinvasion are more likely to give rise to distant metastases.[89] Any tumor that exhibits areas of dedifferentiation should be considered for more aggressive therapy. It remains important to balance the risks of total thyroidectomy and radioactive iodine therapy with the benefit that is likely to be gained, and this requires insight into the many and various factors that alter the predicted outcome.

IMPACT ON CYTOLOGY AND SCREENING

The classification and reclassification of thyroid neoplasms have resulted in many changes to the preoperative diagnosis based on interpretation of biopsies. Most experts have moved away from the need for core biopsies that provide histology, including information about architecture and possibly even encapsulation, and instead rely on cytologic examination of fine-needle aspirations biopsies; however, both techniques can be used.[132–139]

When nuclear morphology is the key feature of malignancy, cytology can be very good at triaging malignancy from benign conditions. This technique is excellent for the diagnosis of benign thyroid lesions and for identifying unequivocal malignancies. However, the challenge in thyroid is the identification of follicular lesions with borderline cytologic atypia. In the past, thyroid cytology also was subject to variable terminologies and descriptive diagnosis. The Bethesda system and several other international initiatives were undertaken to provide categorical classifications for thyroid cytology.[140–143] These guidelines provide acceptable ranges of sensitivity and specificity. However, it is widely recognized that the performance of these criteria varies from laboratory to laboratory, and it is recommended that each laboratory provide their specific performance data to allow clinicians to interpret the results within the context of the individual laboratory.

The move to reclassify lesions as borderline has also created confusion. The sensitivity and specificity of cytologic diagnosis are dependent on how one classifies the "correct" diagnosis, which is the gold-standard, histologic final diagnosis. Laboratories are now struggling with the implications of a diagnosis of NIFT-P (or UMP)[144–147]; because these are borderline lesions, is a positive cytology a false positive or not?

The application of molecular testing can be used to guide the management of patients with thyroid nodules. The main application is for cases with indeterminate cytology. In some situations, it is remarkably helpful.[148] For example, the identification of a *BRAF^V600E* mutation can confirm the diagnosis of PTC, but this is usually not difficult in classical PTCs that have florid cytologic atypia and is therefore mainly valuable when the material is insufficient for cytologic confirmation. Similarly, the presence of a *TERT* promoter mutation or something more ominous, such as *p53* mutation or other alterations associated with more aggressive malignancy, will modify the approach to a patient with what otherwise might have been considered low-risk disease that could be treated with hemithyroidectomy. Several molecular tests have been created for clinical use, including those based on mutational analysis and others on expression profiles, and epigenetic markers, such as microRNAs.[149] Each test has strengths and limitations, with distinct positive predictive value and negative predictive value. Moreover, the added benefit is dependent on the prevalence of cancer in the cytologic category being investigated, a feature that varies widely from laboratory to laboratory.

SUMMARY

Thyroid cancer of follicular cell derivation is a spectrum of cancers that have been well characterized based on both morphology and molecular genetics. There is excellent correlation between these 2 modalities. The current classification is overly complex and requires simplification to reflect earlier insights that have been confirmed by genetics.

Fundamentally, there are benign lesions that can be follicular or papillary, the latter reflecting the "hot nodule." Well-differentiated thyroid carcinoma is follicular in architecture and expansile in growth and has a range of cytologic atypia as well as invasiveness that can be very low risk, as in NIFT-P, UMP, or minimally invasive carcinomas; these all have excellent prognosis and require surgical resection only in most cases. Once these lesions become widely invasive or angioinvasive, they are more aggressive and warrant total thyroidectomy as preparation for radioactive iodine therapy. One of the challenges in thyroid pathology is the accurate definition and identification of these 2 critical features, capsular and vascular invasion. Papillary carcinoma is a less differentiated carcinoma that includes incidental microscopic lesions that are slow growing and usually are incidental findings; these common microtumors are a source of "overdiagnosis" and "overtreatment." They can be infiltrative or circumscribed and may have calcifications in the form of psammoma bodies. The wise clinician will assess such lesions in the clinical context, and when they are clearly indolent, they are best managed conservatively. In contrast, if they have clinical evidence of growth and/or local spread, they require appropriate management with total thyroid-ectomy and radioactive iodine. Again, the challenge is to define the clinical, morpho-logic, and biomarker features that distinguish the ones that will be cured by surgery alone from those that are likely to spread. Progression is a known event in thyroid cancer, giving rise to poorly differentiated and anaplastic carcinomas that are less common but far more aggressive.

REFERENCES

1. Warren S, Meissner WA. Tumors of the thyroid gland. Atlas of tumor pathology, Series 1, Fascicle 14. Washington, DC: Armed Forces Institute of Pathology; 1953.
2. Lyons J, Landis CA, Harsh G, et al. Two G protein oncogenes in human endocrine tumors. Science 1990;249:655–9.
3. Ackerman LV. Surgical pathology. 1st edition. St Louis (MO): C.V. Mosby; 1953.
4. Ackerman LV. Surgical pathology. 2nd edition. St Louis (MO): C.V. Mosby; 1959.
5. Meissner WA, Adler A. Papillary carcinoma of the thyroid. A study of the pathology of two hundred twenty-six cases. Arch Pathol 1958;66:518–25.
6. Meissner WA, Warren S. Tumors of the thyroid gland. atlas of tumor pathology, Series 2, Fascicle 4. Washington, DC: Armed Forces Institute of Pathology; 1969.
7. Parma J, Duprez L, van Sande J, et al. Somatic mutations in the thyrotropin receptor gene cause hyperfunctioning thyroid adenomas. Nature 1993;365: 649–51.
8. Porcellini A, Ciullo I, Laviola L, et al. Novel mutations of thyrotropin receptor gene in thyroid hyperfunctioning adenomas. Rapid identification by fine needle aspiration biopsy. J Clin Endocrinol Metab 1994;79:657–61.
9. Russo D, Arturi F, Wicker R, et al. Genetic alterations in thyroid hyperfunctioning adenomas. J Clin Endocrinol Metab 1995;80:1347–51.
10. van Sande J, Parma J, Tonacchera M, et al. Genetic basis of endocrine disease. Somatic and germline mutations of the TSH receptor gene in thyroid diseases. J Clin Endocrinol Metab 1995;80:2577–85.
11. Krohn D, Fuhrer D, Holzapfel H, et al. Clonal origin of toxic thyroid nodules with constitutively activating thyrotropin receptor mutations. J Clin Endocrinol Metab 1998;83:180–4.
12. Lindsay S. Carcinoma of the thyroid gland. Springfield (IL): C.C. Thomas; 1960.
13. Lindsay S. Natural history of thyroid carcinoma. Ariz Med 1960;17:623–7.
14. Lindsay S. Carcinoma of the thyroid gland. A clinical and pathological study of 293 patients at the University of California Hospital. Springfield (IL): Charles C. Thomas; 1960.
15. DeLellis RA. Orphan Annie eye nuclei: a historical note. Am J Surg Pathol 1993; 17(10):1067–8.
16. Hapke MR, Dehner LP. The optically clear nucleus. A reliable sign of papillary carcinoma of the thyroid? Am J Surg Pathol 1979;3:31–8.
17. Petrilli G, Fisogni S, Rosai J, et al. Nuclear bubbles (nuclear pseudo-pseudoinclusions): a pitfall in the interpretation of microscopic sections from the thyroid and other human organs. Am J Surg Pathol 2017;41(1):140–1.
18. Chen KTK, Rosai J. Follicular variant of thyroid papillary carcinoma: a clinico-pathologic study of six cases. Am J Surg Pathol 1977;1(2):123–30.

19. Carcangiu ML, Zampi G, Rosai J. Poorly differentiated ("insular") thyroid carcinoma. A reinterpretation of Langhans' "wuchernde Struma". Am J Surg Pathol 1984;8:655–68.

20. Sakamoto A, Kasai N, Sugano H. Poorly differentiated carcinoma of the thyroid. A clinicopathologic entity for a high-risk group of papillary and follicular carcinomas. Cancer 1983;52:1849–55.

21. Rosai J, Carcangiu ML, DeLellis RA. Tumors of the thyroid gland. Atlas of tumor pathology, Third Series, Fascicle 5. Washington, DC: Armed Forces Institute of Pathology; 1992.

22. Hicks MJ, Batsakis JG. Tall cell carcinoma of the thyroid gland. Ann Otol Rhinol Laryngol 1993;102:402–3.

23. Flint A, Davenport RD, Lloyd RV. The tall cell variant of papillary carcinoma of the thyroid gland. Arch Pathol Lab Med 1991;115:169–71.

24. Akslen L, Varhaug JE. Thyroid carcinoma with mixed tall cell and columnar cell features. Am J Clin Pathol 1990;94:442–5.

25. Johnson TL, Lloyd RV, Thompson NW, et al. Prognostic implications of the tall cell variant of papillary thyroid carcinoma. Am J Surg Pathol 1988;12:22–7.

26. Wenig BM, Thompson LD, Adair CF, et al. Thyroid papillary carcinoma of columnar cell type: a clinicopathologic study of 16 cases. Cancer 1998;82(4): 740–53.

27. Evans HL. Columnar-cell carcinoma of the thyroid. A report of two cases of an aggressive variant of thyroid carcinoma. Am J Clin Pathol 1986;85:77–80.

28. Asioli S, Maletta F, Pagni F, et al. Cytomorphologic and molecular features of hobnail variant of papillary thyroid carcinoma: case series and literature review. Diagn Cytopathol 2014;42(1):78–84.

29. Asioli S, Erickson LA, Sebo TJ, et al. Papillary thyroid carcinoma with prominent hobnail features: a new aggressive variant of moderately differentiated papillary carcinoma. A clinicopathologic, immunohistochemical, and molecular study of eight cases. Am J Surg Pathol 2010;34(1):44–52.

30. Motosugi U, Murata S, Nagata K, et al. Thyroid papillary carcinoma with micropapillary and hobnail growth pattern: a histological variant with intermediate malignancy? Thyroid 2009;19(5):535–7.

31. Kondo T, Ezzat S, Asa SL. Pathogenetic mechanisms in thyroid follicular-cell neoplasia. Nat Rev Cancer 2006;6(4):292–306.

32. DeLellis RA, Lloyd RV, Heitz PU, et al. Pathology and genetics of tumours of endocrine organs. Lyons (France): IARC Press; 2004.

33. Papotti M, Manazza AD, Chiarle R, et al. Confocal microscope analysis and tridimensional reconstruction of papillary thyroid carcinoma nuclei. Virchows Arch 2004;444(4):350–5.

34. Asioli S, Maletta F, Pacchioni D, et al. Cytological detection of papillary thyroid carcinomas by nuclear membrane decoration with emerin staining. Virchows Arch 2010;457(1):43–51.

35. Asioli S, Bussolati G. Emerin immunohistochemistry reveals diagnostic features of nuclear membrane arrangement in thyroid lesions. Histopathology 2009; 54(5):571–9.

36. LiVolsi VA, Asa SL. The demise of follicular carcinoma of the thyroid gland. Thyroid 1994;4:233–5.

37. Hirokawa M, Carney JA, Goellner JR, et al. Observer variation of encapsulated follicular lesions of the thyroid gland. Am J Surg Pathol 2002;26(11):1508–14.

38. Lloyd RV, Erickson LA, Casey MB, et al. Observer variation in the diagnosis of follicular variant of papillary thyroid carcinoma. Am J Surg Pathol 2004;28(10): 1336–40.
39. Elsheikh TM, Asa SL, Chan JK, et al. Interobserver and intraobserver variation among experts in the diagnosis of thyroid follicular lesions with borderline nuclear features of papillary carcinoma. Am J Clin Pathol 2008;130(5):736–44.
40. Rosai J. Handling of thyroid follicular patterned lesions. Endocr Pathol 2005; 16(4):279–83.
41. Nikiforov YE, Seethala RR, Tallini G, et al. Nomenclature revision for encapsulated follicular variant of papillary thyroid carcinoma: a paradigm shift to reduce overtreatment of Indolent tumors. JAMA Oncol 2016;2(8):1023–9.
42. Chui MH, Cassol CA, Asa SL, et al. Follicular epithelial dysplasia of the thyroid: morphological and immunohistochemical characterization of a putative preneoplastic lesion to papillary thyroid carcinoma in chronic lymphocytic thyroiditis. Virchows Arch 2013;462(5):557–63.
43. LiVolsi VA, Merino MJ. Worrisome histologic alterations following fine needle aspiration of the thyroid. Pathol Annu 1994;29(2):99–120.
44. Seethala RR, Asa SL, Carty SE, et al. Protocol for the examination of specimens from patientswith carcinomas of the thyroid gland. 2014. Available at: http://www.cap.org/apps/docs/committees/cancer/cancer_protocols/2014/Thyroid_14Protocol_3100.pdf.
45. Fuoco A, Grieco M, Santoro M, et al. A new oncogene in human thyroid papillary carcinomas and their lymph-nodal metastases. Naturo 1987;328:170–2.
46. Bongarzone I, Vigneri P, Mariani L, et al. RET/NTRK1 rearrangements in thyroid gland tumors of the papillary carcinoma family: correlation with clinicopathological features. Clin Cancer Res 1998;4(1):223–8.
47. Kroll TG, Sarraf P, Pecciarini L, et al. PAX8-PPARgamma1 fusion oncogene in human thyroid carcinoma. Science 2000;289(5483):1357–60.
48. Castro P, Rebocho AP, Soares RJ, et al. PAX8-PPARã rearrangement is frequently detected in the follicular variant of papillary thyroid carcinoma. J Clin Endocrinol Metab 2006;91(1):213–20.
49. Robbins J, Schneider AB. Thyroid cancer following exposure to radioactive iodine. Rev Endocr Metab Disord 2000;1(3):197–203.
50. Bounacer A, Schlumberger M, Wicker R, et al. Search for NTRK1 proto-oncogene rearrangements in human thyroid tumours originated after therapeutic radiation. Br J Cancer 2000;82(2):308–14.
51. Ramljak V, Ranogajec I, Novosel I, et al. Thyroid tumour in a child previously treated for neuroblastoma. Cytopathology 2006;17(5):295–8.
52. Sampson RJ, Key CR, Buncher CR, et al. Thyroid carcinoma in Hiroshima and Nagasaki. I. Prevalence of thyroid carcinoma at autopsy. JAMA 1969;209(1): 65–70.
53. Ito T, Seyama T, Iwamoto KS, et al. In vitro irradiation is able to cause RET oncogene rearrangement. Cancer Res 1993;53(13):2940–3.
54. Nikiforov Y, Koshoffer A, Nikiforova M, et al. Chromosomal breakpoint positions sugeest a direct role for radiation in inducing illegitimate recombination between the ELE1 and RET genes in radiation-induced thyroid carcinomas. Oncogene 1999;18:6330–4.
55. Rabes HM, Demidchik EP, Sidorow JD, et al. Pattern of radiation-induced RET and NTRK1 rearrangements in 191 post-chernobyl papillary thyroid carcinomas: biological, phenotypic, and clinical implications. Clin Cancer Res 2000;6(3): 1093–103.

56. Williams D. Radiation carcinogenesis: lessons from Chernobyl. Oncogene 2008; 27(Suppl 2):S9–18.

57. Hamatani K, Mukai M, Takahashi K, et al. Rearranged anaplastic lymphoma kinase (ALK) gene in adult-onset papillary thyroid cancer amongst atomic bomb survivors. Thyroid 2012;22(11):1153–9.

58. Leeman-Neill RJ, Kelly LM, Liu P, et al. ETV6-NTRK3 is a common chromosomal rearrangement in radiation-associated thyroid cancer. Cancer 2014;120(6): 799–807.

59. Xu X, Quiros RM, Gattuso P, et al. High prevalence of BRAF gene mutation in papillary thyroid carcinomas and thyroid tumor cell lines. Cancer Res 2003; 63(15):4561–7.

60. Cohen Y, Xing M, Mambo E, et al. BRAF mutation in papillary thyroid carcinoma. J Natl Cancer Inst 2003;95(8):625–7.

61. Fukushima T, Suzuki S, Mashiko M, et al. BRAF mutations in papillary carcinomas of the thyroid. Oncogene 2003;22(41):6455–7.

62. Soares P, Trovisco V, Rocha AS, et al. BRAF mutations and RET/PTC rearrangements are alternative events in the etiopathogenesis of PTC. Oncogene 2003; 22(29):4578–80.

63. Nikiforova MN, Ciampi R, Salvatore G, et al. Low prevalence of BRAF mutations in radiation-induced thyroid tumors in contrast to sporadic papillary carcinomas. Cancer Lett 2004;209(1):1–6.

64. Giordano TJ, Kuick R, Thomas DG, et al. Molecular classification of papillary thyroid carcinoma: distinct BRAF, RAS, and RET/PTC mutation-specific gene expression profiles discovered by DNA microarray analysis. Oncogene 2005; 24(44):6646–56.

65. Suarez HG, du Villard JA, Caillou B, et al. Detection of activated *ras* oncogenes in human thyroid carcinomas. Oncogene 1988;2:403–6.

66. Lemoine NR, Mayall ES, Wyllie FS, et al. Activated *ras* oncogenes in human thyroid cancers. Cancer Res 1988;48:4459–63.

67. Lemoine NR, Mayall ES, Wyllie FS, et al. High frequency of *ras* oncogene activation in all stages of human thyroid tumorigenesis. Oncogene 1989;4:159–64.

68. Wright PA, Lemoine NR, Mayall ES, et al. Papillary and follicular thyroid carcinomas show a different pattern of *ras* oncogene mutation. Br J Cancer 1989; 60:576–7.

69. Namba H, Rubin SA, Fagin JA. Point mutations of ras oncogenes are an early event in thyroid tumorigenesis. Mol Endocrinol 1990;4:1474–9.

70. Suarez HG, du Villard JA, Severino M, et al. Presence of mutations in all three *ras* genes in human thyroid tumors. Oncogene 1990;5:565–70.

71. Namba H, Gutman RA, Matsuo K, et al. H-*ras* protooncogene mutations in human thyroid neoplasms. J Clin Endocrinol Metab 1990;71:223–9.

72. Karga H, Lee J-K, Vickery AL Jr, et al. *Ras* oncogene mutations in benign and malignant thyroid neoplasms. J Clin Endocrinol Metab 1991;73:832–6.

73. Schark C, Fulton N, Yashiro T, et al. The value of measurement of RAS oncogenes and nuclear DNA analysis in the diagnosis of Hürthle cell tumors of the thyroid. World J Surg 1992;16:745–52.

74. Ezzat S, Zheng L, Kolenda J, et al. Prevalence of activating ras mutations in morphologically characterized thyroid nodules. Thyroid 1996;6(5):409–16.

75. Garcia-Rostan G, Zhao H, Camp RL, et al. ras mutations are associated with aggressive tumor phenotypes and poor prognosis in thyroid cancer. J Clin Oncol 2003;21(17):3226–35.

76. The Cancer Genome Atlas Research Network. Integrated genomic characterization of papillary thyroid carcinoma. Cell 2014;159(3):676–90.

77. Asa SL, Giordano TJ, LiVolsi VA. Implications of the TCGA genomic characterization of papillary thyroid carcinoma for thyroid pathology: does follicular variant papillary thyroid carcinoma exist? Thyroid 2015;25(1):1–2.

78. Fagin JA, Wells SA Jr. Biologic and clinical perspectives on thyroid cancer. N Engl J Med 2016;375(11):1054–67.

79. Cho U, Mete O, Kim MH, et al. Molecular correlates and rate of lymph node metastasis of non-invasive follicular thyroid neoplasm with papillary-like nuclear features and invasive follicular variant papillary thyroid carcinoma: the impact of rigid criteria to distinguish non-invasive follicular thyroid neoplasm with papillary-like nuclear features. Mod Pathol 2017;30(6):810–25.

80. Parente DN, Kluijfhout WP, Bongers PJ, et al. Clinical Safety of renaming encapsulated follicular variant of papillary thyroid carcinoma: is NIFTP truly benign? World J Surg 2018;42(2):321–6.

81. Haugen BR, Alexander EK, Bible KC, et al. 2015 American Thyroid Association Management guidelines for adult patients with thyroid nodules and differentiated thyroid cancer: the american thyroid association guidelines task force on thyroid nodules and differentiated thyroid cancer. Thyroid 2016;26(1):1–133.

82. Bychkov A, Hirokawa M, Jung CK, et al. Low rate of noninvasive follicular thyroid neoplasm with papillary-like nuclear features in asian practice. Thyroid 2017; 27(7):983–4.

83. Lloyd RV, Asa SL, LiVolsi VA, et al. The evolving diagnosis of noninvasive follicular thyroid neoplasm with papillary-like nuclear features (NIFTP). Hum Pathol 2018;74:1–4.

84. Bychkov A, Jung CK, Liu Z, et al. Noninvasive follicular thyroid neoplasm with papillary-like nuclear features in asian practice: perspectives for surgical pathology and cytopathology. Endocr Pathol 2018;29(3):276–88.

85. Ahn HS, Kim HJ, Welch HG. Korea's thyroid-cancer "epidemic"–screening and overdiagnosis. N Engl J Med 2014;371(19):1765–7.

86. Ito Y, Miyauchi A, Kudo T, et al. Trends in the implementation of active surveillance for low-risk papillary thyroid microcarcinomas at kuma hospital: gradual increase and heterogeneity in the acceptance of this new management option. Thyroid 2018;28(4):488–95.

87. Lloyd RV, Osamura RY, Kloppel G, et al. WHO classification of tumours of endocrine organs. 4th edition. Lyon (France): IARC; 2017.

88. Yamashina M. Follicular neoplasms of the thyroid. Total circumferential evaluation of the fibrous capsule. Am J Surg Pathol 1992;16:392–400.

89. Mete O, Asa SL. Pathological definition and clinical significance of vascular invasion in thyroid carcinomas of follicular epithelial derivation. Mod Pathol 2011; 24(12):1545–52.

90. Wreesmann VB, Nixon IJ, Rivera M, et al. Prognostic value of vascular invasion in well-differentiated papillary thyroid carcinoma. Thyroid 2015;25(5):503–8.

91. Shi X, Liu R, Basolo F, et al. Differential clinicopathological risk and prognosis of major papillary thyroid cancer variants. J Clin Endocrinol Metab 2016;101(1): 264–74.

92. Cheng S, Serra S, Mercado M, et al. A high-throughput proteomic approach provides distinct signatures for thyroid cancer behavior. Clin Cancer Res 2011;17(8):2385–94.

93. Lubitz CC, Economopoulos KP, Pawlak AC, et al. Hobnail variant of papillary thyroid carcinoma: an institutional case series and molecular profile. Thyroid 2014; 24(6):958–65.

94. Rhoden KJ, Johnson C, Brandao G, et al. Real-time quantitative RT-PCR identifies distinct c-RET, RET/PTC1 and RET/PTC3 expression patterns in papillary thyroid carcinoma. Lab Invest 2004;84(12):1557–70.

95. Thomas GA, Bunnell H, Cook HA, et al. High prevalence of RET/PTC rearrangements in Ukrainian and Belarussian post-Chernobyl thyroid papillary carcinomas: a strong correlation between RET/PTC3 and the solid-follicular variant. J Clin Endocrinol Metab 1999;84:4232–8.

96. Powell DJJr, Russell J, Nibu K, et al. The RET/PTC3 oncogene: metastatic solid-type papillary carcinomas in murine thyroids. Cancer Res 1998;58:5523–8.

97. Prasad ML, Vyas M, Horne MJ, et al. NTRK fusion oncogenes in pediatric papillary thyroid carcinoma in northeast United States. Cancer 2016;122(7): 1097–107.

98. Greco A, Miranda C, Pierotti MA. Rearrangements of NTRK1 gene in papillary thyroid carcinoma. Mol Cell Endocrinol 2010;321(1):44–9.

99. Armstrong MJ, Yang H, Yip L, et al. PAX8/PPARgamma rearrangement in thyroid nodules predicts follicular-pattern carcinomas, in particular the encapsulated follicular variant of papillary carcinoma. Thyroid 2014;24(9):1369–74.

100. Fujimoto Y, Obara T, Ito Y, et al. Diffuse sclerosing variant of papillary carcinoa of the thyroid. Cancer 1990;66:2306–12.

101. Soares J, Limbert E, Sobrinho-Simoes M. Diffuse sclerosing variant of papillary thyroid carcinoma. A clinicopathologic study of 10 cases. Pathol Res Pract 1989;185:200–6.

102. Carcangiu ML, Bianchi S. Diffuse sclerosing variant of papillary thyroid carcinoma: clinicopathologic study of 15 cases. Am J Surg Pathol 1989;13:1041–9.

103. Chan JKC, Tsui MS, Tse CH. Diffuse sclerosing variant of papillary carcinoma of the thyroid: a histological and immunohistochemical study of three cases. Histopathology 1987;11:191–201.

104. Pillai S, Gopalan V, Smith RA, et al. Diffuse sclerosing variant of papillary thyroid carcinoma–an update of its clinicopathological features and molecular biology. Crit Rev Oncol Hematol 2015;94(1):64–73.

105. Sheu SY, Schwertheim S, Worm K, et al. Diffuse sclerosing variant of papillary thyroid carcinoma: lack of BRAF mutation but occurrence of RET/PTC rearrangements. Mod Pathol 2007;20(7):779–87.

106. Chou A, Fraser S, Toon CW, et al. A detailed clinicopathologic study of ALK-translocated papillary thyroid carcinoma. Am J Surg Pathol 2015;39(5):652–9.

107. Dettmer MS, Schmitt A, Steinert H, et al. Tall cell papillary thyroid carcinoma: new diagnostic criteria and mutations in BRAF and TERT. Endocr Relat Cancer 2015;22(3):419–29.

108. Watutantrige-Fernando S, Vianello F, Barollo S, et al. The hobnail variant of papillary thyroid carcinoma: clinical/molecular characteristics of a large monocentric series and comparison with conventional histotypes. Thyroid 2018;28(1): 96–103.

109. Cameselle-Teijeiro JM, Rodriguez-Perez I, Celestino R, et al. Hobnail variant of papillary thyroid carcinoma: clinicopathologic and molecular evidence of progression to undifferentiated carcinoma in 2 cases. Am J Surg Pathol 2017; 41(6):854–60.

110. Papotti M, Botto Micca F, Favero A, et al. Poorly differentiated thyroid carcinomas with primordial cell component. A group of aggressive lesions sharing insular, trabecular, and solid patterns. Am J Surg Pathol 1993;17:291–301.

111. Hiltzik D, Carlson DL, Tuttle RM, et al. Poorly differentiated thyroid carcinomas defined on the basis of mitosis and necrosis: a clinicopathologic study of 58 patients. Cancer 2006;106(6):1286–95.

112. Cheung CC, Ezzat S, Ramyar L, et al. Molecular basis of Hurthle cell papillary thyroid carcinoma. J Clin Endocrinol Metab 2000;85(2):878–82.

113. Maximo V, Sobrinho-Simoes M. Hurthle cell tumours of the thyroid. A review with emphasis on mitochondrial abnormalities with clinical relevance. Virchows Arch 2000;437(2):107–15.

114. Maximo V, Soares P, Lima J, et al. Mitochondrial DNA somatic mutations (point mutations and large deletions) and mitochondrial DNA variants in human thyroid pathology: a study with emphasis on Hurthle cell tumors. Am J Pathol 2002; 160(5):1857–65.

115. Chiappetta G, Toti P, Cetta F, et al. The RET/PTC oncogene is frequently activated in oncocytic thyroid tumors (Hurthle cell adenomas and carcinomas), but not in oncocytic hyperplastic lesions. J Clin Endocrinol Metab 2002;87(1): 364–9.

116. Maximo V, Botelho T, Capela J, et al. Somatic and germline mutation in GRIM-19, a dual function gene involved in mitochondrial metabolism and cell death, is linked to mitochondrion-rioh (Hurthle cell) tumours of the thyroid. Br J Cancer 2005;92(10):1892–8.

117. Bonora E, Porcelli AM, Gasparre G, et al. Defective oxidative phosphorylation in thyroid oncocytic carcinoma is associated with pathogenic mitochondrial DNA mutations affecting complexes I and III. Cancer Res 2006;66(12):6087–96.

118. Gasparre G, Porcelli AM, Bonora E, et al. Disruptive mitochondrial DNA mutations in complex I subunits are markers of oncocytic phenotype in thyroid tumors. Proc Natl Acad Sci U S A 2007;104(21):9001–6.

119. Mete O, Asa SL. Oncocytes, oxyphils, Hurthle, and Askanazy cells: morphological and molecular features of oncocytic thyroid nodules. Endocr Pathol 2010; 21(1):16–24.

120. Asa SL. My approach to oncocytic tumours of the thyroid. J Clin Pathol 2004; 57(3):225–32.

121. Bai S, Baloch ZW, Samulski TD, et al. Poorly differentiated oncocytic (hurthle cell) follicular carcinoma: an institutional experience. Endocr Pathol 2015; 26(2):164–9.

122. Hurthle K. Beitrage zur Kenntiss der Secretionsvorgangs in der Schilddruse. Arch Gesamte Physiol 1894;56:1–44.

123. Gopal RK, Kubler K, Calvo SE, et al. Widespread chromosomal losses and mitochondrial DNA alterations as genetic drivers in hurthle cell carcinoma. Cancer Cell 2018;34(2):242–55.

124. Ganly I, Makarov V, Deraje S, et al. Integrated genomic analysis of hurthle cell cancer reveals oncogenic drivers, recurrent mitochondrial mutations, and unique chromosomal landscapes. Cancer Cell 2018;34(2):256–70.

125. Asa SL, Ezzat S. The epigenetic landscape of differentiated thyroid cancer. Mol Cell Endocrinol 2018;469:3–10.

126. Papp S, Asa SL. When thyroid carcinoma goes bad: a morphological and molecular analysis. Head Neck Pathol 2015;9(1):16–23.

127. Semrad TJ, Keegan THM, Semrad A, et al. Predictors of neck reoperation and mortality after initial total thyroidectomy for differentiated thyroid cancer. Thyroid 2018;28(9):1143–52.

128. van Heerden JA, Hay ID, Goellner JR, et al. Follicular thyroid carcinoma with capsular invasion alone: a nonthreatening malignancy. Surgery 1992;112: 1130–8.

129. Goffredo P, Cheung K, Roman SA, et al. Can minimally invasive follicular thyroid cancer be approached as a benign lesion?: a population-level analysis of survival among 1,200 patients. Ann Surg Oncol 2013;20(3):767–72.

130. Hughes DT, Rosen JE, Evans DB, et al. Prophylactic central compartment neck dissection in papillary thyroid cancer and effect on locoregional recurrence. Ann Surg Oncol 2018;25(9):2526–34.

131. McHenry CR. Is prophylactic central compartment neck dissection indicated for clinically node-negative papillary thyroid cancer: the answer is dependent on how the data are interpreted and the weight given to the risks and benefits. Ann Surg Oncol 2018;25(11):3123–4.

132. Renshaw AA, Pinnar N. Comparison of thyroid fine-needle aspiration and core needle biopsy. Am J Clin Pathol 2007;128(3):370–4.

133. Strauss EB, Iovino A, Upender S. Simultaneous fine-needle aspiration and core biopsy of thyroid nodules and other superficial head and neck masses using sonographic guidance. AJR Am J Roentgenol 2008;190(6):1697–9.

134. Lieu D. Cytopathologist-performed ultrasound-guided fine-needle aspiration and core-needle biopsy: a prospective study of 500 consecutive cases. Diagn Cytopathol 2008;36(5):317–24.

135. Khoo TK, Baker CH, Hallanger-Johnson J, et al. Comparison of ultrasound-guided fine-needle aspiration biopsy with core-needle biopsy in the evaluation of thyroid nodules. Endocr Pract 2008;14(4):426–31.

136. Jung CK, Min HS, Park HJ, et al. Pathology reporting of thyroid core needle biopsy: a proposal of the Korean Endocrine Pathology Thyroid Core Needle Biopsy Study Group. J Pathol Transl Med 2015;49(4):288–99.

137. Yi KS, Kim JH, Na DG, et al. Usefulness of core needle biopsy for thyroid nodules with macrocalcifications: comparison with fine-needle aspiration. Thyroid 2015;25(6):657–64.

138. Chen BT, Jain AB, Dagis A, et al. Comparison of the efficacy and safety of ultrasound-guided core needle biopsy versus fine-needle aspiration for evaluating thyroid nodules. Endocr Pract 2015;21(2):128–35.

139. Trimboli P, Crescenzi A. Thyroid core needle biopsy: taking stock of the situation. Endocrine 2015;48(3):779–85.

140. Baloch ZW, Cibas ES, Clark DP, et al. The National Cancer Institute Thyroid fine needle aspiration state of the science conference: a summation. Cytojournal 2008;5:6.

141. Pagni F, Prada M, Goffredo P, et al. Indeterminate for malignancy' (Tir3/Thy3 in the Italian and British systems for classification) thyroid fine needle aspiration (FNA) cytology reporting: morphological criteria and clinical impact. Cytopathology 2014;25(3):170–6.

142. Pusztaszeri M, Rossi ED, Auger M, et al. The Bethesda system for reporting thyroid cytopathology: proposed modifications and updates for the second edition from an international panel. Acta Cytol 2016;60(5):399–405.

143. Satoh S, Yamashita H, Kakudo K. Thyroid cytology: the japanese system and experience at Yamashita Thyroid Hospital. J Pathol Transl Med 2017;51(6): 548–54.

144. Baloch ZW, Seethala RR, Faquin WC, et al. Noninvasive follicular thyroid neoplasm with papillary-like nuclear features (NIFTP): a changing paradigm in thyroid surgical pathology and implications for thyroid cytopathology. Cancer Cytopathol 2016;124(9):616–20.
145. Poller DN, Glaysher S. Molecular pathology and thyroid FNA. Cytopathology 2017;28(6):475–81.
146. Amendoeira I, Maia T, Sobrinho-Simoes M. Non-invasive follicular thyroid neoplasm with papillary-like nuclear features (NIFTP): impact on the reclassification of thyroid nodules. Endocr Relat Cancer 2018;25(4):R247–58.
147. Bychkov A, Keolawat S, Agarwal S, et al. Impact of non-invasive follicular thyroid neoplasm with papillary-like nuclear features on the Bethesda system for reporting thyroid cytopathology: a multi-institutional study in five Asian countries. Pathol 2018;50(4):411–7.
148. Nikiforov YE, Carty SE, Chiosea SI, et al. Impact of the multi-gene ThyroSeq next-generation sequencing assay on cancer diagnosis in thyroid nodules with Atypia of undetermined significance/follicular lesion of undetermined significance cytology. Thyroid 2015;25(11):1217–23.
149. Ferris RL, Baloch Z, Bernet V, et al. American Thyroid Association statement on surgical application of molecular profiling for thyroid nodules: current impact on perioperative decision making. Thyroid 2015;25(7):760–8.

Evolving Understanding of the Epidemiology of Thyroid Cancer

Carolyn Dacey Seib, MD, MAS[a], Julie Ann Sosa, MD, MA[b,c],*

KEYWORDS

- Thyroid cancer • Papillary thyroid cancer • Epidemiology • Incidence
- Environmental exposure

KEY POINTS

- Thyroid cancer has increased in incidence in the past 3 decades, driven largely by new cases of papillary thyroid cancer.
- The detection of small, low-risk tumors as a result of increased diagnostic imaging has contributed significantly to this rising incidence.
- Thyroid cancers of all sizes and stages are increasing in number, as is incidence-based mortality; this is consistent with there also being a true increase in the occurrence of thyroid cancer.
- Environmental exposures may be contributing to the observed increase in thyroid cancer.
- Priority should be placed on research to identify modifiable risk factors for thyroid cancer, novel therapies for advanced disease, as well as tools for risk stratification to inform individualized treatment.

INTRODUCTION

Thyroid cancer is the most common endocrine malignancy and the fastest increasing cancer in the United States.[1] It is more common in women, with a 3:1 female-to-male ratio in most geographic regions and demographic groups,[2] and it is the fifth most common cancer in women.[3] Thyroid cancer affects a younger population than most

Disclosures: Dr J.A. Sosa is a member of the Data Monitoring Committee of the Medullary Thyroid Cancer Consortium Registry supported by GlaxoSmithKline, Novo Nordisk, AstraZeneca and Eli Lilly. Dr C.D. Seib has no relevant disclosures.
[a] Department of Surgery, University of California, San Francisco, 1600 Divisadero Street, 4th Floor, Box 1674, San Francisco, CA 94143, USA; [b] Department of Surgery, University of California, San Francisco, 513 Parnassus Avenue, Suite S320, Box 0104, San Francisco, CA 94143, USA; [c] Department of Medicine, University of California, San Francisco, 513 Parnassus Avenue, Suite S320, Box 0104, San Francisco, CA 94143, USA
* Corresponding author. Department of Surgery, University of California, San Francisco, 513 Parnassus Avenue, Suite S320, Box 0104, San Francisco, CA 94143.
E-mail address: julie.sosa@ucsf.edu

Endocrinol Metab Clin N Am 48 (2019) 23–35
https://doi.org/10.1016/j.ecl.2018.10.002
0889-8529/19/© 2018 Elsevier Inc. All rights reserved.

endo.theclinics.com

malignancies, with a median age at diagnosis of 51 years, and 43% of incident cases occur in patients between 45 and 64 years.[4] Differentiated thyroid cancer refers to thyroid neoplasms derived from follicular cells, including papillary thyroid cancer (PTC), follicular thyroid cancer (FTC), and Hurthle cell cancer. PTC is the most common histologic subtype of thyroid cancer, accounting for 90% of new cases, and has the best prognosis. Thyroid cancer has an estimated 5-year survival of 98.1% overall: 99.9% for localized disease and 55.5% for distant disease.[1]

The incidence of thyroid cancer in the United States and worldwide has increased 300% over the past 3 decades, due predominantly to an increase in PTC (**Fig. 1**).[2] There has been substantial debate about whether the increase in PTC represents a true increase in incidence or whether it is attributable to increased detection and "overdiagnosis" of small, indolent PTCs that would never otherwise cause symptoms or require treatment.[5,6] An accurate assessment of factors contributing to the increased incidence of thyroid cancer is necessary to guide the evaluation of thyroid nodules and management of thyroid cancer in the future. In this review, the authors present data supporting the contribution of both increased diagnosis and a true increase in incidence of PTC. In addition, they review the main risk factors for thyroid cancer and evidence supporting the association of specific patient factors and risks in the exposome with the development of thyroid cancer.

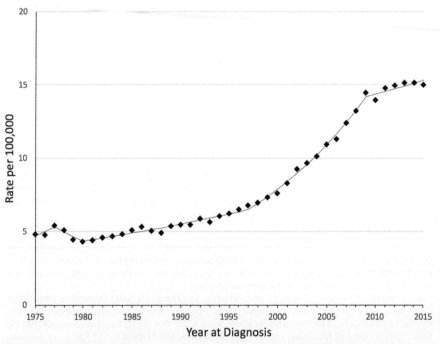

Fig. 1. Trends in total thyroid cancer age-adjusted incidence (SEER-9) from 1975 to 2015. Rates are per 100,000 and age-adjusted to the 2000 US Standard Population (Census P25 – 1130). Regression lines are calculated using the Joinpoint Regression Program Version 4.6, February 2018, National Cancer Institute. *Data from* Noone AM, Howlader N, Krapcho M, et al, editors. SEER cancer statistics review, 1975-2015. Bethesda (MD): National Cancer Institute. 2018. Available at: https://seer.cancer.gov/csr/1975_2015/, based on November 2017 SEER data submission, posted to the SEER Web site.

INCIDENCE
Thyroid Nodules

Thyroid nodules are radiographically distinct lesions within the thyroid gland that can be benign or malignant. The overwhelming majority of thyroid nodules are benign, with a malignancy rate of approximately 5% in adult patients without a history of radiation exposure.[7] The prevalence of thyroid nodules is dependent on the patient population and the method with which they are identified. Palpable thyroid nodules were historically reported in 4% to 7% of patients based on detection via physical examination,[8] but the use of ultrasonography is more sensitive and allows increased detection. Ezzat and colleagues[9] performed a prospective study of 100 patients without a history of thyroid disease and found that 21 had thyroid nodules based on physical examination, but 67 had thyroid nodules identified on ultrasound. Brander and colleagues[10] screened 253 men and women aged 19 to 50 years of age in Finland for thyroid nodules on examination and with ultrasound. The investigators found that 13 out of 253 (5.1%) had abnormal thyroid examinations based on palpation, 5 of which had normal ultrasounds; 69 out of 253 (27.3%) had ≥1 thyroid nodules,[10] demonstrating the low sensitivity of palpation as a screening tool for identifying nodules. Nodules are more common among patients of older age, female sex, and those with a history of iodine deficiency or exposure to ionizing radiation.[11–13] Bartolotta and colleagues[11] examined 704 patients without a history of thyroid disease and found incidental thyroid nodules in 31% of patients, with the highest prevalence observed in women (36% with thyroid nodules) and older patients, with nodules observed in 38.5% of men and women aged 60 to 80 years. Imaizumi and colleagues[14] evaluated the prevalence of thyroid nodules among survivors of the atomic bombings in Hiroshima and Nagasaki and identified thyroid nodules in 14% of patients overall, with a linear dose-response relationship based on estimated radiation exposure. The investigators estimated that 28% of nodules were associated with radiation exposure, but noted that survival bias relating to the delay in their analysis until more than 50 years after the nuclear incidents may have underestimated the attributable risk in this population.[14]

Improvement in the resolution of medical imaging and its increased use has contributed to an increase in the identification of thyroid nodules and, as a result, thyroid cancer.[15] Thyroid nodules are incidentally identified on up to 67% of neck ultrasounds,[9] 16% of computed tomography (CT) and MRI studies that include the neck,[16] 9% of carotid duplex studies,[17] and 2% of PET with ^{18}F-fluorodeoxyglucose (FDG-PET) scans.[18] Incidental thyroid nodules present a difficult clinical challenge because they can have a low risk of malignancy in the general population without a history of thyroid disease (range from 1.6% to 12.5% malignant[19–21]) and are often identified in older adults who are more likely to have coexisting acute or chronic illness.[22] In addition, there are not reliable or standardized methods for reporting features concerning for malignancy in nodules detected on imaging other than ultrasound, which results in variation in the workup and management of nodules identified in this manner.[23] However, the number of incidental thyroid nodules identified on diagnostic imaging studies of the head and neck in routine clinical practice is likely much less than is reported in the literature. Uppal and colleagues[24] reviewed more than 97,000 ultrasound, CT, FDG-PET, and MRI studies of the head, neck, and chest performed at a single institution from 2007 to 2012 and found 387 (0.4%) of studies reported incidental thyroid nodules. Of these nodules, 163 (42.1%) were worked up with fine-needle aspiration (FNA) biopsies, diagnosing 27 thyroid cancers (0.03% of all studies and 7.0% of reported incidentalomas).[24] When dedicated review was performed of

500 randomly selected CT scans from this sample, 10% were found to have incidental thyroid nodules, demonstrating inconsistent reporting of incidental thyroid nodules by radiologists in clinical practice.[24] Autopsy studies have shown that 50% or more of adults have thyroid nodules on postmortem examination.[25] Occult PTCs have been documented in as many as 35% of adults over the age of 60 years,[26] with a prevalence estimate of 11% based on pooled analyses.[27] The findings of these studies suggest that there is a reservoir of patients with thyroid nodules and thyroid cancers that is clinically occult, many of which are papillary thyroid microcarcinomas (measuring ≤1 cm).[23]

The increased identification of nodules on diagnostic imaging studies has coincided with increased use of thyroid FNA biopsies to obtain cytopathology for the purpose of guiding treatment recommendations, and a concurrent increase in the number of thyroid operations performed in the United States.[28] Sosa and colleagues[28] used private and public insurance claims data to document that the use of thyroid FNA doubled from 2006 to 2011, showing 16% annual growth, and coinciding with a 31% increase in the number of thyroid operations performed for thyroid nodules over the same time period. A large number of patients with incidentally discovered thyroid nodules undergo surgery as part of their workup and management, related in part to FNA results documenting indeterminate cytology results ("atypia/follicular lesion of undetermined significance" [Bethesda III] or "suspicious for follicular neoplasm" [Bethesda IV]). However, the majority are found to be benign on final pathology. Shrestha and colleagues[29] analyzed the results of all thyroid FNAs performed at a single institution over a 10-year period and found that 667 of 3013 patients (22%) underwent surgery, and only 129 of those (17.1%) were found to have thyroid cancer on final surgical pathology. Increased attention has been paid recently to reducing the need for diagnostic lobectomy, and, therefore, associated morbidity, through the use of molecular testing for indeterminate thyroid nodules.

True Incidence Versus Overdiagnosis of Thyroid Cancer

In 2006, Davies and Welch[15] published an analysis of Surveillance, Epidemiology, and End Results (SEER) data showing that from 1973 to 2002, the incidence of thyroid cancer increased 2.4-fold, from 3.6 per 100,000 to 8.7 per 100,000 people, whereas disease-specific mortality remained unchanged. The increased incidence was driven almost entirely by a 2.9-fold increase in the occurrence of PTC. In addition, they reported that between 1998 and 2002, during which data on tumor size were available, most cases involved small PTCs, with 49% of newly diagnosed cancers measuring ≤1 cm and 87% measuring ≤2 cm.[15] These results were interpreted by the investigators to ascribe the increasing numbers of thyroid cancers to the overdiagnosis of small, indolent tumors, many of which were not clinically significant and likely the result of surveillance bias.[15] One year later, Kent and colleagues[30] published a population-based study of the incidence of differentiated thyroid cancer using the Ontario Cancer Registry, including review of a random 10% sample of pathology reports from each year studied.[30] The investigators found a steady increase in the incidence of DTC from 1990 to 2001, with an overall increase per year of 13%, and significant increases seen in tumors that were ≤2 cm compared with no significant increase in the number of tumors measuring 2 to 4 cm or greater than 4 cm.[30] As a result, the investigators concurred with Davies and Welch in their assertion that the increased incidence of thyroid cancer was related to increased detection of small, subclinical tumors, which they suggested was due to increased utilization of medical imaging.[30] Significant debate has ensued regarding whether overdiagnosis alone, due in part to surveillance bias, is driving the increase in thyroid cancer incidence; resolution of this discussion has important implications for how patients with thyroid nodules and biopsy-proven thyroid cancer are managed.

The most striking example of the impact of surveillance bias on the overdiagnosis of thyroid cancer has been demonstrated in South Korea, where a national program instituted in 1999 geared toward screening for other common malignancies contributed to concurrent widespread screening for thyroid cancer by fee-for-service providers. As a result of wide implementation of screening thyroid ultrasounds, the rate of diagnosis for thyroid cancer increased 15 times from 1993 to 2011, all of which was due to PTC, and large numbers of patients received surgical management with total thyroidectomy for tumors ≤1 cm.[31] However, thyroid cancer mortality did not increase during this same time period, and the geographic distribution of the increase in incidence was highly correlated with the regional performance of screening, consistent with overdiagnosis of indolent thyroid cancers.[31] This phenomenon received wide media attention in South Korea, and in the international scientific community with a publication by Ahn and colleagues[31] in the *New England Journal of Medicine*. A follow-up publication in 2015 demonstrated a 30% reduction in the incidence of thyroid cancer and a 35% reduction in the annual number of thyroid operations, suggesting that educating patients and providers about the risks of overdiagnosis can decrease screening and reduce the number of new diagnoses of thyroid cancer.[32] Long-term data around patient outcomes will be needed to monitor the impact of these practice pattern changes in South Korea.

In 2017, the US Preventive Services Task Force (USPSTF) reviewed the evidence for thyroid cancer screening and gave the practice a grade D recommendation, indicating a moderate degree of certainty that screening with neck palpation or ultrasound has no net benefit or that its harms outweigh those benefits.[33] In their statement, the investigators acknowledged the dramatic increase in incidence of thyroid cancer but highlighted the excellent prognosis of differentiated thyroid cancer; specifically, the task force called out the results of observational studies showing no change in thyroid cancer disease-specific mortality over the same time period as evidence against screening.[33] The USPSTF literature review did not identify any randomized or high-quality trials that compared outcomes of patients who underwent thyroid cancer screening versus those who did not.[34] The USPFTF referenced the population-based observational data published by Davies and Welch[5,15,35] using SEER data and by La Vecchia and colleagues[36] using the Cancer Incidence in Five Continents database, in addition to the previously mentioned reports on occult PTCs in autopsy studies and outcomes following de facto screening in South Korea as strong support for the overdiagnosis of thyroid cancer as a problem.[34] Concern was expressed that screening would result in unnecessary operations and, as a result, complications, such as hypoparathyroidism and recurrent laryngeal nerve injury, without a survival advantage.[34]

Criticisms of this statement included a lack of emphasis placed on the importance of screening high-risk patient populations, such as those with a history of radiation exposure, a family history of thyroid cancer, or genetic syndromes associated with thyroid malignancies, as well as a failure to qualify that neck and thyroid evaluations remain important components of a general physical examination.[37] In addition, the overall conclusions of the updated USPSTF recommendation did not include data published from SEER challenging the prevailing theory that overdiagnosis is responsible for the entire increased incidence of thyroid cancer in the United States. Enewold and colleagues[38] performed a study using SEER data from 1980 to 2005 and found that although there was significant expansion in the number of small PTCs, there was also an increase in larger and more advanced stage PTCs. The investigators found that 50% of the increase in PTCs was due to tumors ≤1 cm, but that tumors greater than 2 cm accounted for 20% of the increased incidence.[38] In addition, among white women, they found a 222% increase in the incidence of tumors greater than 5 cm.[38] If the documented increase in incidence was wholly the result of overdiagnosis, it would be anticipated that all excess incidence to be attributed to small and clinically insignificant PTCs. Therefore, the key factor suggesting a true increase in the occurrence of thyroid cancer is documentation of an increase in the diagnosis of tumors of all sizes. As a result, the investigators interpreted their findings to indicate overdiagnosis alone was unlikely to account for all of the increase in incidence of thyroid cancer. Li and colleagues[39] used socioeconomic status (SES) as a surrogate for access to diagnostic technology that would increase the detection of indolent thyroid cancers in their assessment of thyroid cancer incidence using SEER data linked to the US Census database. The investigators found that there was a greater increase in the incidence of thyroid cancers measuring less than 4 cm in high SES areas compared with low SES areas (suggesting overdiagnosis in this group), but that there were similar and steady increases in the incidence of tumors greater than 4 cm in both groups when taking SES into account, suggesting a true increase in incidence of large thyroid cancers that was not related to surveillance bias.[39]

More recently, Lim and colleagues[6] evaluated trends in thyroid cancer incidence and, importantly, incidence-based mortality using data from the SEER-9 cancer registry program, which contains data that are representative of 10% of the US population, combined with mortality information from the National Center for Health Statistics. The investigators found that thyroid cancer incidence increased by 3.6% per year between 1974 and 2013, primarily due to an increase in PTC. Importantly, the investigators documented increases in PTCs of all sizes and stages, including small, localized tumors (increase in incidence of 4.6% per year) as well as larger tumors (tumors >4 cm increased by 6.1% per year).[6] In addition, PTCs with regional and distant spread both increased significantly over the time period, by 4.3% per year and 2.4% per year, respectively.[6] Incidence-based mortalities increased 1.1% per year overall, with an increase of 2.9% per year for distant stage PTCs. The investigators also documented that the incidence-based mortality of patients with smaller tumors was increasing too (≤2 cm tumors increased by 6.8% per year), suggesting a shift in the biologic profile of thyroid cancers toward a more aggressive profile in recent years.[6] Based on these data, the investigators concluded that overdiagnosis was not the only explanation for rising thyroid cancer incidence and suggested that focus be paid to understanding the drivers of increasing numbers of advanced-stage PTCs.[6] The findings of this study led to a call for further examination of the potential impact of environmental exposure on the development of thyroid cancer and focus on transdisciplinary care of patients with high-risk disease to curtail increasing mortality in this population.

Clinical Implications

Based on the above data, it can be concluded that the increasing incidence of thyroid cancer is due in large part to increasing surveillance and overdiagnosis, but that there is also a true increase in the occurrence of thyroid cancer that warrants further investigation. Recognizing that overdiagnosis is playing a contributory role, it is important that providers exercise appropriate clinical judgment in deciding when to recommend FNA of thyroid nodules. The 2015 American Thyroid Association Management Guidelines for Adult Patients with Thyroid Nodules and Differentiated Thyroid Cancer include evidence-based recommendations on this topic that should be familiar to clinicians, including recommendations to refrain from FNA of nodules less than 1 cm unless patient or other factors suggest additional risk, such as family history or radiation exposure.[40] In addition, surgeons should be up-to-date on the evidence supporting thyroid lobectomy in low-risk PTC based on long-term data showing no difference in disease-specific mortality, with the goal of minimizing complications in those with a favorable prognosis.[41] The increasing incidence of advanced thyroid cancers and associated disease-specific mortality suggests changing biology of thyroid cancer or potentially unrecognized risk factors contributing to the burden of disease. These findings also highlight the need for aggressive, transdisciplinary management of these patients, continued investigation of novel therapies for locally advanced and distant metastatic disease, and further research of environmental exposures associated with thyroid cancer. In addition, a priority should be placed on research around the identification of markers of indolent versus aggressive disease to improve the ability to prognosticate and tailor treatment strategies to the biology of an individual's thyroid cancer.

THYROID CANCER RISK FACTORS

Another factor that would be consistent with a true increase in the occurrence on thyroid cancer is the increase in known risk factors for the condition, including environmental exposures. Therefore, it is important to document changes in exposures known to be associated with thyroid cancer and new evidence for previously unknown exposures. Established risk factors for thyroid cancer include exposure to ionizing radiation, family history, sex, obesity, and alcohol and tobacco use. Recent studies also have documented an association between exposure to flame retardants and PTC.[42]

Ionizing Radiation

Exposure to environmental, diagnostic, and therapeutic ionizing radiation in childhood and adolescence is a well-established risk factor for PTC. This association was evaluated in population-based case-control studies of adolescents exposed to radiation following the Chernobyl accident, in which a dose-dependent response of exposure to risk of thyroid carcinoma was demonstrated,[43] and in those exposed as a result of the atomic bombings of Hiroshima and Nagasaki.[44] The risk of developing thyroid cancer is increased with younger age of exposure, peaks 15 to 19 years following exposure, and persists for more than 40 years after the exposure event.[45] The effect of radiation exposure on the risk of thyroid cancer has been a concern with regard to the use of diagnostic imaging in young patients. Use of CT scans for diagnostic purposes in children less than 16 years of age ranges from 3% to 16% in international studies, with imaging of the head and neck being the most common.[46] Exposure to diagnostic imaging in adults is also increasing, predominantly due to CT and nuclear medicine studies.[44] A recent meta-analysis including 9 studies from 12 publications investigating the association between exposure to ionizing radiation through diagnostic imaging and thyroid cancer risk demonstrated overall radiation exposure from CTs and dental X rays was associated with an increased risk of thyroid cancer with an odds ratio of 1.52 (05% confidence interval [CI] 1.13–2.04).[47] Limitations of this analysis and other retrospective studies include the inability to determine causation or eliminate the potential contribution of confounding related to the underlying conditions prompting imaging. However, these results suggest that increased risk of thyroid cancer should be weighed when considering diagnostic imaging that would include the thyroid in its field.

Exposure to therapeutic radiation before the age of 21 years is associated with a dose-dependent increased risk of thyroid cancer. The Childhood Cancer Survivor

Study included long-term follow-up of a cohort of patients less than 21 years of age who underwent cancer treatment between 1970 and 1986 in the United States and Canada. Evaluation of patients in this study who received radiotherapy showed an increased risk of subsequent thyroid cancer in a linear fashion up to 20 Gy, with a peak excess relative risk of 14.6.[48] In addition, the risk of thyroid cancer was highest in patients who were women and younger at the time of exposure.[48] Although a history of exposure to radiation via therapeutic or excess diagnostic imaging should certainly be incorporated into risk stratification for patients being evaluated with thyroid nodules, it is unclear whether this cause accounts for a significant proportion of the increased incidence of thyroid cancer based on changes in the genetic profile of PTCs over time. Studies analyzing PTCs that resulted from post-Chernobyl and external beam therapeutic radiation exposure have documented a large proportion of *RET/PTC* rearrangements in these cancers.[49–51] Romei and colleagues[52] compared the prevalence of BRAF V600E mutations and *RET/PTC* rearrangements in 401 PTCs from 1996 to 2000, 2001 to 2005, and 2006 to 2010 and found decreasing frequency of *RET/PTC* rearrangements over time (33%, 17%, and 9.8%, respectively) and increasing frequency of BRAF V600E mutations (28%, 48.9%, and 58.1%, respectively). The decrease in *RET/PTC* mutations suggests radiation-induced thyroid cancer does not account for the large increase in PTC incidence, suggesting the presence of additional, alternative risk factors.

Patient and Environmental Exposures

There are several patient factors and exposures that are associated with an increased risk of thyroid cancer, some of which are potentially relevant to its increasing incidence. A family history of thyroid cancer in first-degree relatives is associated with a 10-fold increased risk of nonmedullary thyroid cancer based on a large case-control study from Canada.[53] Population-based data from Sweden document a standardized incidence ratio for PTC of 3.2 for a parent and 6.2 for a sibling with a history of thyroid cancer, further documenting that this risk was increased to 11.2 for sisters.[54] Women are about 3 times more likely to develop thyroid cancer than men. However, the impact of hormonal factors that may explain the mechanism of this dominant risk factor has not been consistent or especially informative.[55] In a pooled analysis of 14 case-control studies looking at patient and environmental factors associated with thyroid cancer, the presence of a goiter and hyperthyroidism was the most strongly associated with the incidence of thyroid cancer, following the expected strong association with the presence of thyroid nodules.[55] Current tobacco use has an inverse association with thyroid cancer in a dose-dependent manner, with pooled analysis demonstrating a hazard ratio (HR) of 0.68 (95% CI 0.55–0.85) compared with never-smokers.[56] There is also an inverse association between alcohol consumption and risk of PTC, although it is less pronounced than that seen with tobacco use. Although the mechanism of these associations is unknown, further research is needed to determine if the recent decrease in prevalence of smoking and alcohol use is causally related to the increased incidence of PTC.

The prevalence of obesity has increased significantly in the United States over the last 3 decades, coinciding with trends in the incidence of thyroid cancer.[51] Population-based studies have documented that 39.8% of adults and 18.5% of children are obese.[57] The most rapid increase in rates of obesity occurred between 1992 and 2002, with rates leveling out in 2006, especially in developing countries.[58] Observational studies have shown that obesity is consistently associated with an increased risk of thyroid cancer, including PTC, FTC, and anaplastic thyroid cancer.[59] Kitahara and colleagues[60] performed a pooled analysis of 22 prospective, international studies and found that a higher baseline body mass index (BMI) was associated with an increased risk of thyroid cancer (HR per 5 kg/m^2 increase = 1.06, 95% CI 1.02-1.10), with the risk in young adulthood being more pronounced (HR per 5 kg/m^2 increase = 1.13, 95% CI 1.02–1.25). The investigators also demonstrated a more significant association between adiposity and thyroid cancer mortality, with an HR per 5 kg/m^2 increase in baseline BMI = 1.29 (95% CI 1.07–1.55).[60] In retrospective, cross-sectional studies of patients with PTC, obesity has been associated with advanced stage disease with aggressive features, and, in some cases, an increased risk of thyroid cancer recurrence.[61–63] The mechanism by which obesity and related factors contribute to thyroid cancer risk is unknown, but continued laboratory-based studies may provide more insight into the hormonal pathways involved.[64,65]

There is new evidence to suggest that exposure to specific flame retardants is associated with an increased risk of PTC. The use of flame retardants, such as polybrominated diphenyl ethers (PBDEs) and newer brominated and organophasphate flame retardants, has increased over time due to fire safety standards of furniture, electronics, and construction materials, and these compounds are commonly encountered in household dust.[42] Many flame retardants have chemical structures similar to thyroid hormone and, as a result, have been shown to alter thyroid hormone homeostasis, which led to hypothesis generation regarding their potential impact on the risk of thyroid cancer.[66,67] Hoffman and colleagues[42] performed a matched case-control study to assess the association between serum levels of 27 flame retardants and the amount of flame retardants identified in household dust and the odds of PTC. The investigators found that increased exposure to decabromodiphenyl ether (BDE-209) in household dust was associated with more than 2 times the odds of PTC, with a stronger association with smaller, less aggressive tumors, and specific organophosphate flame retardants associated with larger, more aggressive tumors. One prior study investigating the association between thyroid cancer and serum levels of a smaller subset of PBDEs alone found no significant associations.[68] However, given the contemporaneous increase in flame-retardant use and the incidence of small PTCs, further targeted investigations of this association are warranted to determine the contribution of this environmental exposure.

SUMMARY

With the increasing incidence of thyroid cancer come increased urgency to understand the factors driving this trend and evidence for how best to manage the large number of patients who will seek care. Current population-based data are consistent with a significant contribution from overdiagnosis in addition to a small but real true increase in the occurrence of PTC as well as increased incidence-based mortality. Continued investment is needed to improve the treatment of advanced disease. In addition, patient and environmental factors that may contribute to the development of thyroid cancer should be further investigated such that eliminating and mitigating exposure becomes a public health priority in at risk populations. Improved risk stratification tools will be essential to inform appropriate and individualized treatment of the increasing number of patients with thyroid cancer.

REFERENCES

1. Surveillance Research Program NCI. Fast stats: an interactive tool for access to SEER cancer statistics. Available at: https://seer.cancer.gov/faststats. Accessed August 21, 2018.

2. Kilfoy BA, Zheng T, Holford TR, et al. International patterns and trends in thyroid cancer incidence, 1973–2002. Cancer Causes Control 2009;20(5):525–31.
3. Siegel RL, Miller KD, Jemal A. Cancer statistics, 2017. CA Cancer J Clin 2017; 67(1):7–30.
4. Institute NC. SEER cancer stat facts: thyroid cancer. Available at: https://seer.cancer.gov/statfacts/html/thyro.html. Accessed August 21, 2018.
5. Davies L, Welch HG. Current thyroid cancer trends in the United States. JAMA Otolaryngol Head Neck Surg 2014;140(4):317–22.
6. Lim H, Devesa SS, Sosa JA, et al. Trends in thyroid cancer incidence and mortality in the United States, 1974-2013. JAMA 2017;317(13):1338–48.
7. Belfiore A, Giuffrida D, La Rosa GL, et al. High frequency of cancer in cold thyroid nodules occurring at young age. Acta Endocrinol (Copenh) 1989;121(2): 197–202.
8. Vander JB, Gaston EA, Dawber TR. The significance of nontoxic thyroid nodules: final report of a 15-year study of the incidence of thyroid malignancy. Ann Intern Med 1968;69(3):537–40.
9. Ezzat S, Sarti DA, Cain DR, et al. Thyroid incidentalomas: prevalence by palpation and ultrasonography. Arch Intern Med 1994;154(16):1838–40.
10. Brander A, Viikinkoski P, Nickels J, et al. Thyroid gland: US screening in a random adult population. Radiology 1991;181(3):683–7.
11. Bartolotta T, Midiri M, Runza G, et al. Incidentally discovered thyroid nodules: inoidonce, and greyscale and colour Doppler pattern in an adult population screened by real-time compound spatial sonography. Radiol Med 2006;111(7): 989–98.
12. Laurberg P, Jørgensen T, Perrild H, et al. The Danish investigation on iodine intake and thyroid disease, DanThyr: status and perspectives. Eur J Endocrinol 2006;155(2):219–28.
13. Schneider AB, Ron E, Lubin J, et al. Dose-response relationships for radiation-induced thyroid cancer and thyroid nodules: evidence for the prolonged effects of radiation on the thyroid. J Clin Endocrinol Metab 1993;77(2):362–9.
14. Imaizumi M, Tominaga T, Neriishi K, et al. Radiation dose-response relationships for thyroid nodules and autoimmune thyroid diseases in Hiroshima and Nagasaki atomic bomb survivors 55-58 years after radiation exposure. JAMA 2006;295(9): 1011–22.
15. Davies L, Welch HG. Increasing incidence of thyroid cancer in the United States, 1973-2002. JAMA 2006;295(18):2164–7.
16. Youserm D, Huang T, Loevner LA, et al. Clinical and economic impact of incidental thyroid lesions found with CT and MR. AJNR Am J Neuroradiol 1997; 18(8):1423–8.
17. Steele SR, Martin MJ, Mullenix PS, et al. The significance of incidental thyroid abnormalities identified during carotid duplex ultrasonography. Arch Surg 2005; 140(10):981–5.
18. Cohen MS, Arslan N, Dehdashti F, et al. Risk of malignancy in thyroid incidentalomas identified by fluorodeoxyglucose-positron emission tomography. Surgery 2001;130(6):941–6.
19. Smith-Bindman R, Lebda P, Feldstein VA, et al. Risk of thyroid cancer based on thyroid ultrasound imaging characteristics: results of a population-based study. JAMA Intern Med 2013;173(19):1788–95.
20. Yoon DY, Chang SK, Choi CS, et al. The prevalence and significance of incidental thyroid nodules identified on computed tomography. J Comput Assist Tomogr 2008;32(5):810–5.

21. Hoang JK, Grady AT, Nguyen XV. What to do with incidental thyroid nodules identified on imaging studies? Review of current evidence and recommendations. Curr Opin Oncol 2015;27(1):8–14.
22. Nguyen X, Choudhury KR, Eastwood J, et al. Incidental thyroid nodules on CT: evaluation of 2 risk-categorization methods for work-up of nodules. AJNR Am J Neuroradiol 2013;34(9):1812–7.
23. Grady A, Sosa J, Tanpitukpongse T, et al. Radiology reports for incidental thyroid nodules on CT and MRI: high variability across subspecialties. AJNR Am J Neuroradiol 2015;36(2):397–402.
24. Uppal A, White MG, Nagar S, et al. Benign and malignant thyroid incidentalomas are rare in routine clinical practice: a review of 97,908 imaging studies. Cancer Epidemiol Biomarkers Prev 2015;24(9):1327–31.
25. Mortensen J, Woolner LB, Bennett WA. Gross and microscopic findings in clinically normal thyroid glands. J Clin Endocrinol Metab 1955;15(10):1270–80.
26. Harach HR, Franssila KO, Wasenius VM. Occult papillary carcinoma of the thyroid. A "normal" finding in Finland. A systematic autopsy study. Cancer 1985; 56(3):531–8.
27. Furuya-Kanamori L, Bell KJL, Clark J, et al. Prevalence of differentiated thyroid cancer in autopsy studies over six decades: a meta-analysis. J Clin Oncol 2016;34(30):3672–9.
28. Sosa JA, Hanna JW, Robinson KA, et al. Increases in thyroid nodule fine-needle aspirations, operations, and diagnoses of thyroid cancer in the United States. Surgery 2013;154(6):1420–7.
29. Shrestha M, Crothers BA, Burch HB. The impact of thyroid nodule size on the risk of malignancy and accuracy of fine-needle aspiration: a 10-year study from a single institution. Thyroid 2012;22(12):1251–6.
30. Kent WD, Hall SF, Isotalo PA, et al. Increased incidence of differentiated thyroid carcinoma and detection of subclinical disease. Can Med Assoc J 2007; 177(11):1357–61.
31. Ahn HS, Kim HJ, Welch HG. Korea's thyroid-cancer "epidemic"—screening and overdiagnosis. N Engl J Med 2014;371(19):1765–7.
32. Ahn HS, Welch HG. South Korea's thyroid-cancer "epidemic"—turning the tide. N Engl J Med 2015;373(24):2389–90.
33. Bibbins-Domingo K, Grossman DC, Curry SJ, et al. Screening for thyroid cancer: US Preventive Services Task Force recommendation statement. JAMA 2017; 317(18):1882–7.
34. Lin JS, Bowles E, Williams SB, et al. Screening for thyroid cancer: updated evidence report and systematic review for the us preventive services task force. JAMA 2017;317(18):1888–903.
35. Davies L, Welch H. Thyroid cancer survival in the united states: observational data from 1973 to 2005. Arch Otolaryngol Head Neck Surg 2010;136(5):440–4.
36. La Vecchia C, Malvezzi M, Bosetti C, et al. Thyroid cancer mortality and incidence: a global overview. Int J Cancer 2015;136(9):2187–95
37. Sosa J, Duh Q, Doherty G. Striving for clarity about the best approach to thyroid cancer screening and treatment: is the pendulum swinging too far? JAMA Surg 2017;152(8):721–2.
38. Enewold L, Zhu K, Ron E, et al. Rising thyroid cancer incidence in the United States by demographic and tumor characteristics, 1980-2005. Cancer Epidemiol Biomarkers Prev 2009;18(3):784–91.
39. Li N, Du XL, Reitzel LR, et al. Impact of enhanced detection on the increase in thyroid cancer incidence in the United States: review of incidence trends by

socioeconomic status within the surveillance, epidemiology, and end results registry, 1980–2008. Thyroid 2013;23(1):103–10.

40. HaugenBryan R, AlexanderErik K, BibleKeith C, et al. 2015 American Thyroid Association management guidelines for adult patients with thyroid nodules and differentiated thyroid cancer: the American Thyroid Association guidelines task force on thyroid nodules and differentiated thyroid cancer. Thyroid 2016;26(1): 1–133.

41. Welch HG, Doherty GM. Saving thyroids — overtreatment of small papillary cancers. N Engl J Med 2018;379(4):310–2.

42. Hoffman K, Lorenzo A, Butt CM, et al. Exposure to flame retardant chemicals and occurrence and severity of papillary thyroid cancer: a case-control study. Environ Int 2017;107:235–42.

43. Cardis E, Kesminiene A, Ivanov V, et al. Risk of thyroid cancer after exposure to 131 I in childhood. J Natl Cancer Inst 2005;97(10):724–32.

44. Parker LN, Belsky JL, Yamamoto T, et al. Thyroid carcinoma after exposure to atomic radiation: a continuing survey of a fixed population, Hiroshima and Nagasaki, 1958-1971. Ann Intern Med 1974;80(5):600–4.

45. Ron E, Lubin JH, Shore RE, et al. Thyroid cancer after exposure to external radiation: a pooled analysis of seven studies. Radiat Res 1995;141(3):259–77.

46. Linet MS, pyo Kim K, Rajaraman P. Children's exposure to diagnostic medical radiation and cancer risk: epidemiologic and dosimetric considerations. Pediatr Radiol 2009;39(1):4–26.

47. Han MA, Kim JH. Diagnostic x-ray exposure and thyroid cancer risk: systematic review and meta-analysis. Thyroid 2018;28(2):220–8.

48. Bhatti P, Veiga LH, Ronckers CM, et al. Risk of second primary thyroid cancer after radiotherapy for a childhood cancer in a large cohort study: an update from the childhood cancer survivor study. Radiat Res 2010;174(6a):741–52.

49. Elisei R, Romei C, Vorontsova T, et al. RET/PTC rearrangements in thyroid nodules: studies in irradiated and not irradiated, malignant and benign thyroid lesions in children and adults. J Clin Endocrinol Metab 2001;86(7):3211–6.

50. Thomas G, Bunnell H, Cook H, et al. High prevalence of RET/PTC rearrangements in Ukrainian and Belarussian post-Chernobyl thyroid papillary carcinomas: a strong correlation between RET/PTC3 and the solid-follicular variant. J Clin Endocrinol Metab 1999;84(11):4232–8.

51. Kitahara CM, Sosa JA. The changing incidence of thyroid cancer. Nat Rev Endocrinol 2016;12(11):646.

52. Romei C, Fugazzola L, Puxeddu E, et al. Modifications in the papillary thyroid cancer gene profile over the last 15 years. J Clin Endocrinol Metab 2012;97(9): E1758–65.

53. Pal T, Vogl FD, Chappuis PO, et al. Increased risk for nonmedullary thyroid cancer in the first degree relatives of prevalent cases of nonmedullary thyroid cancer: a hospital-based study. J Clin Endocrinol Metab 2001;86(11):5307–12.

54. Hemminki K, Eng C, Chen B. Familial risks for nonmedullary thyroid cancer. J Clin Endocrinol Metab 2005;90(10):5747–53.

55. Preston-Martin S, Franceschi S, Ron E, et al. Thyroid cancer pooled analysis from 14 case–control studies: what have we learned? Cancer Causes Control 2003; 14(8):787–9.

56. Kitahara CM, Linet MS, Freeman LEB, et al. Cigarette smoking, alcohol intake, and thyroid cancer risk: a pooled analysis of five prospective studies in the United States. Cancer Causes Control 2012;23(10):1615–24.

57. Hales CM, Carroll MD, Fryar CD, et al. Prevalence of obesity among adults and youth: United States, 2015-2016. NCHS data brief, no 288. Hyattsville, MD: National Center for Health Statistics; 2017.
58. Ng M, Fleming T, Robinson M, et al. Global, regional, and national prevalence of overweight and obesity in children and adults during 1980–2013: a systematic analysis for the Global Burden of Disease Study 2013. Lancet 2014;384(9945): 766–81.
59. Schmid D, Ricci C, Behrens G, et al. Adiposity and risk of thyroid cancer: a systematic review and meta-analysis. Obes Rev 2015;16(12):1042–54.
60. Kitahara CM, McCullough ML, Franceschi S, et al. Anthropometric factors and thyroid cancer risk by histological subtype: pooled analysis of 22 prospective studies. Thyroid 2016;26(2):306–18.
61. Kim HJ, Kim NK, Choi JH, et al. Associations between body mass index and clinico-pathological characteristics of papillary thyroid cancer. Clin Endocrinol 2013; 78(1):134–40.
62. Trésallet C, Seman M, Tissier F, et al. The incidence of papillary thyroid carcinoma and outcomes in operative patients according to their body mass indices. Surgery 2014;156(5):1145–52.
63. Harari A, Endo B, Nishimoto S, et al. Risk of advanced papillary thyroid cancer in obese patients. Arch Surg 2012;147(9):805–11.
64. Pazaitou-Panayiotou K, Polyzos S, Mantzoros C. Obesity and thyroid cancer: epidemiologic associations and underlying mechanisms. Obes Rev 2013; 14(12):1006–22.
65. Malaguarnera R, Vella V, Nicolosi ML, et al. Insulin resistance: any role in the changing epidemiology of thyroid cancer? Front Endocrinol (Lausanne) 2017;8: 314.
66. Mughal BB, Demeneix BA. Endocrine disruptors: flame retardants and increased risk of thyroid cancer. Nat Rev Endocrinol 2017;13(11):627.
67. Liu S, Zhao G, Li J, et al. Association of polybrominated diphenylethers (PBDEs) and hydroxylated metabolites (OH-PBDEs) serum levels with thyroid function in thyroid cancer patients. Environ Res 2017;159:1–8.
68. Aschebrook-Kilfoy B, DellaValle CT, Purdue M, et al. Polybrominated diphenyl ethers and thyroid cancer risk in the Prostate, Colorectal, Lung, and Ovarian Cancer Screening Trial cohort. Am J Epidemiol 2015;181(11):883–8.

Coding Molecular Determinants of Thyroid Cancer Development and Progression

Veronica Valvo, PhD[a,b], Carmelo Nucera, MD, PhD[a,b,c],*

KEYWORDS

- BRAF[V600E] • Thyroid carcinoma • hTERT • PAX8/PPRγ • CDKN2A • RAS
- Microenvironment

KEY POINTS

- BRAF[V600E], RAS, RET/PTC, and PAX8/PPARγ are the most characterized genetic alterations responsible for thyroid tumorigenesis, causing deregulation of MAPK (MEK1/2 and ERK1/2) and PI3K-AKT intracellular signaling.
- In the past years, other genetic alterations have been reported, including hTERT mutations.
- Accumulation of multiple mutations involving different pathways can lead to thyroid cancer progression.
- Whole genome sequencing has shed light on unknown genetic landscape, unraveling novel genomic alterations.

INTRODUCTION

Thyroid cancer not only is the most common malignancy of the endocrine system but also shows an increased incidence rate,[1] overall increasing 3% annually.[2] The incidence-based mortality is typically low; however, from 1994 to 2013 an increase of approximately 1.1% per year[2] has been observed.

[a] Laboratory of Human Thyroid Cancers Preclinical and Translational Research, Division of Experimental Pathology, Department of Pathology, Cancer Research Institute (CRI), Cancer Center, Beth Israel Deaconess Medical Center, Harvard Medical School, 99 Brookline Avenue, Boston, MA 02215, USA; [b] Department of Pathology, Center for Vascular Biology Research (CVBR), Beth Israel Deaconess Medical Center, Harvard Medical School, 99 Brookline Avenue, Boston, MA 02215, USA; [c] Broad Institute of MIT and Harvard, 415 Main Street, Cambridge, MA 02142, USA
* Corresponding author. Laboratory of Human Thyroid Cancers Preclinical and Translational Research, Division of Experimental Pathology, Department of Pathology, Cancer Research Institute (CRI), Cancer Center, Center for Vascular Biology Research (CVBR), Beth Israel Deaconess Medical Center, Harvard Medical School, RN270G, 99 Brookline Avenue, Boston, MA 02215.
E-mail address: cnucera@bidmc.harvard.edu

Endocrinol Metab Clin N Am 48 (2019) 37–59
https://doi.org/10.1016/j.ecl.2018.10.003
0889-8529/19/© 2018 Elsevier Inc. All rights reserved.

According to the cellular origin, thyroid cancer is classified in 2 main histologic types. Parafollicular or C cells have a neuroendocrine function, the production and secretion of calcitonin hormone, and originate medullary thyroid cancer, a small fraction of all malignancies (3%–5%), whereas most malignancies arise from follicular cells, responsible for thyroid hormone synthesis. Follicular cell-derived tumors are subsequently divided into subtypes according to their differentiation: differentiated thyroid cancer (DTC) that includes papillary thyroid cancer (PTC) (80%–85%) and follicular thyroid cancer (FTC) (10%–15%); poorly differentiated thyroid cancer (PDTC); and anaplastic thyroid cancer (ATC) (collectively 1%–2%).[3] Conventional treatment of thyroid malignancy is characterized by surgical thyroidectomy followed by adjuvant radioiodine ablation in the case of radioiodine uptake in the tumor foci.[4] Unfortunately, recurrences are not infrequent, with high risk of long distance metastasis.[4] In the past 10 years, the understanding of the molecular mechanisms that occur to thyroid cancer pathogenesis has greatly increased, which has led to the continuous discovery of new therapeutic strategies. This article addresses the important developments toward greater knowledge of genetic alterations of molecular determinants with coding capabilities (oncogenic proteins, mutant tumor suppressors) in follicular-derived thyroid cancers.

GENETIC ALTERATIONS IN EARLY THYROID TUMORIGENESIS
Gene Mutations

BRAF
BRAF belongs to a family of serine/threonine kinases and works as downstream effector of RAS. BRAF transmits the signal through the mitogen-activated protein kinase (MAPK) pathway that has a fundamental role in promoting cell proliferation and survival.[5] In physiologic conditions, MAPK signaling has a negative feedback mechanism mediated by ERK1/2, the principal downstream effector.[6] In 2002, the T1799A point mutation located in the exon 15 *BRAF* gene was first described in several human malignancies.[7] In the presence of this missense nucleotide substitution, the residue 600 switches from glutamic acid to valine and causes the constitutive serine/threonine kinase activity with loss of inhibition loop. BRAF^{V600E} is the most frequent genetic alteration in melanoma,[8] hairy cell leukemia,[9] and PTC.[10,11] PDTC and ATC also harbor BRAF^{V600E} with high prevalence (~33% and ~45%, respectively),[12] but the mutation is absent in FTC.[13] A less prevalent BRAF point mutation has been described in K601E residue in follicular thyroid adenoma (FTA)[14] and follicular variant of PTC.[15,16] Generally, tumors harboring this mutation show a follicular pattern and have a better clinical outcome.[16]

The presence of BRAF^{V600E} in micro-PTC suggests its role as driver in thyroid tumor initiation.[13] In fact, BRAF^{V600E} conditional expression is able to induce dedifferentiation and genomic instability in rat normal thyroid cells.[17] Moreover, BRAF^{V600E} detection in PTC has been significantly associated with increased mortality[18] and poorer clinicopathologic outcomes, including increased aggressiveness, risk of recurrence, loss of radioiodine avidity, and eventually, therapy failure.[19] Transgenic mice carrying BRAF^{V600E} mutation and xenograft tumor models confirmed its essential role in the carcinogenic process and development of aggressive features.[20,21] Given the high relevance of this genetic alteration, the clonality of BRAF^{V600E} has been debated, because studies were reporting discordant results.[22,23] A more conclusive evidence from TCGA genome sequencing has provided that BRAF^{V600E} is a driving mutation clonally present in the PTC cells.[10,23]

Importantly, BRAF^{V600E} is also deeply involved in the modulation of microenvironment to promote tumor progression and aggressiveness.[24] BRAF^{V600E} modifies immune cells infiltration in PTC and correlated with increased levels of some chemokines.[25,26] Furthermore, BRAF[V600E] PTC more often express high levels of immunosuppressive ligands programmed death ligand 1 (53% vs 12.5%) and human leukocyte antigen G (41% vs 12.5%) compared with BRAF wild-type tumors.[27] Importantly, RNAseq analysis has linked BRAF[V600E] with overall decreased expression of immune and inflammatory response genes compared with BRAF[WT], leading to the hypothesis of a general immune escape mechanism operated by this oncogene.[28] Moreover, the overexpression of vascular endothelial growth factor A (VEGFA),[29] metalloproteinase,[30] fibronectin and vimentin,[31] transforming growth factor beta (TGF-β),[24,32,33] thrombospondin 1 (TSP-1),[24] and p21-activated kinase[34] have been correlated to BRAF[V600E]. It is clear that the interplay between thyroid tumor cells and microenvironment is crucial to determine tumor aggressiveness and progression. Tumor cells and microenvironment stromal cells can interact through paracrine and autocrine signaling loops stimulating tumor progression. A recent study showed that tumor microenvironment pericytes play an essential role in protecting human thyroid cancer cells against therapy targeting BRAF[V600E] (ie, vemurafenib) and tyrosine kinases (TKs) (ie, sorafenib) via TSP-1/TGF-β1 axis[35] (**Fig. 1**). Specifically, pericytes were able to secrete both TSP-1 and TGF-β1, triggering drug resistance. BRAF[WT/V600E]-PTC clinical samples were enriched in pericytes, and TSP-1 and TGF-β1 expression evoked gene-regulatory networks and pathways in the microenvironment essential for BRAF[V600E]-PTC cell survival. Critically, antagonism of the TSP-1/TGF-β1 axis reduced tumor cell growth and overcomes drug resistance.[35] Antagonizing this molecular pathway may represent a novel therapeutic translational approach against BRAF[WT/V600E]-PTC resistant to targeted therapies.

BRAF[V600E] could also be responsible for some clinical symptoms: in ATC, the production and secretion of different angiogenic and proinflammatory key factors (eg, VEGFA, VEGFC, interleukin-6 [IL-6]) may contribute to the worsening of pathologic features, such as cachexia (the result of complex metabolic alterations that cause morbidity).[36] Overall, these results highlight the complexity of tumor interaction with the microenvironment, and how this interplay can affect thyroid cancer progression and consequently patient prognosis.

RAS

RAS is a G protein or guanosine-nucleotide-binding protein; specifically, RAS proteins belong to the small GTPases family, and they are upstream to several intracellular signaling pathways.[37] The GTP bounding promotes their activation; RAS proteins

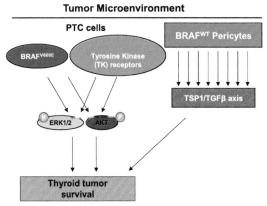

Fig. 1. Role of pericytes in tumor microenvironment in promoting thyroid cancer cell survival via the TSP1/TGF-β1 axis.

have an intrinsic hydrolysis activity that hydrolyzes a bound GTP molecule into GDP, which brings it back to the inactive state.[38] RAS mutations occur in thyroid carcinomas.[39–41] Point mutations in 3 different codons (12, 13, and 61) are associated constitutive aberrant activation of downstream effectors.[42] This protein family is composed of 3 genes: HRAS, KRAS, and NRAS. All 3 mutant RAS are associated with cancer, including thyroid cancer.[39,43–45] Both MAPK and PI3K (phosphatidylinositol-3-kinase)-AKT pathways are regulated by RAS, and thyroid tumors with RAS mutations also show overactivation of PI3K-AKT.[46,47] Intriguingly, RAS mutations are more frequent in follicular variant of PTC or FTC than classical PTC.[10,44,47–51] Follicular variant of PTC can harbor RAS mutations.[52] However, noninvasive follicular thyroid neoplasm with papillary-like nuclear features, which have a very low risk of adverse outcome, also showed RAS mutations.[53] RAS oncogene activation might play a role in early events of thyroid tumorigenesis, inducing proliferation in normal human thyroid epithelial cells without loss of differentiation cells.[54,55] Interestingly, studies from a transgenic mouse model confirmed that mutant KRAS requires additional genetic alterations (such as PTEN deletion) to develop thyroid cancer, leading to invasive and metastatic FTC.[56]

Gene Translocations

RET/PTC

The most common gene translocation in PTC is RET/PTC. The RET gene is encoded for a transmembrane TK receptor, and [57] the 3′ portion can be fused with more than 10 other genes at their 5′. The most frequent rearrangements are RET/PTC1 and RET/PTC3,[58,59] respectively, nuclear receptor coactivator 4 (also known ELE1 or RFG) and coiled-coil domain-containing gene 6 (also known as H4).[59,60] In the presence of RET/PTC translocation, the fused protein keeps the kinase domains in the C-terminal and acquires a new N-terminal that provides to ligand-independent dimerization and constitutive TK activity. The pathogenic cause to this translocation event has been associated with the colocalization of chromosomal fragile sites, genome regions prone to DNA breakage.[61] Variability in RET/PTC prevalence is due to clonal or subclonal presence in the thyroid tumor. Clonal rearrangements are specific for PTC and occur in 10% to 20% of cases,[62] while the presence of RET/PTC in a small fraction of tumor mass has been detected in other thyroid cancer variants and also in benign thyroid lesions.[63–66] Interestingly, RET fusions have a small prevalence in PDTC (6%) but are absent in ATC, not showing overlap with point mutations.[12]

Paired box 8/proliferator activated receptor γ

Another relevant gene rearrangement (somatic translocation) in thyroid cancer is the fusion between the paired box 8 (PAX8) and proliferator activated receptor gamma (PPARγ) (PAX8/PPARγ). PAX8 is an essential transcription factor for thyroid gland development,[67,68] and in the mature organ, it is responsible for thyroid-specific gene expression.[68] Instead, PPARγ, a nuclear hormone receptor, has no known physiologic role in the thyroid, but is well described as promoter of anti-inflammatory phenotype in macrophage[69] and as master regulator of adipogenesis.[70] First described in 2000,[71] the PAX8-PPARγ translocation has been detected with high prevalence in FTC (∼50%), in a small fraction of follicular variant of PTC (1%–5%), and also in FTA (2%–13%).[72,73] PAX8/PPARγ rarely overlaps with RAS point mutation, another common alteration of FTC, probably indicating distinct pathogenic pathways involved in tumorigenesis.[39] In PTCs, the detection of PAX8/PPARγ is strongly associated with follicular features: tumors are encapsulated and likely have an indolent clinical course.[74] PAX8/PPARγ has intact DNA binding domain, and it is able to target

DNA binding sites of transcriptional factors with a proadipogenic expression profile, preferentially activated in thyroid cells with this rearrangement.[75] In thyroid cells, PAX8/PPARγ expression can induce activation of the WNT/TCF pathway, causing an increase of invasiveness and aggressiveness features, like anchorage-independent growth.[76]

A transgenic mouse model showed that PAX8/PPARγ (PPFP) itself was not sufficient to induce tumor initiation without other mutation such as PTEN deletion. Mice with combined PPFP and PTEN deletion developed metastatic thyroid cancer, consistent with patient data that PPFP is occasionally found in benign thyroid adenomas and that PPFP carcinomas have instead increased phosphorylated AKT/protein kinase B.[77] Chip-seq analysis on the mentioned mouse model (PPFPxPten⁻) showed enrichment in binding on genes involved in fatty acid metabolism, cell-cycle regulation, and WNT signaling.[78] Furthermore, treatment with a PPARγ agonist (pioglitazone) showed a significant increase of immune cells infiltration compared with the control, suggesting a potential therapeutic effect for this type of thyroid cancer[78] (**Fig. 2**).

Neurotrophic tyrosine kinase receptor

The neurotrophic tyrosine kinase receptor family is involved in sporadic rearrangements in thyroid cancer. NTRK1 gene, which resides in chromosome 1q, can have different partners, such as TPR[79,80] TMP3,[81,82] and TFG.[83] The fused protein has constitutive kinase activity, with promotion of downstream pathways. The prevalence of this genetic alteration is still debated, with previous studies showing about 11.8% in PTC[84] and more recent analysis decreasing up to 1% to 2%[85]; even there is accordance in a higher frequency among young patients. NTRK3/ETV6 fusions were

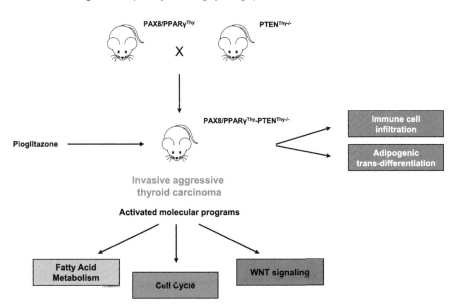

Fig. 2. Transgenic mouse model with thyroid-specific PPFP and PTEN deletion develops follicular thyroid carcinoma. At a molecular level, PPFP weakly induces a subset of adipocyte PPARγ target genes, promotes cell-cycle progression, and activates the WNT/TCF pathway. Pioglitazone (a PPARγ agonist that also binds PPFP) causes PPFP to strongly activate adipocyte PPARγ target genes, resulting in transdifferentiation of the thyroid cancer cells into adipocyte-like cells. In addition, pioglitazone-activated PPFP recruits immune cells in the tumor microenvironment.

exclusively found in 13% of follicular variant of PTC, in both encapsulated and infiltrative variants, but were not found in FTAs and FTCs.[86] NTRK3/RBPMS is another fusion that occurs in 1.2% of PTC.[10] Importantly, ETV6/NTRK3 fusion is more common (14.5%) in radiation-exposed population (post-Chernobyl PTCs) and in 2% sporadic PTCs.[87]

Striatin/anaplastic lymphoma kinase

RNAseq analysis has recently allowed the identification of a novel gene fusion in thyroid cancer, involving the anaplastic lymphoma kinase (ALK) gene and the striatin (STRN) gene.[88] This event is the result of a complex rearrangement involving the short arm of chromosome 2. The fusion between exon 3 of STRN and exon 20 of ALK leads to protein dimerization (mediated by the coiled-coil domain) of STRN and subsequent ALK constitutive kinase activity. In thyroid cancer cells, STRN/ALK rearrangement stimulates proliferation independently from TSH signaling, further inducing tumor transformation.[88] STRN/ALK has been detected in PTC,[86,88,89] in follicular variant of PTC,[86,88] in PDPTC, and in ATC.[88] Interestingly, STRN/ALK fusion tumors are negative for other driver mutations, indicating its role in thyroid tumorigenesis and suggesting that it may represent a therapeutic target for patients with this type of tumors.

AKAP9/BRAF

AKAP9/BRAF is a rare gene fusion in radiation-induced PTC via paracentric inversion of chromosome 7q resulting in an in-frame fusion between exons 1 and 8 of the AKAP9 gene and exons 9 to 18 of BRAF. The fusion protein contains the protein kinase domain and lacks the autoinhibitory N-terminal portion of BRAF.[90] The prevalence of this fusion protein in sporadic PTC is very low and can be considered a rare event.[91,92] This molecular fusion has elevated kinase activity and transforms NIH3T3 cells.

GENETIC ALTERATIONS AND PATHWAYS DEREGULATION ASSOCIATED WITH THYROID CANCER PROGRESSION

Additional mutations that occur in thyroid cancer are very often associated with cancer progression and tumor aggressive features.

WNT/β-Catenin Signaling Pathway

The WNT/β-catenin pathway has a key role in multiple cell processes, such as cell growth and proliferation, cell adhesion, and stem cell differentiation. If altered (eg, mutation on WNT receptors), it can commonly lead to constitutive activation in human tumors.[93] In thyroid cancer, this process is caused by mutations on the CTNNB1 gene (encoding for β-catenin) that occurs with high prevalence in PDPTC and ATC (up to 60%).[94–96] The consequence is the impairment of physiologic β-catenin degradation, thus allowing cytoplasmic accumulation and translocation into the nucleus and eventually promoting transcription of genes involved in tumorigenesis, for example, cell-cycle regulators.[97,98] In addition, no β-catenin mutations have been detected in DTCs, leading to the association of this pathway to increased aggressiveness. However, β-catenin nuclear aberrant translocation and localization can be caused by other mechanisms, including posttranslational modifications.[93] It is well known that PI3K/AKT pathway deactivates (by AKT direct phosphorylation) GSK3β, a key promoter of β-catenin ubiquitination and of further degradation.[99] AKT phosphorylates β-catenin at serine (Ser, S) 552, which leads to its disassociation from cell-cell contacts, increases its binding to 14-3-3 and its transcriptional activity, and enhances invasion by tumor cells activity.[100] Furthermore, ERK1/2 can inhibit GSK3β resulting in upregulation of β-catenin.[101] In thyroid cells, β-catenin is activated physiologically by PI3K signaling in response to TSH and IGF1,[102] but it has also been demonstrated that RET/PTC translocation and HRAS mutation (but not BRAF) activate β-catenin in cancer cells.[103–106] This BRAF[V600E] independency is still controversial, because upregulation of β-catenin has been found in PTC and ATC cells with BRAF[V600E].[107] However, another study based on immunohistochemical and microarray analysis showed differential β-catenin upregulation in BRAF[WT] versus BRAF[V600E] PTCs.[108] Additional work is probably needed to understand what drives abnormal activation of WNT-β-catenin in a physiologic context and which molecular partners are involved.

TP53

Mutations leading loss of function of the tumor suppressor and cell-cycle regulator p53 were first described as a unique characteristic of thyroid cancer dedifferentiation with high prevalence (50%–80%) in ATC.[109–111] Further analysis with mouse model generation and targeted next-generation sequencing has confirmed the correlation between TP53 alterations and worse pathologic features of ATC.[112,113]

TERT

In 2013, 2 point mutations on the TERT gene promoter were detected in thyroid carcinoma, C228T and C250T.[114,115] The TERT gene encodes the reverse transcriptase subunit of the telomerase complex, the specialized DNA polymerase that elongates the telomere portion of chromosomes adding repeated sequences. Its expression and activity are usually absent/low in normal cells, whereas is strongly increased in cancer cells,[116] including aggressive thyroid cancers.[117,118] The mutations in the promoter of TERT gene were found in different cancers,[119–121] determining a consensus binding site for E-twenty-six (ETS) transcription factors. C228T and C250T are both present with lower prevalence in PTCs (~10%) compared with PDTCs (40%) and ATCs (~70%).[12] A significant cooccurrence with mutations of BRAF and RAS suggested the TERT role as an acquired genetic alteration that allows extended survival to clones with preexisting driver mutations and subsequently leads to cancer progression.[114] This hypothesis has been confirmed by different studies showing TERT promoter mutations: (i) with higher prevalence in FTCs and aggressive BRAF[V600E]-positive PTCs[122] and no TERT mutation was found in benign thyroid lesions; (ii) correlated with a worse clinical outcome in patients with DTCs[123]; (iii) coexistence with BRAF[V600E] has a robust synergistic impact on tumor aggressiveness of PTCs, including poor clinicopathologic characteristics[122,124] and increased patient mortality[125]; and (iv) significantly correlated with BRAF[V600E], older patient age, and tumor distant metastasis in ATC.[126] Importantly, the molecular mechanism of synergistic coexistence between BRAF[V600E] and TERT promoter mutations in cancer has been recently elucidated: BRAF[V600E] through its effector ERK1/2 enhances MYC expression and FOS phosphorylation and the latter promotes GA binding protein (GABPB) expression. MYC and GABPB are both transcriptional factors that bind TERT promoter and trigger its overexpression, with the effect of GABPB being in a TERT mutation-dependent manner[127] (**Fig. 3**).

EIF1AX

The eukaryotic translation initiation factor EIF1AX was first discovered mutated in uveal melanomas,[128] and this genetic alteration has been reported as largely mutually exclusive with BRAF and RAS in 1% of PTCs.[10] The prevalence increases in PDTCs (11%) and in ATCs (9%), and EIF1AX is strongly correlated with RAS.[12] The most

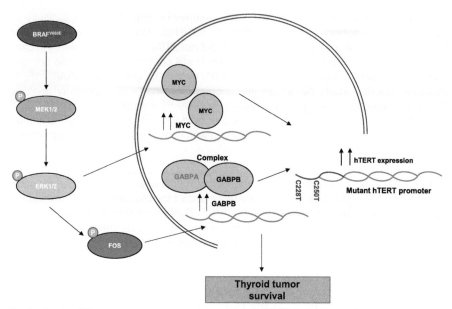

Fig. 3. Human (h) TERT promoter mutations and BRAF^{V600E} elicit synergistic pathways in thyroid carcinoma cells. BRAF^{V600E} via ERK1/2 phosphorylation promotes MYC expression and FOS phosphorylation. FOS is a transcription factor that regulates GABPB expression. MYC and GABPB are both transcriptional factors responsive to TERT promoter mutations and enhance mutant hTERT expression.

prevalent mutational event consists of a splice mutation causing C-terminal 12-amino-acid in-frame. EIF1AX mutations are also predictive of low survival in PDTC.[10,12]

PI3K-AKT Pathway Mutations and Deregulations

The PI3K pathway is composed of a large group of proteins that control several cellular processes, including cell proliferation, survival, and motility.[129] In physiologic conditions, PI3K is recruited in the internal layer of plasma membrane by protein adaptors that can be activated by multiple transmembrane TK receptors. Moreover, some isoforms have a binding domain that permits activation from RAS. PI3K phosphorylates phosphatidylinositol-4,5-bisphosphate in phosphatidylinositol-3,4,5-trisphosphate (PIP3). PIP3 is a second messenger promoting the activation of effectors such as PDK1 and AKT. Genetic alterations carried by partners in the PI3K-AKT pathway are strongly correlated to thyroid cancer progression. Overall, PI3K-AKT signaling shows an important role in thyroid oncogenesis.[130]

PTEN, a protein tyrosine phosphatase with homology to tensin, is a tumor-suppressor gene that encodes a protein and lipid phosphatase. Specifically, PTEN inhibits PI3K-AKT pathway promoting PIP3 dephosphorylation. The first evidence that linked PTEN loss-of-function mutations with thyroid cancer came from a study on Cowden syndrome, a congenital disease characterized by germline mutations of PTEN, that shows a strong predisposition for FTA and FTC.[131] Subsequently, the importance of PTEN as a tumor suppressor has been demonstrated in a heterozygous PTEN$^{+/-}$ mouse model that spontaneously develops, among the others, thyroid and colon cancer.[132] However, the complete PTEN loss in the thyroid is not sufficient to originate invasive tumors as has been shown in a tissue-specific transgenic mouse model, suggesting the importance of additional genetic alterations in order to promote thyroid transformation.[133] In human thyroid tumors, the most common genetic alteration associated is somatic deletions of the PTEN gene (~5%–25%) due to loss of heterozygosity on chromosome 10.[134,135] PTEN frameshift mutations can occur in ATC[113]; also, PTEN mutations are more frequent in ATC (15%) compared with PDTC.[12]

Somatic mutations in exon 9 and exon 20 of PIK3CA, encoding the PI3K catalytic subunit p110a, are frequent in many human tumors,[136] including DTC (~8%)[137] and ATC (~25%),[138,139] with an interesting cooccurrence with BRAF[V600E] in the undifferentiated tumors.[12] In the presence of these genetic alterations, the kinase is not sensitive to its regulatory subunit and is not deactivated.[140] Mutations on other PI3K subunits have been observed in PDTCs and ATCs but with lower prevalence.[12]

AKT is the downstream effector of PI3K signaling and is recruited by PIP3 and subsequently phosphorylated and activated by PDK1 and mechanistic target of rapamycin (mTOR). AKT is a serine/threonine kinase and has 3 different isoforms, encoded by different genes all regularly expressed in thyroid tissue that differ mainly for their regulatory and adaptor domains. In metastatic thyroid cancer, AKT1 can be mutated.[141] mTOR is another serine/threonine kinase that exists in 2 complexes: mTORC1 (or mTOR-Raptor), activated by AKT, that promotes, among other functions, cell growth and biosynthesis of macromolecules, and mTORC2 (or mTOR-Rictor) that phosphorylates AKT (as mentioned above) and triggers cell survival processes.[142] MTOR gene mutation has been described in PDTC and ATC at low frequency (1% and 6%, respectively).[12] Overall it has been shown that more than 50% of FTC and ATC harbored at least one PI3K-AKT pathway–related genetic alteration.[137]

In addition, PI3K-AKT signaling can be abnormally active in the absence of mutation. AKT1 and AKT2 are overexpressed and overactivated particularly in FTC.[143] AKT1 nuclear translocation has been also linked to capsular invasiveness, cell invasion, and migration.[144] AKT1 deletion in PTEN[+/−] mouse model sufficiently inhibits tumor development,[145] and AKT2 deficiency does not have the same ubiquitous effect as AKT in PTEN[+/−] mice, but still shows a decreased incidence of thyroid tumors.[146]

Gene Copy-Number Variations

Copy-number variations (CNV) (including gene amplification) are additional mechanisms that critically contribute to carcinogenesis.[147,148] They are due to chromosome instability and aneuploidy that permits the acquisition of a genetic advantage promoting pathogenic signaling.[148,149] Genes encoding for various types of TK receptors, including EGFR, PDGFRA, PDGFRB, VEGFR1, VEGFR2, and so forth, have been detected in FTCs and ATCs, in association with increased activation of phosphorylated AKT and ERK1/2.[47] Genes of the PI3K-AKT pathway that are also amplified include PIK3CA, PIK3CB, AKT1, and AKT2.[47,137,139] Interestingly, PIK3CA mutation and PIK3CA amplification are mutually exclusive in DTCs,[137,150] suggesting that one specific genetic alteration of PI3K-AKT pathway is sufficient for promoting thyroid tumorigenesis. Whereas accumulation of different genetic alterations occurs in ATC,[47,137] increasing potential of metastasis and tumor progression.

In PTC, CNV include loss on chromosome 22 (q arm)[10,146] in a region that shows sequence of the NF2 and CHEK2 gene and reported to be lost with significant frequency; amplification on chromosome 1q; and gain of 5p and 5q often in association with BRAF[V600E] mutation.[10] NF2 gene encodes for a tumor suppressor protein, which inhibits cell growth in response to cell-to-cell contact. NF2 loss augments mutant RAS signaling, strengthening MAPK signaling, in part through inactivation of Hippo, which activates a YAP-TEAD transcriptional program in murine model of PDTC.[151] Moreover,

BRAF^{V600E}-PTCs with metastasis showed amplification of 26 genes on chromosome 1q, including MCL1 (antiapoptotic gene belonging to BCL2 family) and P16 gene (CDKN2A) loss on chromosome 9p.[152] P16 is a cell-cycle negative regulator, impairing CDK4/6 complexes formation and Rb phosphorylation during G1 phase[153] (**Fig. 4**). For this reason, CDK4/6 inhibitors in combination with BRAF^{V600E} inhibitor (vemurafenib) have been demonstrated to strongly induce apoptosis in PTC and ATC cells with the heterozygous BRAF^{V600E} mutation and with P16 loss.[154] DNA CNVs might occur on chromosome 7, 12, and 17 in thyroid lesions.[155] Overall, CNV frequency is higher in aggressive thyroid tumors and ATC, indicating a role in tumor progression.

NF-κB Signaling Pathway

(Nuclear factor-kappa B (NF-κB) signaling plays an important role in cancer development and progression, providing a mechanistic link between inflammation and cancer.[156] NF-κB is able to induce tumor proliferation, block apoptosis, and promote angiogenesis and invasion.[156] From many years, it has been known that in thyroid cancer cells NF-κB pathway has a pro-oncogenic role.[157–159] More specifically, it has been demonstrated that the genetic alterations mainly occurring in thyroid carcinogenesis converging in activation of NF-κB are: BRAF^{V600E} in an MEK-independent manner[160]; RET/PTC3, through stabilization of NF-κB-inducing kinase[161]; PAX8/PPARγ, due to reduced PPARγ protein abundance.[162] Moreover, constitutive activation of the PI3K-AKT pathway due to PTEN inactivation increases NF-κB activity, thus accelerating thyroid cancer progression.[163] The NF-κB role in angiogenesis and metastasis promotion has been further characterized in a mouse model of ATC and PDTC harboring BRAF^{V600E}, providing an association with IL-8 secretion.[164] However, NF-κB inhibitors administered in combination with classical chemotherapy and radiation are not sufficient to target thyroid cancer cells,[165] suggesting that further investigations are needed to understand which subset of patients/tumors could respond to this therapeutic target.

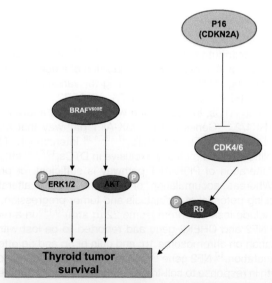

Fig. 4. BRAF^{V600E} and P16 loss cooperate to promote thyroid tumor survival through phosphorylation of ERK1/2 and AKT, activating CDK4/6 and inactivating Rb by phosphorylation.

RCAN1-4

RCAN1 (regulator of calcineurin 1, also known as Down syndrome candidate region 1) is a gene located in chromosome 21 with multiple transcriptional start sites that expresses 2 main isoforms, RCAN1-1 and RCAN1-4.[166] RCAN1-4 is a competitive inhibitor for the phosphatase calcineurin and thereby suppresses calcineurin-mediated dephosphorylation and activation of nuclear factor of activated T cells (NFAT).[167] Because NFAT is a transcriptional factor promoting RCAN1-4 gene expression, RCAN1-4 can be considered a mediator of a negative feedback loop on this pathway.[168]

Interestingly, RCAN1 has been correlated with tumor growth protection in individuals with Down syndrome,[169] and its tumor suppressor activity is probably exerted by blocking the angiogenesis process (impairing endothelial cell migration, neovascularization, and tumor growth) through NFAT inhibition.[170–172]

RCAN1 expression is increased in primary tumors versus normal tissue, but the expression is lost in metastases, a pattern consistent with a metastasis suppressor.[173] Moreover, in different cancer cell lines (including FTC cells) RCAN1 reduces migration and alters cell adhesion.[174] Recently, it has been reported that stable downregulation of RCAN1-4 in human thyroid cancer cell lines increased cell viability and invasion in vitro and promoted tumor growth and metastasis in mouse xenograft models.[175] These phenotypes were dependent on NFE2L3 (nuclear factor, erythroid 2-like 3), a transcription factor overexpressed in human thyroid cancer samples.[175]

BRAF, RAS, RET/PTC Overlapping and Signaling Cooperation Between MAPK and PI3K-AKT

It has already been discussed how progressive mutations on the PI3K-AKT pathway accelerate and lead to thyroid tumor progression. In DTCs, genetic alterations on main oncogenic drivers, such as BRAF, RAS, and RET/PTC, are mutually exclusive.[10,14,176] Instead, in aggressive thyroid tumors, a potential overlap is still debated: BRAF^{V600E} mutation and RET/PTC translocations cooccurred in recurrent PTC,[177] next-generation sequencing on PDTC and ATC showed mutual exclusivity for BRAF^{V600E}, RAS mutations, and gene fusions rearrangements.[12] Intriguingly, driver mutations that potentially activate both MAPK and PI3K were reported,[47,139,141] suggesting a precise time course of thyroid tumor initiation and progression. Therefore, the most common genetic alterations are mainly responsible for initial tumor transformation and lead tumor cells to a "cancer-prone environment" more susceptible to additional mutations (secondary or passenger mutations). With the progressive accumulation of deregulated signaling pathways and aberrant functional proteins (not only MAPK and PI3K-AKT, but also β-catenin, hTERT, TP53, and so on), the aggressiveness features (angiogenesis, cell adhesion, migration, invasion, and metastasis) worsens toward undifferentiated/anaplastic thyroid tumors, which are well known for having the highest mortalities.[178]

THYROID HORMONE RECEPTOR-β: A KEY PLAYER IN ROBUST PRECLINICAL MODELS OF INVASIVE FOLLICULAR THYROID CANCER

Thyroid hormone receptors are ligand-dependent transcription factors that regulate cell growth, development, and differentiation in response to thyroid hormone (T3). This protein family is entirely encoded from 2 genes, TRα and TRβ. In 2000, a mouse model carrying a targeted mutation on TRβ (TRβPV) was established to understand the molecular basis of resistance to thyroid hormone syndrome, characterized by reduced sensitivity of tissues to the action of thyroid hormone.[179] Those mice exhibited impaired growth and resistance to thyroid hormone. A couple of years later, it was reported that mice homozygotes for PV mutation (TRβ$^{PV/PV}$) spontaneously develop metastatic FTC, showing aggressive features, such as anaplasia and metastasis.[180] Many studies later focused on elucidating the pathways contributing to tumor initiation in TRβ$^{PV/PV}$ mice. PPARγ mRNA expression is downregulated[181] due to transcription repressive activity of TRβPV on the peroxisome proliferator response element.[182] More importantly, TRβPV has been linked to PI3K-AKT pathway activation via interaction with p85a (regulatory subunit of PI3K), well known for being a key regulator in thyroid tumorigenesis.[183] Cancer progression and occurrence of metastasis are increased if combined with PTEN deficiency, causing AKT overexpression and overactivation, with significant effects on AKT downstream targets: increased mTOR-p70S6K signaling and inhibition of FOXO3a, a member of the forkhead family of transcription factor FOXO, promoter of proapoptotic factors transcription, and repressor of cyclin D1.[163] In addition, it has been demonstrated that T3 has a role in β-catenin suppression. T3 binding on TRβ induces dissociation and subsequent degradation of β-catenin in cells via proteosomal pathways,[184] and direct repression of CTNNB1 gene through interaction with negative thyroid hormone response elements in the promoter.[185] TRβPV is refractory to this mechanism, stabilizing β-catenin and promoting oncogenesis. TRβ$^{PV/PV}$ mouse model has further been developed following some strategy: high fat diet in TRβ$^{PV/PV}$Pten$^{+/-}$ showed an increased level of circulating leptin with activation of JAK2-STAT3 pathway with higher occurrence of metastasis.[186] STAT3 is a transcription factor promoter of cyclin D1, Myc, and Bcl2 and crucial for metastasis; importantly, the leptin JAK-STAT3 signaling role was confirmed using a STAT3 selective inhibitor[187] that reduced vascular invasion, anaplasia, and metastasis. Moreover, metformin treatments in high fat diet-TRβ$^{PV/PV}$Pten$^{+/-}$ reduced capsular invasion and blocked anaplasia and vascular invasion but not thyroid tumor growth.[188] The genetically targeted KRAS (G12D) mutation in thyroid epithelial cells of TRβ$^{PV/PV}$ mice develop a more aggressive tumor, with frequent anaplastic foci showing lack of PAX8 expression, MYC upregulation. Thus, MYC might serve as a potential target for therapeutic intervention and may suggest a signaling cross-talk between RAS, PI3K/AKT, and β-catenin pathways.[189] An MYC inhibitor (JQ1) showed successful inhibition of tumor growth in TRβ$^{PV/PV}$-KRAS^{G12D} mice.[190] Also, combined treatment with JQ1 and metformin has been recently performed on high fat diet-TRβ$^{PV/PV}$Pten$^{+/-}$ mice, reducing tumor growth by attenuating STAT3, decreasing antiapoptotic key regulators and suppressing vascular invasion, anaplasia, and lung metastasis.[191]

SUMMARY

In these past years, there has been remarkable progress in the understanding of the molecular signature (molecular determinants with coding capabilities) of thyroid cancer. Novel genetic alterations associated with clinicopathologic features of thyroid carcinomas have been discovered. The characterization of these genetic alterations revealed the essential role of MAPK and PI3K/AKT signaling in promoting thyroid tumor initiation and progression. These results have greatly led to the development of targeted therapies for precision medicine, inhibiting key players of these pathways. Unfortunately, selective drug resistance has been constantly reported, explaining the need to identify new potential therapeutic targets in order to overcome tumor resistance. The interplay between different pathways in advanced thyroid cancers refractory to standard therapies (including radioiodine) has been recently better characterized, opening new possibilities of early treatment and improved prognosis.

ACKNOWLEDGMENTS

C. Nucera (Principal Investigator, Human Thyroid Cancers Preclinical and Translational Research at the Beth Israel Deaconess Medical Center [BIDMC]/Harvard Medical School) was awarded grants by the National Cancer Institute/National Institutes of Health (1R21CA165039-01A1 and 1R01CA181183-01A1), the American Thyroid Association and ThyCa:Thyroid Cancer Survivors Association Inc for Thyroid Cancer Research. C. Nucera was also a recipient of the Guido Berlucchi "Young Investigator" research award 2013 (Brescia, Italy) and BIDMC/CAO Grants (Boston, MA). V. Valvo is recipient of a PhD fellowship from the MIUR and UCSC (Rome, Italy).

REFERENCES

1. Cancer Statistics Review, 1975-2015 - SEER Statistics. Available at: https://seer.cancer.gov/csr/1975_2015/. Accessed June 12, 2018.
2. Lim H, Devesa SS, Sosa JA, et al. Trends in thyroid cancer incidence and mortality in the United States, 1974-2013. JAMA 2017;317:1338.
3. Lloyd RV, Osamura RY, Klöppel G, et al. WHO classification of tumours of endocrine organs WHO classification of tumours. vol. 10. Lyon (France): IARC press; 2017.
4. Baudin E, Schlumberger M. New therapeutic approaches for metastatic thyroid carcinoma. Lancet Oncol 2007;8:148–56.
5. Fanger GR. Regulation of the MAPK family members: role of subcellular localization and architectural organization. Histol Histopathol 1999;14:887–94.
6. Kyriakis JM, App H, Zhang XF, et al. Raf-1 activates MAP kinase-kinase. Nature 1992;358:417–21.
7. Davies H, Bignell GR, Cox C, et al. Mutations of the BRAF gene in human cancer. Nature 2002;417:949–54.
8. Sosman JA, Kim KB, Schuchter L, et al. Survival in BRAF V600–mutant advanced melanoma treated with vemurafenib. N Engl J Med 2012;366:707–14.
9. Tiacci E, Trifonov V, Schiavoni G, et al. BRAF mutations in hairy-cell leukemia. N Engl J Med 2011;364:2305–15.
10. Cancer Genome Atlas Research Network. Integrated genomic characterization of papillary thyroid carcinoma. Cell 2014;159:676–90.
11. Cohen Y, Xing M, Mambo E, et al. BRAF mutation in papillary thyroid carcinoma. J Natl Cancer Inst 2003;95:625–7.
12. Landa I, Ibrahimpasic T, Boucai L, et al. Genomic and transcriptomic hallmarks of poorly differentiated and anaplastic thyroid cancers. J Clin Invest 2016;126: 1052–66.
13. Nikiforova MN, Kimura ET, Gandhi M, et al. BRAF mutations in thyroid tumors are restricted to papillary carcinomas and anaplastic or poorly differentiated carcinomas arising from papillary carcinomas. J Clin Endocrinol Metab 2003;88: 5399–404.
14. Soares P, Trovisco V, Rocha AS, et al. BRAF mutations and RET/PTC rearrangements are alternative events in the etiopathogenesis of PTC. Oncogene 2003; 22:4578–80.
15. Trovisco V, Vieira de Castro I, Soares P, et al. BRAF mutations are associated with some histological types of papillary thyroid carcinoma. J Pathol 2004; 202:247–51.
16. Afkhami M, Karunamurthy A, Chiosea S, et al. Histopathologic and clinical characterization of thyroid tumors carrying the BRAF(K601E) Mutation. Thyroid 2016; 26:242–7.

17. Mitsutake N, Knauf JA, Mitsutake S, et al. Conditional BRAFV600E expression induces DNA synthesis, apoptosis, dedifferentiation, and chromosomal instability in thyroid PCCL3 cells. Cancer Res 2005;65:2465–73.
18. Xing M, Alzahrani AS, Carson KA, et al. Association between BRAF V600E mutation and mortality in patients with papillary thyroid cancer. JAMA 2013;309: 1493.
19. Xing M, Westra WH, Tufano RP, et al. BRAF mutation predicts a poorer clinical prognosis for papillary thyroid cancer. J Clin Endocrinol Metab 2005;90:6373–9.
20. Knauf JA, Ma X, Smith EP, et al. Targeted expression of BRAF V600E in thyroid cells of transgenic mice results in papillary thyroid cancers that undergo dedifferentiation. Cancer Res 2005;65:4238–45.
21. Liu D, Liu Z, Condouris S, et al. BRAF V600E maintains proliferation, transformation, and tumorigenicity of BRAF-mutant papillary thyroid cancer cells. J Clin Endocrinol Metab 2007;92:2264–71.
22. Guerra A, Sapio MR, Marotta V, et al. The primary occurrence of BRAF(V600E) is a rare clonal event in papillary thyroid carcinoma. J Clin Endocrinol Metab 2012; 97:517–24.
23. Ghossein RA, Katabi N, Fagin JA. Immunohistochemical detection of mutated BRAF V600E supports the clonal origin of BRAF-induced thyroid cancers along the spectrum of disease progression. J Clin Endocrinol Metab 2013;98: E1414–21.
24. Nucera C, Porrello A, Antonello ZA, et al. B-Raf(V600E) and thrombospondin-1 promote thyroid cancer progression. Proc Natl Acad Sci U S A 2010;107. 10649–54.
25. Oler G, Camacho CP, Hojaij FC, et al. Gene expression profiling of papillary thyroid carcinoma identifies transcripts correlated with BRAF mutational status and lymph node metastasis. Clin Cancer Res 2008;14:4735–42.
26. Ryder M, Gild M, Hohl TM, et al. Genetic and pharmacological targeting of CSF-1/CSF-1R inhibits tumor-associated macrophages and impairs BRAF-induced thyroid cancer progression. PLoS One 2013;8:e54302.
27. Angell TE, Lechner MG, Jang JK, et al. BRAF V600E in papillary thyroid carcinoma is associated with increased programmed death ligand 1 expression and suppressive immune cell infiltration. Thyroid 2014;24:1385–93.
28. Smallridge RC, Chindris AM, Asmann YW, et al. RNA sequencing identifies multiple fusion transcripts, differentially expressed genes, and reduced expression of immune function genes in BRAF (V600E) mutant vs BRAF wild-type papillary thyroid carcinoma. J Clin Endocrinol Metab 2014;99:E338–47.
29. Jo YS, Li S, Song JH, et al. Influence of the BRAF V600E mutation on expression of vascular endothelial growth factor in papillary thyroid cancer. J Clin Endocrinol Metab 2006;91:3667–70.
30. Mesa C, Mirza M, Mitsutake N, et al. Conditional activation of RET/PTC3 and BRAFV600E in thyroid cells is associated with gene expression profiles that predict a preferential role of BRAF in extracellular matrix remodeling. Cancer Res 2006;66:6521–9.
31. Watanabe R, Hayashi Y, Sassa M, et al. Possible involvement of BRAFV600E in altered gene expression in papillary thyroid cancer. Endocr J 2009;56:407–14.
32. Riesco-Eizaguirre G, Rodríguez I, De la Vieja A, et al. The BRAFV600E oncogene induces transforming growth factor beta secretion leading to sodium iodide symporter repression and increased malignancy in thyroid cancer. Cancer Res 2009;69:8317–25.

33. Knauf JA, Sartor MA, Medvedovic M, et al. Progression of BRAF-induced thyroid cancer is associated with epithelial-mesenchymal transition requiring concomitant MAP kinase and TGFβ signaling. Oncogene 2011;30:3153–62.

34. McCarty SK, Saji M, Zhang X, et al. BRAF activates and physically interacts with PAK to regulate cell motility. Endocr Relat Cancer 2014;21:865–77.

35. Prete A, Lo AS, Sadow PM, et al. Pericytes elicit resistance to vemurafenib and sorafenib therapy in thyroid carcinoma via the TSP-1/TGFβ1 axis. Clin Cancer Res 2018. https://doi.org/10.1158/1078-0432.CCR-18-0693.

36. Husain A, Hu N, Sadow PM, et al. Expression of angiogenic switch, cachexia and inflammation factors at the crossroad in undifferentiated thyroid carcinoma with BRAF(V600E). Cancer Lett 2016;380:577–85.

37. Khosravi-Far R, Der CJ. The Ras signal transduction pathway. Cancer Metastasis Rev 1994;13:67–89.

38. Gibbs JB, Sigal IS, Poe M, et al. Intrinsic GTPase activity distinguishes normal and oncogenic ras p21 molecules. Proc Natl Acad Sci U S A 1984;81:5704–8.

39. Nikiforova MN, Lynch RA, Biddinger PW, et al. RAS point mutations and PAX8-PPAR gamma rearrangement in thyroid tumors: evidence for distinct molecular pathways in thyroid follicular carcinoma. J Clin Endocrinol Metab 2003;88: 2318–26.

40. Namba H, Rubin SA, Fagin JA. Point mutations of ras oncogenes are an early event in thyroid tumorigenesis. Mol Endocrinol 1990;4:1474–9.

41. Xing M. Clinical utility of RAS mutations in thyroid cancer: a blurred picture now emerging clearer. BMC Med 2016;14:12.

42. Prior IA, Lewis PD, Mattos C. A comprehensive survey of Ras mutations in cancer. Cancer Res 2012;72:2457–67.

43. Suárez HG, Suárez HG, Du Villard JA, et al. Detection of activated ras oncogenes in human thyroid carcinomas. Oncogene 1988;2:403–6.

44. Suarez HG, du Villard JA, Severino M, et al. Presence of mutations in all three ras genes in human thyroid tumors. Oncogene 1990;5:565–70.

45. Lemoine NR, Mayall ES, Wyllie FS, et al. High frequency of ras oncogene activation in all stages of human thyroid tumorigenesis. Oncogene 1989;4:159–64.

46. Abubaker J, Jehan Z, Bavi P, et al. Clinicopathological analysis of papillary thyroid cancer with PIK3CA alterations in a Middle Eastern population. J Clin Endocrinol Metab 2008;93:611–8.

47. Liu Z, Hou P, Ji M, et al. Highly prevalent genetic alterations in receptor tyrosine kinases and phosphatidylinositol 3-kinase/akt and mitogen-activated protein kinase pathways in anaplastic and follicular thyroid cancers. J Clin Endocrinol Metab 2008;93:3106–16.

48. Esapa CT, Johnson SJ, Kendall-Taylor P, et al. Prevalence of Ras mutations in thyroid neoplasia. Clin Endocrinol (Oxf) 1999;50:529–35.

49. Manenti G, Pilotti S, Re FC, et al. Selective activation of ras oncogenes in follicular and undifferentiated thyroid carcinomas. Eur J Cancer 1994;30A:987–93.

50. Ezzat S, Zheng L, Kolenda J, et al. Prevalence of activating ras mutations in morphologically characterized thyroid nodules. Thyroid 1996;6:409–16.

51. Ellis RJ, Wang Y, Stevenson HS, et al. Genome-wide methylation patterns in papillary thyroid cancer are distinct based on histological subtype and tumor genotype. J Clin Endocrinol Metab 2014;99:E329–37.

52. Zhu Z, Gandhi M, Nikiforova MN, et al. Molecular profile and clinical-pathologic features of the follicular variant of papillary thyroid carcinoma. An unusually high prevalence of ras mutations. Am J Clin Pathol 2003;120:71–7.

53. Ferris RL, Nikiforov Y, Terris D, et al. AHNS Series: Do you know your guidelines? AHNS Endocrine Section Consensus Statement: State-of-the-art thyroid surgical recommendations in the era of noninvasive follicular thyroid neoplasm with papillary-like nuclear features. Head Neck 2018. https://doi.org/10.1002/hed.25141.

54. Bond JA, Wyllie FS, Rowson J, et al. In vitro reconstruction of tumour initiation in a human epithelium. Oncogene 1994;9:281–90.

55. Gire V, Wynford-Thomas D. RAS oncogene activation induces proliferation in normal human thyroid epithelial cells without loss of differentiation. Oncogene 2000;19:737–44.

56. Miller KA, Yeager N, Baker K, et al. Oncogenic Kras requires simultaneous PI3K signaling to induce ERK activation and transform thyroid epithelial cells in vivo. Cancer Res 2009;69:3689–94.

57. Nikiforova MN, Stringer JR, Blough R, et al. Proximity of chromosomal loci that participate in radiation-induced rearrangements in human cells. Science 2000;290:138–41.

58. Grieco M, Santoro M, Berlingieri MT, et al. PTC is a novel rearranged form of the ret proto-oncogene and is frequently detected in vivo in human thyroid papillary carcinomas. Cell 1990;60:557–63.

59. Santoro M, Dathan NA, Berlingieri MT, et al. Molecular characterization of RET/PTC3; a novel rearranged version of the RETproto-oncogene in a human thyroid papillary carcinoma. Oncogene 1994;9:509–16.

60. Ciampi R, Nikiforov YE. RET/PTC rearrangements and BRAF mutations in thyroid tumorigenesis. Endocrinology 2007;148:936–41.

61. Gandhi M, Dillon LW, Pramanik S, et al. DNA breaks at fragile sites generate oncogenic RET/PTC rearrangements in human thyroid cells. Oncogene 2010;29:2272–80.

62. Santoro M, Carlomagno F, Hay ID, et al. Ret oncogene activation in human thyroid neoplasms is restricted to the papillary cancer subtype. J Clin Invest 1992;89:1517–22.

63. Elisei R, Romei C, Vorontsova T, et al. RET/PTC rearrangements in thyroid nodules: studies in irradiated and not irradiated, malignant and benign thyroid lesions in children and adults. J Clin Endocrinol Metab 2001;86:3211–6.

64. Chiappetta G, Toti P, Cetta F, et al. The RET/PTC oncogene is frequently activated in oncocytic thyroid tumors (Hurthle cell adenomas and carcinomas), but not in oncocytic hyperplastic lesions. J Clin Endocrinol Metab 2002;87:364–9.

65. Sapio MR, Guerra A, Marotta V, et al. High growth rate of benign thyroid nodules bearing RET/PTC rearrangements. J Clin Endocrinol Metab 2011;96:E916–9.

66. Guerra A, Sapio MR, Marotta V, et al. Prevalence of RET/PTC rearrangement in benign and malignant thyroid nodules and its clinical application. Endocr J 2011;58:31–8.

67. Macchia PE, Lapi P, Krude H, et al. PAX8 mutations associated with congenital hypothyroidism caused by thyroid dysgenesis. Nat Genet 1998;19:83–6.

68. Pasca di Magliano M, Di Lauro R, Zannini M. Pax8 has a key role in thyroid cell differentiation. Proc Natl Acad Sci U S A 2000;97:13144–9.

69. Ricote M, Li AC, Willson TM, et al. The peroxisome proliferator-activated receptor-gamma is a negative regulator of macrophage activation. Nature 1998;391:79–82.

70. Rosen ED, Sarraf P, Troy AE, et al. PPAR gamma is required for the differentiation of adipose tissue in vivo and in vitro. Mol Cell 1999;4:611–7.

71. Kroll TG, Sarraf P, Pecciarini L, et al. PAX8-PPARgamma1 fusion oncogene in human thyroid carcinoma [corrected]. Science 2000;289:1357–60.
72. Nikiforova MN, Biddinger PW, Caudill CM, et al. PAX8-PPARgamma rearrangement in thyroid tumors: RT-PCR and immunohistochemical analyses. Am J Surg Pathol 2002;26:1016–23.
73. Marques AR, Espadinha C, Catarino AL, et al. Expression of PAX8-PPAR gamma 1 rearrangements in both follicular thyroid carcinomas and adenomas. J Clin Endocrinol Metab 2002;87:3947–52.
74. Armstrong MJ, Yang H, Yip L, et al. *PAX8/PPARγ* rearrangement in thyroid nodules predicts follicular-pattern carcinomas, in particular the encapsulated follicular variant of papillary carcinoma. Thyroid 2014;24:1369–74.
75. Zhang Y, Yu J, Lee C, et al. Genomic binding and regulation of gene expression by the thyroid carcinoma-associated PAX8-PPARG fusion protein. Oncotarget 2015;6:40418–32.
76. Vu-Phan D, Grachtchouk V, Yu J, et al. The thyroid cancer PAX8-PPARG fusion protein activates Wnt/TCF-responsive cells that have a transformed phenotype. Endocr Relat Cancer 2013;20:725–39.
77. Dobson ME, Diallo-Krou E, Grachtchouk V, et al. Pioglitazone induces a proadipogenic antitumor response in mice with PAX8-PPARgamma fusion protein thyroid carcinoma. Endocrinology 2011;152:4455–65.
78. Zhang Y, Yu J, Grachtchouk V, et al. Genomic binding of PAX8-PPARG fusion protein regulates cancer-related pathways and alters the immune landscape of thyroid cancer. Oncotarget 2017;8:5761–73.
79. Greco A, Pierotti MA, Bongarzone I, et al. TRK-T1 is a novel oncogene formed by the fusion of TPR and TRK genes in human papillary thyroid carcinomas. Oncogene 1992;7:237–42.
80. Miranda C, Minoletti F, Greco A, et al. Refined localization of the human TPR gene to chromosome 1q25 by in situ hybridization. Genomics 1994;23:714–5.
81. Radice P, Sozzi G, Miozzo M, et al. The human tropomyosin gene involved in the generation of the TRK oncogene maps to chromosome 1q31. Oncogene 1991; 6:2145–8.
82. Butti MG, Bongarzone I, Ferraresi G, et al. A sequence analysis of the genomic regions involved in the rearrangements between TPM3 and NTRK1 genes producing TRK oncogenes in papillary thyroid carcinomas. Genomics 1995;28: 15–24.
83. Greco A, Mariani C, Miranda C, et al. The DNA rearrangement that generates the TRK-T3 oncogene involves a novel gene on chromosome 3 whose product has a potential coiled-coil domain. Mol Cell Biol 1995;15:6118–27.
84. Bongarzone I, Vigneri P, Mariani L, et al. RET/NTRK1 rearrangements in thyroid gland tumors of the papillary carcinoma family: correlation with clinicopathological features. Clin Cancer Res 1998;4:223–8.
85. Prasad ML, Vyas M, Horne MJ, et al. NTRK fusion oncogenes in pediatric papillary thyroid carcinoma in northeast United States. Cancer 2016;122:1097–107.
86. Bastos AU, de Jesus AC, Cerutti JM. ETV6-NTRK3 and STRN-ALK kinase fusions are recurrent events in papillary thyroid cancer of adult population. Eur J Endocrinol 2018;178:85–93.
87. Leeman-Neill RJ, Kelly LM, Liu P, et al. ETV6-NTRK3 is a common chromosomal rearrangement in radiation-associated thyroid cancer: *ETV6-NTRK3* Fusion in Thyroid Cancer. Cancer 2014;120:799–807.

88. Kelly LM, Barila G, Liu P, et al. Identification of the transforming STRN-ALK fusion as a potential therapeutic target in the aggressive forms of thyroid cancer. Proc Natl Acad Sci U S A 2014;111:4233–8.
89. Pérot G, Soubeyran I, Ribeiro A, et al. Identification of a recurrent STRN/ALK fusion in thyroid carcinomas. PLoS One 2014;9:e87170.
90. Ciampi R, Knauf JA, Kerler R, et al. Oncogenic AKAP9-BRAF fusion is a novel mechanism of MAPK pathway activation in thyroid cancer. J Clin Invest 2005; 115:94–101.
91. Gandhi M, Evdokimova V, Nikiforov YE. Frequency of close positioning of chromosomal loci detected by FRET correlates with their participation in carcinogenic rearrangements in human cells. Genes Chromosomes Cancer 2012;51: 1037–44.
92. Lee J-H, Lee ES, Kim YS, et al. BRAF mutation and AKAP9 expression in sporadic papillary thyroid carcinomas. Pathology 2006;38:201–4.
93. Clevers H, Nusse R. Wnt/β-catenin signaling and disease. Cell 2012;149: 1192–205.
94. Garcia-Rostan G, Tallini G, Herrero A, et al. Frequent mutation and nuclear localization of beta-catenin in anaplastic thyroid carcinoma. Cancer Res 1999;59: 1811–5.
95. Garcia-Rostan, Camp RL, Herrero A, et al. Beta-catenin dysregulation in thyroid neoplasms: down-regulation, aberrant nuclear expression, and CTNNB1 exon 3 mutations are markers for aggressive tumor phenotypes and poor prognosis. Am J Pathol 2001;158(3):987–96.
96. Ishigaki K, Namba H, Nakashima M, et al. Aberrant localization of beta-catenin correlates with overexpression of its target gene in human papillary thyroid cancer. J Clin Endocrinol Metab 2002;87:3433–40.
97. Lazzereschi D, Sambuco L, Carnovale Scalzo C, et al. Cyclin D1 and Cyclin E expression in malignant thyroid cells and in human thyroid carcinomas. Int J Cancer 1998;76:806–11.
98. Meirmanov S, Nakashima M, Kondo H, et al. Correlation of cytoplasmic beta-catenin and cyclin D1 overexpression during thyroid carcinogenesis around Semipalatinsk nuclear test site. Thyroid 2003;13:537–45.
99. Cross DA, Alessi DR, Cohen P, et al. Inhibition of glycogen synthase kinase-3 by insulin mediated by protein kinase B. Nature 1995;378:785–9.
100. Fang D, Hawke D, Zheng Y, et al. Phosphorylation of beta-catenin by AKT promotes beta-catenin transcriptional activity. J Biol Chem 2007;282:11221–9.
101. Ding Q, Xia W, Liu JC, et al. Erk associates with and primes GSK-3beta for its inactivation resulting in upregulation of beta-catenin. Mol Cell 2005;19:159–70.
102. Sastre-Perona A, Santisteban P. Wnt-independent role of β-catenin in thyroid cell proliferation and differentiation. Mol Endocrinol Baltim Md 2014;28:681–95.
103. Castellone MD, De Falco V, Rao DM, et al. The beta-catenin axis integrates multiple signals downstream from RET/papillary thyroid carcinoma leading to cell proliferation. Cancer Res 2009;69:1867–76.
104. Cassinelli G, Favini E, Degl'Innocenti D, et al. RET/PTC1-driven neoplastic transformation and proinvasive phenotype of human thyrocytes involve Met induction and beta-catenin nuclear translocation. Neoplasia 2009;11:10–21.
105. Tartari CJ, Donadoni C, Manieri E, et al. Dissection of the RET/β-catenin interaction in the TPC1 thyroid cancer cell line. Am J Cancer Res 2011;1:716–25.
106. Sastre-Perona A, Riesco-Eizaguirre G, Zaballos MA, et al. ß-catenin signaling is required for RAS-driven thyroid cancer through PI3K activation. Oncotarget 2016;7:49435–49.

107. Cho NL, Lin CI, Whang EE, et al. Sulindac reverses aberrant expression and localization of beta-catenin in papillary thyroid cancer cells with the BRAFV600E mutation. Thyroid 2010;20:615–22.
108. Cho SW, Kim YA, Sun HJ, et al. Therapeutic potential of Dickkopf-1 in wild-type BRAF papillary thyroid cancer via regulation of β-catenin/E-cadherin signaling. J Clin Endocrinol Metab 2014;99:E1641–9.
109. Ito T, Seyama T, Mizuno T, et al. Unique association of p53 mutations with undifferentiated but not with differentiated carcinomas of the thyroid gland. Cancer Res 1992;52:1369–71.
110. Fagin JA, Matsuo K, Karmakar A, et al. High prevalence of mutations of the p53 gene in poorly differentiated human thyroid carcinomas. J Clin Invest 1993;91:179–84.
111. Donghi R, Longoni A, Pilotti S, et al. Gene p53 mutations are restricted to poorly differentiated and undifferentiated carcinomas of the thyroid gland. J Clin Invest 1993;91:1753–60.
112. McFadden DG, Vernon A, Santiago PM, et al. p53 constrains progression to anaplastic thyroid carcinoma in a Braf-mutant mouse model of papillary thyroid cancer. Proc Natl Acad Sci U S A 2014;111:E1600–9.
113. Sadow PM, Dias-Santagata D, Zheng Z, et al. Identification of insertions in PTEN and TP53 in anaplastic thyroid carcinoma with angiogenic brain metastasis. Endocr Relat Cancer 2015;22:L23–8.
114. Landa I, Ganly I, Chan TA, et al. Frequent somatic TERT promoter mutations in thyroid cancer: higher prevalence in advanced forms of the disease. J Clin Endocrinol Metab 2013;98:E1562–6.
115. Liu X, Bishop J, Shan Y, et al. Highly prevalent TERT promoter mutations in aggressive thyroid cancers. Endocr Relat Cancer 2013;20:603–10.
116. Meyerson M, Counter CM, Eaton EN, et al. hEST2, the putative human telomerase catalytic subunit gene, is up-regulated in tumor cells and during immortalization. Cell 1997;90:785–95.
117. Brousset P, Chaouche N, Leprat F, et al. Telomerase activity in human thyroid carcinomas originating from the follicular cells. J Clin Endocrinol Metab 1997;82:4214–6.
118. Saji M, Xydas S, Westra WH, et al. Human telomerase reverse transcriptase (hTERT) gene expression in thyroid neoplasms. Clin Cancer Res 1999;5:1483–9.
119. Horn S, Figl A, Rachakonda PS, et al. TERT promoter mutations in familial and sporadic melanoma. Science 2013;339:959–61.
120. Huang FW, Hodis E, Xu MJ, et al. Highly recurrent TERT promoter mutations in human melanoma. Science 2013;339:957–9.
121. Vinagre J, Almeida A, Pópulo H, et al. Frequency of TERT promoter mutations in human cancers. Nat Commun 2013;4:2185.
122. Liu X, Qu S, Liu R, et al. TERT promoter mutations and their association with BRAF V600E mutation and aggressive clinicopathological characteristics of thyroid cancer. J Clin Endocrinol Metab 2014;99:E1130–6.
123. Melo M, da Rocha AG, Vinagre J, et al. TERT promoter mutations are a major indicator of poor outcome in differentiated thyroid carcinomas. J Clin Endocrinol Metab 2014;99:E754–65.
124. Xing M, Liu R, Liu X, et al. BRAF V600E and TERT promoter mutations cooperatively identify the most aggressive papillary thyroid cancer with highest recurrence. J Clin Oncol 2014;32:2718–26.

125. Liu R, Bishop J, Zhu G, et al. Mortality risk stratification by combining BRAF V600E and TERT promoter mutations in papillary thyroid cancer: genetic duet of BRAF and TERT promoter mutations in thyroid cancer mortality. JAMA Oncol 2016. https://doi.org/10.1001/jamaoncol.2016.3288.

126. Shi X, Liu R, Qu S, et al. Association of TERT promoter mutation 1,295,228 C>T with BRAF V600E mutation, older patient age, and distant metastasis in anaplastic thyroid cancer. J Clin Endocrinol Metab 2015;100:E632-7.

127. Liu R, Zhang T, Zhu G, et al. Regulation of mutant TERT by BRAF V600E/MAP kinase pathway through FOS/GABP in human cancer. Nat Commun 2018;9:579.

128. Martin M, Maßhöfer L, Temming P, et al. Exome sequencing identifies recurrent somatic mutations in EIF1AX and SF3B1 in uveal melanoma with disomy 3. Nat Genet 2013;45:933-6.

129. Cantley LC. The phosphoinositide 3-kinase pathway. Science 2002;296:1655-7.

130. Xing M. Genetic alterations in the phosphatidylinositol-3 kinase/Akt pathway in thyroid cancer. Thyroid 2010;20:697-706.

131. Liaw D, Marsh DJ, Li J, et al. Germline mutations of the PTEN gene in Cowden disease, an inherited breast and thyroid cancer syndrome. Nat Genet 1997;16: 64-7.

132. Di Cristofano A, Pesce B, Cordon-Cardo C, et al. Pten is essential for embryonic development and tumour suppression. Nat Genet 1998;19:348-55.

133. Yeager N, Klein-Szanto A, Kimura S, et al. Pten loss in the mouse thyroid causes goiter and follicular adonomas: insights into thyroid function and Cowden disease pathogenesis. Cancer Res 2007;67:959-66.

134. Dahia PLM, Marsh DJ, Zheng Z, et al. Somatic deletions and mutations in the cowden disease gene, PTEN, in sporadic thyroid tumors. Cancer Res 1997; 57:4710-3.

135. Halachmi N, Halachmi S, Evron E, et al. Somatic mutations of the PTEN tumor suppressor gene in sporadic follicular thyroid tumors. Genes Chromosomes Cancer 1998;23:239-43.

136. Samuels Y, Wang Z, Bardelli A, et al. High frequency of mutations of the PIK3CA gene in human cancers. Science 2004;304:554.

137. Hou P, Liu D, Shan Y, et al. Genetic alterations and their relationship in the phosphatidylinositol 3-kinase/Akt pathway in thyroid cancer. Clin Cancer Res 2007; 13:1161-70.

138. García-Rostán G, Costa AM, Pereira-Castro I, et al. Mutation of the PIK3CA gene in anaplastic thyroid cancer. Cancer Res 2005;65:10199-207.

139. Santarpia L, El-Naggar AK, Cote GJ, et al. Phosphatidylinositol 3-kinase/akt and ras/raf-mitogen-activated protein kinase pathway mutations in anaplastic thyroid cancer. J Clin Endocrinol Metab 2008;93:278-84.

140. Burke JE, Perisic O, Masson GR, et al. Oncogenic mutations mimic and enhance dynamic events in the natural activation of phosphoinositide 3-kinase p110α (PIK3CA). Proc Natl Acad Sci U S A 2012;109:15259-64.

141. Ricarte-Filho JC, Ryder M, Chitale DA, et al. Mutational profile of advanced primary and metastatic radioactive iodine-refractory thyroid cancers reveals distinct pathogenetic roles for BRAF, PIK3CA, and AKT1. Cancer Res 2009; 69:4885-93.

142. Laplante M, Sabatini DM. mTOR signaling in growth control and disease. Cell 2012;149:274-93.

143. Ringel MD, Hayre N, Saito J, et al. Overexpression and overactivation of Akt in thyroid carcinoma. Cancer Res 2001;61:6105-11.

144. Vasko V, Saji M, Hardy E, et al. Akt activation and localisation correlate with tumour invasion and oncogene expression in thyroid cancer. J Med Genet 2004;41:161–70.

145. Chen ML, Xu PZ, Peng XD, et al. The deficiency of Akt1 is sufficient to suppress tumor development in Pten+/− mice. Genes Dev 2006;20:1569–74.

146. Xu P-Z, Chen ML, Jeon SM, et al. The effect Akt2 deletion on tumor development in Pten(+/-) mice. Oncogene 2012;31:518–26.

147. Beroukhim R, Mermel CH, Porter D, et al. The landscape of somatic copy-number alteration across human cancers. Nature 2010;463:899–905.

148. Tang YC, Amon A. Gene copy-number alterations: a cost-benefit analysis. Cell 2013;152:394–405.

149. Knouse KA, Davoli T, Elledge SJ, et al. Aneuploidy in cancer: seq-ing answers to old questions. Annu Rev Cancer Biol 2017;1:335–54.

150. Wang Y, Hou P, Yu H, et al. High prevalence and mutual exclusivity of genetic alterations in the phosphatidylinositol-3-kinase/akt pathway in thyroid tumors. J Clin Endocrinol Metab 2007;92:2387–90.

151. Garcia-Rendueles ME, Ricarte-Filho JC, Untch BR, et al. NF2 loss promotes oncogenic RAS-induced thyroid cancers via YAP-dependent transactivation of RAS proteins and sensitizes them to MEK inhibition. Cancer Discov 2015;5:1178–93.

152. Duquette M, Sadow PM, Husain A, et al. Metastasis-associated MCL1 and P16 copy number alterations dictate resistance to vemurafenib in a BRAF V600E patient-derived papillary thyroid carcinoma preclinical model. Oncotarget 2015;6:42445–67.

153. Anders L, Ke N, Hydbring P, et al. A systematic screen for CDK4/6 substrates links FOXM1 phosphorylation to senescence suppression in cancer cells. Cancer Cell 2011;20:620–34.

154. Antonello ZA, Hsu N, Bhasin M, et al. Vemurafenib-resistance via de novo RBM genes mutations and chromosome 5 aberrations is overcome by combined therapy with palbociclib in thyroid carcinoma with BRAF^{V600E}. Oncotarget 2017;8:84743–60.

155. Liu Y, Cope L, Sun W, et al. DNA copy number variations characterize benign and malignant thyroid tumors. J Clin Endocrinol Metab 2013;98:E558–66.

156. Karin M. Nuclear factor-kappaB in cancer development and progression. Nature 2006;441:431–6.

157. Visconti R, Cerutti J, Battista S, et al. Expression of the neoplastic phenotype by human thyroid carcinoma cell lines requires NFkappaB p65 protein expression. Oncogene 1997;15:1987–94.

158. Starenki D, Namba H, Saenko V, et al. Inhibition of nuclear factor-kappaB cascade potentiates the effect of a combination treatment of anaplastic thyroid cancer cells. J Clin Endocrinol Metab 2004;89:410–8.

159. Pacifico F, Mauro C, Barone C, et al. Oncogenic and anti-apoptotic activity of NF-kappa B in human thyroid carcinomas. J Biol Chem 2004;279:54610–9.

160. Bommarito A, Richiusa P, Carissimi E, et al. BRAF-V600E mutation, TIMP-1 upregulation, and NF-κB activation: closing the loop on the papillary thyroid cancer trilogy. Endocr Relat Cancer 2011;18:669–85.

161. Neely RJ, Brose MS, Gray CM, et al. The RET/PTC3 oncogene activates classical NF-κB by stabilizing NIK. Oncogene 2011;30:87–96.

162. Kato Y, Ying H, Zhao L, et al. PPARgamma insufficiency promotes follicular thyroid carcinogenesis via activation of the nuclear factor-kappaB signaling pathway. Oncogene 2006;25:2736–47.

163. Guigon CJ, Zhao L, Willingham MC, et al. PTEN deficiency accelerates tumour progression in a mouse model of thyroid cancer. Oncogene 2009;28:509–17.
164. Bauerle KT, Schweppe RE, Lund G, et al. Nuclear factor κB-dependent regulation of angiogenesis, and metastasis in an in vivo model of thyroid cancer is associated with secreted interleukin-8. J Clin Endocrinol Metab 2014;99: E1436–44.
165. Pozdeyev N, Berlinberg A, Zhou Q, et al. Targeting the NF-κB pathway as a combination therapy for advanced thyroid cancer. PLoS One 2015;10: e0134901.
166. Davies KJ, Ermak G, Rothermel BA, et al. Renaming the DSCR1/Adapt78 gene family as RCAN: regulators of calcineurin. FASEB J 2007;21:3023–8.
167. Martínez-Martínez S, Genescà L, Rodríguez A, et al. The RCAN carboxyl end mediates calcineurin docking-dependent inhibition via a site that dictates binding to substrates and regulators. Proc Natl Acad Sci U S A 2009;106:6117–22.
168. Hogan PG, Chen L, Nardone J, et al. Transcriptional regulation by calcium, calcineurin, and NFAT. Genes Dev 2003;17:2205–32.
169. Baek KH, Zaslavsky A, Lynch RC, et al. Down's syndrome suppression of tumour growth and the role of the calcineurin inhibitor DSCR1. Nature 2009; 459:1126–30.
170. Hesser BA, Liang XH, Camenisch G, et al. Down syndrome critical region protein 1 (DSCR1), a novel VEGF target gene that regulates expression of inflammatory markers on activated endothelial cells. Blood 2004;104:149–58.
171. Iizuka M, Abe M, Shiiba K, et al. Down syndrome candidate region 1,a downstream target of VEGF, participates in endothelial cell migration and angiogenesis. J Vasc Res 2004;41:334–44.
172. Minami T, Horiuchi K, Miura M, et al. Vascular endothelial growth factor- and thrombin-induced termination factor, Down syndrome critical region-1, attenuates endothelial cell proliferation and angiogenesis. J Biol Chem 2004;279: 50537–54.
173. Stathatos N, Bourdeau I, Espinosa AV, et al. KiSS-1/G protein-coupled receptor 54 metastasis suppressor pathway increases myocyte-enriched calcineurin interacting protein 1 expression and chronically inhibits calcineurin activity. J Clin Endocrinol Metab 2005;90:5432–40.
174. Espinosa AV, Shinohara M, Porchia LM, et al. Regulator of calcineurin 1 modulates cancer cell migration in vitro. Clin Exp Metastasis 2009;26:517–26.
175. Wang C, Saji M, Justiniano SE, et al. RCAN1-4 is a thyroid cancer growth and metastasis suppressor. JCI Insight 2017;2:e90651.
176. Kimura ET, Nikiforova MN, Zhu Z, et al. High prevalence of BRAF mutations in thyroid cancer: genetic evidence for constitutive activation of the RET/PTC-RAS-BRAF signaling pathway in papillary thyroid carcinoma. Cancer Res 2003;63:1454–7.
177. Henderson YC, Shellenberger TD, Williams MD, et al. High rate of BRAF and RET/PTC dual mutations associated with recurrent papillary thyroid carcinoma. Clin Cancer Res 2009;15:485–91.
178. Smallridge RC, Ain KB, Asa SL, et al. American Thyroid Association guidelines for management of patients with anaplastic thyroid cancer. Thyroid 2012;22: 1104–39.
179. Kaneshige M, Kaneshige K, Zhu X, et al. Mice with a targeted mutation in the thyroid hormone beta receptor gene exhibit impaired growth and resistance to thyroid hormone. Proc Natl Acad Sci U S A 2000;97(24):13209–14.

180. Suzuki H, Willingham MC, Cheng SY. Mice with a mutation in the thyroid hormone receptor beta gene spontaneously develop thyroid carcinoma: a mouse model of thyroid carcinogenesis. Thyroid 2002;12:963–9.
181. Ying H, Suzuki H, Zhao L, et al. Mutant thyroid hormone receptor beta represses the expression and transcriptional activity of peroxisome proliferator-activated receptor gamma during thyroid carcinogenesis. Cancer Res 2003;63:5274–80.
182. Araki O, Ying H, Furuya F, et al. Thyroid hormone receptor beta mutants: dominant negative regulators of peroxisome proliferator-activated receptor gamma action. Proc Natl Acad Sci U S A 2005;102:16251–6.
183. Furuya F, Hanover JA, Cheng S. Activation of phosphatidylinositol 3-kinase signaling by a mutant thyroid hormone beta receptor. Proc Natl Acad Sci U S A 2006;103:1780–5.
184. Guigon CJ, Zhao L, Lu C, et al. Regulation of beta-catenin by a novel nongenomic action of thyroid hormone beta receptor. Mol Cell Biol 2008;28:4598–608.
185. Guigon CJ, Kim DW, Zhu X, et al. Tumor suppressor action of liganded thyroid hormone receptor beta by direct repression of beta-catenin gene expression. Endocrinology 2010;151:5528–36.
186. Kim WG, Park JW, Willingham MC, et al. Diet-induced obesity increases tumor growth and promotes anaplastic change in thyroid cancer in a mouse model. Endocrinology 2013;154:2936–47.
187. Park JW, Han CR, Zhao L, et al. Inhibition of STAT3 activity delays obesity-induced thyroid carcinogenesis in a mouse model. Endocr Relat Cancer 2016;23:53–63.
188. Park J, Kim WG, Zhao L, et al. Metformin blocks progression of obesity-activated thyroid cancer in a mouse model. Oncotarget 2016;7:34832–44.
189. Zhu X, Zhao L, Park JW, et al. Synergistic signaling of KRAS and thyroid hormone receptor β mutants promotes undifferentiated thyroid cancer through MYC up-regulation. Neoplasia N Y N 2014;16:757–69.
190. Zhu X, Enomoto K, Zhao L, et al. Bromodomain and extraterminal protein inhibitor JQ1 suppresses thyroid tumor growth in a mouse model. Clin Cancer Res 2017;23:430–40.
191. Park S, Willingham M, Qi J, et al. Metformin and JQ1 synergistically inhibit obesity-activated thyroid cancer. Endocr Relat Cancer 2018. https://doi.org/10.1530/ERC-18-0071.

Clinical Diagnostic Evaluation of Thyroid Nodules

Carolyn Maxwell, MD[a], Jennifer A. Sipos, MD[b],*

KEYWORDS

• Thyroid • Thyroid nodule • Ultrasound • Lymph node • Fine-needle aspiration

KEY POINTS

• Evaluation of patients with thyroid nodules should include a neck ultrasound.
• The determination of the need for fine-needle aspiration of a thyroid nodule is based on the clinical presentation, the serum thyroid-stimulating hormone, and the sonographic pattern of the nodule.
• Sonographic assessment of the lymph nodes in the neck is an important component of the evaluation of patients with thyroid nodules.

INTRODUCTION

Thyroid nodules are a common clinical entity, occurring in up to 70% of patients older than 70 years.[1] The preponderance of these lesions represents a benign neoplasm, with only 5% to 15% of nodules harboring a malignancy.[2,3] Fortunately, thyroid carcinoma is highly treatable, with most of the patients enjoying an excellent long-term survival. Indeed, observational studies of small, low-risk thyroid cancers without surgical intervention have determined that less than 10% of patients demonstrate disease progression after a median follow-up of 6 years.[4] However, not all thyroid malignancies are associated with such a favorable prognosis; larger, higher-stage tumors may be seen in up to 20% of patients at initial diagnosis.[5,6] Therefore, it is incumbent on the clinician to have a triaging system to sort through the abundance of benign thyroid nodules efficiently and accurately so that the infrequent but potentially lethal tumors may be identified and removed, without exposing the patient to excessive risk.

The authors have nothing to disclose.
[a] Division of Endocrinology and Metabolism, Stony Brook University School of Medicine, 26 Research Way, East Setauket, NY 11733, USA; [b] Division of Endocrinology and Metabolism, The Ohio State University Wexner Medical Center, 1581 Dodd Drive, 5th Floor McCampbell Hall, South, Columbus, OH 43210, USA
* Corresponding author.
E-mail address: Jennifer.sipos@osumc.edu

Endocrinol Metab Clin N Am 48 (2019) 61–84
https://doi.org/10.1016/j.ecl.2018.11.001
0889-8529/19/© 2018 Elsevier Inc. All rights reserved.

endo.theclinics.com

EPIDEMIOLOGY

The prevalence of thyroid nodules depends on the method of detection. By palpation, nodules are identified in approximately 5% to 10% of patients.[1] The use of a sensitive imaging modality such as ultrasound (US), however, reveals nodular thyroid disease in as many as 34.2% of patients.[7] Nodularity within the thyroid increases linearly with age. Thyroid nodules are seen in 12.9% of those younger than 30 years, whereas 50% to 70% of those older than 70 years have one or more nodules.[7-9] The risk is further modified by gender, with women having a 3 to 4 times higher likelihood of nodularity than men.[7,10] The cause for this disparity is unclear; referral bias,[11] metabolic parameters,[12] and estrogen effects[13,14] have been offered as possible reasons.

RISK FACTORS

Iodine intake, in both insufficient and excessive quantities, confers a higher risk for the development of thyroid nodules.[15] Another important risk factor is exposure to ionizing radiation in childhood.[16,17] In a large retrospective study of patients treated for childhood Hodgkin disease, those with radiation exposure to the thyroid were 27 times more likely to develop nodules than their sibling controls.[18] And, in a recent study of 119 childhood cancer survivors, those exposed to ionizing radiation and chemotherapy (n = 60) were twice as likely to harbor a thyroid nodule (36.7%) compared with those exposed to chemotherapy alone (18.6%, $P = .03$).[19] Quantification of the excess risk for development of thyroid nodules with adult exposure to therapeutic radiation remains elusive.[16]

SYMPTOMS
History and Physical Examination

Although the history and physical examination alone cannot reliably distinguish the nature of the nodule, certain clinical features may elevate the concern for a thyroid malignancy.[20] It is important, therefore, to inquire about personal history of radiation exposure and a family history of thyroid cancer or thyroid cancer syndromes (multiple endocrine neoplasia, Cowden syndrome, familial adenomatous hyperplasia, or Gardner syndrome) and assess for rapid growth of the neck mass (if identified by the patient) because these features increase the likelihood of harboring a thyroid cancer. Further, the identification of a fixed nodule, enlarged locoregional lymph nodes, or the presence of vocal cord paralysis escalates the risk of malignancy to more than 70%.[20]

Patients with a thyroid nodule also should be questioned regarding the presence of local compressive symptoms. Specifically, the clinician should determine whether the patient is experiencing difficulty swallowing solids, dysphonia, or neck tightness. The presence of such symptoms does not necessarily elevate the concern for malignancy but may alter the decision to operate.[21]

DIAGNOSTIC TESTS AND IMAGING LABORATORY EVALUATION

All patients suspected of harboring a thyroid nodule should undergo measurement of a serum thyroid-stimulating hormone (TSH).[21] A low TSH suggests subclinical or overt hyperthyroidism and necessitates further laboratory testing, US, and possibly scintigraphic evaluation to evaluate for a "hot" nodule (see Thyroid Scintigraphy).[22] A normal or elevated TSH, on the other hand, is unlikely to be associated with an autonomous nodule; scinitigraphic imaging is of limited value and the diagnostic evaluation should proceed to sonography.

Thyrotropin is a known growth factor for thyroid follicular cells; suppression of serum TSH is associated with improved survival in patients with advanced thyroid cancer.[23] Further, an elevated TSH increases the likelihood of malignancy in a thyroid nodule[24]; one prospective study demonstrated a 3-fold higher risk of thyroid cancer in patients with a serum TSH greater than or equal to 2.26 μU/mL compared with those with lower TSH levels.[25] In addition, higher preoperative TSH levels in those diagnosed with thyroid cancer predict advanced tumor stage, presence of gross extrathyroidal extension, and lymph node metastases.[26,27]

Measurement of serum calcitonin, a marker for medullary thyroid cancer (MTC), in all patients with thyroid nodules is controversial.[21] A large, prospective study of more than 10,000 patients with nodular thyroid disease found that routine measurement of serum calcitonin provided improved diagnostic sensitivity and specificity compared with fine-needle aspiration (FNA) alone. Those patients who were screened were diagnosed with MTC at an earlier stage and had a higher likelihood of achieving complete remission compared with those diagnosed before routine calcitonin measurement.[28] This and other studies demonstrating a benefit from routine calcitonin measurement used pentagastrin stimulation to confirm MTC in those with an elevated initial value. Such stimulation testing is not currently available in the United States, however. A basal calcitonin of 50 to 100 pg/mL has a specificity of only 25%; false elevations may be seen in many conditions, including renal failure, smoking, chronic autoimmune thyroiditis, and other neuroendocrine tumors.[29] The absence of confirmatory testing therefore poses the risk of significant overtreatment of many patients.[29] Acknowledging the lack of definitive data supporting or controverting the role of screening, the current American Thyroid Association (ATA) guidelines could not recommend for against routine calcitonin measurement.[21]

Serum thyroglobulin is not a useful test to determine malignancy risk.[21] Although typically high in patients with thyroid cancer, thyroglobulin also can be markedly elevated in patients with a benign multinodular goiter.[30]

Thyroid Scintigraphy

Radionuclide scintigraphy provides information about the functional status of a nodule. Iodine isotopes (typically 123-I) or technetium-99m pertechnetate are administered followed by planar imaging via gamma camera with a pinhole collimator. The poor resolution of these scans limits its utility to the detection of nodules larger than 1 cm. In patients with multinodular goiter, the 2-dimensional imaging may confound accurate characterization of the functional status of overlapping nodules.

Malignant nodules typically concentrate the radioisotopes less avidly than normal thyroid tissue and will appear as "cold" or nonfunctioning. Most benign nodules also are nonfunctioning, however, diminishing the specificity of this finding. The sonographic features therefore dictate the need for further cytologic evaluation in cold nodules. The clinical value of scintigraphy lies instead with the identification of nodules that concentrate iodine more avidly than the adjacent thyroid tissue. These autonomous (or "hot") nodules rarely harbor malignancy and as such, do not require FNA.[22]

ULTRASOUND

US should be performed in all patients suspected of having a thyroid nodule.[21] Sonography changes management in up to 63% of patients.[31] In one retrospective study of 114 patients with clinically detected thyroid nodules, a sonographic examination demonstrated no nodules in 16% of cases.[31] Furthermore, US identified another nonpalpable lesion elsewhere in the thyroid gland in 23% of patients.[31] Sonographic assessment of the lateral neck during initial evaluation of a patient with a thyroid nodule helps define the extent of surgery when cancer is ultimately identified. Indeed, several studies have found that preoperative US of the neck changes the surgical approach in up to 40% of patients.[32,33]

Benefits of Office-Based Ultrasound

Office-based sonogram offers numerous advantages to the clinician and patient. Point-of-care US acts as an extension of the physical examination by allowing the clinician to place the probe directly at the site of concern and aids in the determination of a treatment plan. Many gray scale sonographic features are more easily identified when viewed in real time rather than in still images, particularly in the delineation of hyperechoic foci as either colloid or microcalcifications, which have opposing clinical implications.[34]

How to Perform a Neck Ultrasound Examination

A comprehensive cervical US is best performed with the patient laying supine, with the neck fully extended. This can be achieved by placing a pillow or rolled towel between the shoulders. The use of a high-frequency probe (5–13 MHz) enables high-resolution imaging.

To ensure a comprehensive study, the authors use a standardized list of areas to inspect. The thyroid itself is examined in 3 parts: isthmus, left lobe, and right lobe, and it is viewed in both transverse and sagittal views (**Fig. 1**). The size of the lobes is documented in 3 dimensions as well as overall features of the gland (**Table 1**).

Documentation of thyroid nodules should be standardized (see **Table 1**) to improve decision-making at the time of the study as well as enhance the sensitivity of surveillance examinations.

Careful inspection of the central compartment (posterior to the thyroid) as well as the lateral neck is a key component of a comprehensive neck US; identification of abnormal cervical lymph nodes contributes to risk stratification and informs surgical planning. The central compartment, or level VI, contains the paratracheal lymph nodes and extends from the hyoid bone superiorly to the sternal notch inferiorly. Sensitivity of the examination of the central compartment is limited in the presence of an intact thyroid gland.[35]

The lateral neck should also be examined in a systematic fashion, from level IV to level II, which is bordered inferiorly at the clavicle and medially at the carotid sheath,

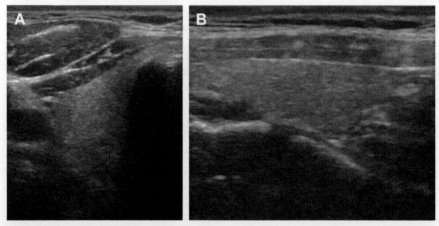

Fig. 1. (A) Normal right thyroid lobe and isthmus in transverse view. (B) Normal sagittal (longitudinal) view of the thyroid.

Table 1
Features of sonographic examination report

Thyroid Gland Features	Nodule Features	Lymph Node Features
Size of each lobe	Size	Size
Echogenicity	Location	Shape
Texture (smooth/heterogeneous)	Echogenicity	Calcifications/cystic change
Vascularity	Composition	Location
Tracheal deviation	Echogenic foci	Vascular pattern
Isthmus thickness	Margins	Echogenicity
	Vascular pattern	

laterally at the posterior edge of the sternocleidomastoid, and superiorly at the mandible. Level V, lateral to the sternocleidomastoid muscle, comprises nodes in the posterior compartment of the neck and is subdivided into upper (VA) and lower (VB) levels by the cricoid cartilage.

Sonographic Risk Stratification

Several sonographic features of thyroid nodules have been long associated with an increased risk of papillary thyroid cancer (PTC), and several multivariate analyses have established that the risk increases when these features are observed in aggregate in a single nodule.[36,37] Six essential components of the sonographic appearance of a nodule are assessed to determine malignancy potential: composition, echogenicity, shape, margins, echogenic foci, and intranodular vascularity.

Composition

Nodules are classified as entirely solid, entirely cystic, or mixed cystic and solid. Most thyroid cancers are solid; one retrospective review of 360 malignant nodules found that 88% were either entirely solid or less than 5% cystic.[38] Solid composition, however, is not specific, because most solid nodules are benign. Entirely cystic, or anechoic nodules, are nearly always benign[39] and being acellular, typically have no diagnostic yield from sampling. Nodules with mixed cystic and solid composition have a lower likelihood of malignancy than entirely solid nodules[38,40] but may require further analysis in the presence of suspicious US features. For example, a spongiform pattern (**Fig. 2**A), in which greater than 50% of the nodule is composed of microcystic

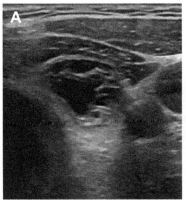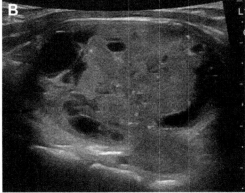

Fig. 2. (A) Spongiform nodule. (B) Complex nodule with suspicious sonographic findings (irregular margins, microcalcifications).

change, has a very low risk of being malignant.[36,39,41,42] In other mixed solid and cystic nodules there is an increased risk of malignancy when the solid component meets the wall of the nodule at an acute angle, is eccentric in shape, or contains microcalcifications[38,40,43] (**Fig. 2**B).

Echogenicity

The echogenicity of a nodule is described in 2 categories: *hyperechoic/isoechoic* and *hypoechoic*, as it appears relative to normal thyroid parenchyma. Nodules that are hyper/isoechoic (brighter than or of the same echogenicity of normal thyroid tissue) are typically benign but when malignant are more likely to represent a follicular-patterned tumor[44,45](**Fig. 3**A). Hypoechogenicity, darker than normal thyroid parenchyma, is associated with increased risk of malignancy, although it is not a specific finding, because more than half of hypoechoic nodules are benign (**Fig. 3**B). Nodules that are markedly hypoechoic, or as dark or darker than the surrounding musculature, are associated with an increased risk for malignancy[37,41] (**Fig. 3**C).

Shape

The natural growth plane of a benign thyroid nodule is in the horizontal direction when the patient is supine (**Fig. 4**A); growth opposite that plane, or a taller-than-wide shape, suggests a more aggressive neoplasm and is concerning for a malignancy[46](**Fig. 4**B). Several studies have reported that the taller-than-wide shape in either transverse or longitudinal imaging confers an increased risk of malignancy[47,48] but is only seen in

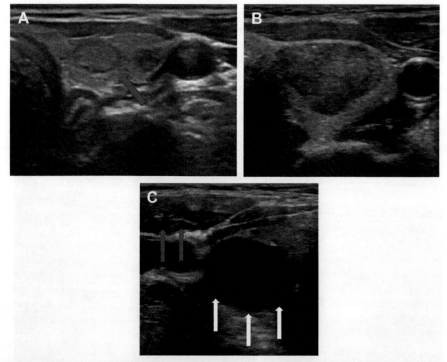

Fig. 3. (*A*) Isoechoic nodule (*red arrow*). (*B*) Hypoechoic nodule. (*C*) Markedly hypoechoic nodule; note the nodule echogenicity (*white arrows*) is darker than the anterior strap muscles (*red arrows*).

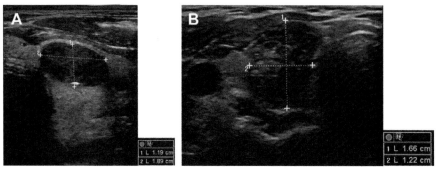

Fig. 4. (*A*) Oval-shaped nodule (horizontal growth plane). (*B*) Taller than wide shape.

12% of thyroid nodules.[36] The specificity of this finding has been reported to be up to 94%.[48] The utility of this finding may be size-dependent, because one study found that the specificity of shape is increased for lesions measuring less than 1 cm compared with larger nodules.[46]

Margins

Irregular (infiltrative, speculated, or microlobulated) thyroid nodule margins are associated with increased risk of malignancy; although this feature lacks sensitivity, 33% to 93% of malignancies may have a smooth or regular border[49](**Fig. 5A**). It is important to distinguish an irregular margin from an ill-defined margin, in which the borders of the nodule are not clearly delineated from the surrounding thyroid. Ill-defined margins are frequently seen in benign isoechoic or mildly hypoechoic nodules and do not increase the risk of malignancy (**Fig. 5B**).[41] The presence of a halo, an anechoic (sonolucent) rim surrounding the nodule (**Fig. 5C**), was previously thought to be associated with a benign nodule. Recent US stratification systems have not incorporated this feature into assessment of risk because it may be difficult to discriminate or define, can exist in the presence of irregular margins, and is seen in some cancers.[37,49] Extension of a nodule through the capsule of the thyroid and into adjacent muscle or vasculature is very concerning for malignancy.[37,50,51]

Echogenic Foci

Echogenic areas within a nodule contribute to risk stratification, but accurate classification is critical, because some, but not all, forms of calcifications increase risk of malignancy. A macrocalcification is a coarse hyperechoic inclusion measuring greater than 1 mm associated with posterior acoustic shadowing[36] (**Fig. 6A**). Intranodular macrocalcifications have been reported as increasing likelihood of cancer in some[52,53] studies, but several analyses have found that isolated macrocalcifications in the absence of other suspicious features are not reliable predictors of malignancy.[36,54,55] Similarly, peripheral linear calcifications, also referred to as rim, or eggshell calcifications (**Fig. 6B**), have conflicting data regarding malignancy risk. However, an interrupted rim with soft tissue extrusion has a high likelihood of malignancy.[56]

Small, less than 1 mm punctate echogenic foci may represent either colloid or microcalcifications. Representing opposite ends of the risk spectrum, proper distinction of these disparate findings is important but can be challenging. The hallmark feature of a colloid inclusion is demonstration of a posterior reverberation artifact, also commonly referred to as a comet-tail sign or V-shaped artifacts (**Fig. 6C**). These are more easily identified using real-time sonography than on static images. Punctate

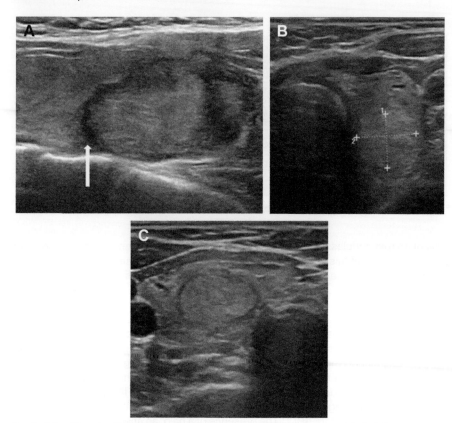

Fig. 5. (*A*) Infiltrative/lobulated margin denoted by the white arrow. (*B*) Ill-defined margin, echogenicity of the nodule and the thyroid are very similar, making definition of the nodule challenging. (*C*) Halo—sonolucent rim around the isoechoic nodule.

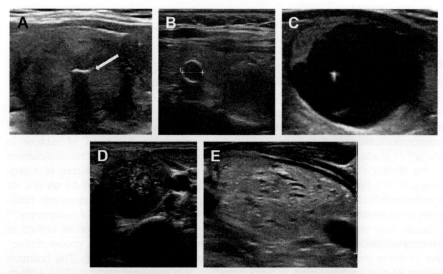

Fig. 6. (*A*) Macrocalcification (*white arrow*) with posterior acoustic shadow (*red arrow*). (*B*) Uninterrupted egg-shell calcification. (*C*) Comet tail sign. (*D*) Microcalcifications. (*E*) Bright linear reflectors posterior to cystic content.

foci that lack the comet-tail sign (**Fig. 6**D) are more likely to represent microcalcifications, which are typically associated with papillary thyroid cancer.[36,41] Finally, small linear hyperechoic inclusions located posterior to microcystic areas, as seen in spongiform nodules, are an artifact of posterior acoustic enhancement within the solid components of complex nodules and do not raise the malignancy risk (**Fig. 6**E).

Intranodular Vascularity

Increased nodular vascularity was previously identified as a risk factor for malignancy[57,58] but more recently has been shown to have no predictive capability.[59,60] One study of nearly 700 thyroid neoplasms found that more than half of the malignant nodules, 63%, lacked intranodular vascularity on preoperative imaging.[60] Indeed, the most current risk stratification guidelines from the ATA[21] and the American College of Radiology (TIRADS)[37] do not incorporate vascularity status into their sonographic stratification systems. It should be noted, however, that intranodular vascularity may correlate with malignancy risk in neoplasms and malignancies other than classic PTC including noninvasive follicular thyroid neoplasm with papillary-like nuclear features (NIFTP), follicular variant of papillary thyroid carcinoma (FVPTC), follicular thyroid carcinoma (FTC), and MTC.[39,60–62]

Nonpapillary Thyroid Carcinoma

The classic suspicious sonographic features, such as taller-than-wide shape, microcalcifications, and hypoechogenicity, are well established predictors of PTC but are less frequently associated with other forms of thyroid carcinoma. FTC and FVPTC are more likely to be sonographically indeterminate: isoechoic, lacking microcalcifications, and having an oval shape (rather than tall).[44,45,63] For this reason, nodules without these suspicious features are still monitored and aspirated.[21] The size threshold for FNA in these sonographically indeterminate nodules is larger, however, because follicular cancers measuring less than 2 cm have very low metastatic rates.[64]

Few studies have addressed specific sonographic features of MTC. Available data suggest that MTC shares certain suspicious characteristics with PTC such as marked hypoechogenicity and coarse calcifications but is more likely to be round (not taller than wide), have regular borders, and features intranodular vascularity than PTC.[62,65–67] One study reports that sonographic features of subcentimeter MTC tend to mimic PTC, with a taller-than-wide shape and spiculated borders; however, larger (>1 cm) medullary cancers tended to feature less suspicious elements such as a round shape with regular borders.[68]

Pseudonodules

Certain sonographic features within the thyroid parenchyma may give a false appearance of a nodule or a "pseudonodule." This occurs most frequently in patients with autoimmune thyroiditis, in which chronic inflammation renders the thyroid parenchyma heterogeneous, with large deposits of lymphocytes appearing as hypoechoic patches that may be mistaken for nodules. This finding, often referred to as a "giraffe" (**Fig. 7**A, B), or "Swiss cheese" (**Fig. 7**C) pattern, should not prompt sampling of the hypoechoic areas, which simply represent lymphocytic infiltrate. In addition, chronic inflammation causes fibrosis that appears as hyperechoic linear bands, which may give the false impression of a thyroid nodule within their borders (**Fig. 7**D). These areas typically can be distinguished from true nodules by demonstrating that they lack the appearance of a distinct nodule in both transverse and sagittal imaging and do not track with movement of the probe.

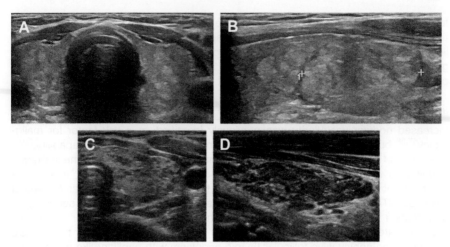

Fig. 7. (*A*) "Giraffe" pattern in autoimmune thyroiditis, transverse view. (*B*) "Giraffe" pattern in autoimmune thyroiditis, sagittal view. (*C*) Microcystic change ("Swiss cheese") in early Hashimoto thyroiditis. (*D*) Fibrous bands in autoimmune thyroiditis.

Lymph Node Evaluation

Sonographic examination of the central and lateral neck compartments is a key element of a comprehensive neck US, because identification of nonpalpable suspicious lymph nodes affects malignancy risk and alters surgical planning in about a third of patients.[32,33] Benign lymph nodes have a characteristic sonographic appearance— a flat or ovoid shape—and the presence of a hyperechoic hilum, a fluid-filled sinus, and afferent lymphatic vessels[69] (**Fig. 8**A). The hilum may be seen in 30% to 80% of

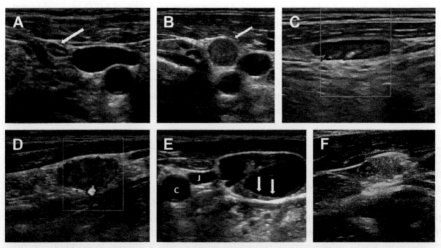

Fig. 8. (*A*) Benign lateral lymph node with hilum, fusiform (*oval*) shaped. The white arrow denotes the hilum. (*B*) Round malignant node anterior to the carotid in the left lateral neck (*white arrow*). (*C*) Benign lymph node with normal Doppler flow in the hilum. (*D*) Malignant node with peripheral vascular flow. (*E*) Malignant node with internal cystic degeneration and small peripheral solid component (*white arrows*). C is carotid, J is jugular. (*F*) Malignant node with microcalcifications (*red arrow*).

normal lymph nodes.[70–73] The absence of a hilum may be seen in both benign and cancerous nodes, but its presence essentially rules out a malignant process.[74]

Enlargement of a lymph node, generally defined as greater than 8 to 10 mm in shortest axis is suggestive of but not specific for malignancy, because enlargement is a normal nodal response to infection or inflammation. The shape of a node, with transformation from oval to rounded, suggests malignancy (**Fig. 8B**). Objectively, round shape is defined as a short:long axis ratio of 0.5 or greater, although this transformation can also occur in a benign reactive process.[75] It is important to examine each lymph node in both the transverse and sagittal views, however. A node may seem rounded based on its positioning in relation to the probe but visualization in a different plane may reveal elongation of the node.

Several more specific sonographic features are associated with the presence of metastatic thyroid cancer within a lymph node. The presence of hyperechoic tissue (of similar appearance to thyroid tissue) within the node, either as small deposits initially or eventually with replacement of the entire node, results from infiltration of the node with malignant follicular cells and colloid.[71,76] Vascular flow within the node can also help distinguish a benign or malignant process. A benign or reactive lymph node typically demonstrates either hilar (**Fig. 8C**) or absent vascular flow, whereas disorganized or peripheral vascularity may be observed in a metastatic node[71,77] (**Fig. 8D**). Also highly predictive of malignant transformation, cystic degeneration can be seen as scattered small cystic areas within the node or the entire replacement of the node with cystic fluid[70,71,76] (**Fig. 8E**). Intranodal calcifications are seen in 46% to 69% of metastatic nodes from PTC[69] and less commonly may be seen in medullary thyroid carcinoma.[78] They are typically found in the periphery of the node and are punctate (**Fig. 8F**). Calcifications may also be seen in nodes after irradiation or chemotherapy.[78]

Risk Stratification Systems

Multiple risk-stratification systems based on the abovementioned sonographic features of thyroid nodules have been created,[21,37,79–84] with the aim to develop a common language to describe and triage nodules at greatest risk for morbidity, while avoiding unnecessary biopsy of those which are benign. Early systems advised biopsy of nodules with a single suspicious feature,[79,80] whereas more recent classification schemes use pattern recognition or adopt a quantitative methodology.[21,37,81,82] Although the likelihood of malignancy escalates with an increasing number of suspicious features,[36,85,86] sensitivity is low for any individual sonographic element. Interobserver agreement is only moderate to fair, even with experienced sonographers, when examining individual sonographic features.[87] The use of a pattern-based classification system, however, is associated with significantly improved interobserver agreement.[88,89]

Thyroid Imaging, Reporting, and Data System

The TIRADS acronym was first proposed by Horvath and colleagues[82] as an adaptation of the American College of Radiology's (ACR) widely used BIRADS classification system of mammography. Multiple thyroid risk stratification systems entitled TIRADS subsequently have been published[90] using a range of 5 to 10 risk tiers. The 10-tiered system first proposed by Horvath and colleagues[82] has been validated in a separate study, with reported 99.6% sensitivity and 74.4% specificity for malignancy in the higher risk patterns.[91]

The TIRADS system endorsed by the American College of Radiology (ACR-TIRADS)[37] consists of a point system assigned for individual features such as taller than wide shape, irregular margins, etc, which are then further classified into 5 TIRADS categories (**Tables 2** and **3**). The ACR-TIRADS has been validated in a large multiinstitutional

Table 2
ACR-TIRADS nodule features and associated points for each characteristic

Composition		Echogenicity		Shape		Margin		Echogenic Foci	
Cystic	0	Anechoic	0	Wider than tall	0	Smooth	0	None	0
Spongiform	0	Hyper/isoechoic	0	Taller than wide	3	Ill-defined	0	Comet-tails	0
Mixed	1	Hypoechoic	1			Lobulated/irregular	2	Macrocalcifications	1
Solid	2	Markedly hypoechoic	2			Extrathyroidal extension	3	Peripheral/rim	2
								Punctate	3

Adapted from Tessler FN, Middleton WD, Grant EG, et al. ACR thyroid imaging, reporting and data system (TI-RADS): white paper of the ACR TI-RADS Committee. J Am Coll Radiol 2017;14(5):589; with permission.

Table 3
ACR-TIRADS scores

Score	0	2	3	4–6	7
TIRADS class	TR1	TR2	TR3	TR4	TR5
Clinical description	Benign	Not Suspicious	Mildly Suspicious	Moderately Suspicious	Highly Suspicious

Adapted from Tessler FN, Middleton WD, Grant EG, et al. ACR thyroid imaging, reporting and data system (TI-RADS): white paper of the ACR TI-RADS Committee. J Am Coll Radiol 2017;14(5):589; with permission.

study,[86] which evaluated 3422 nodules and assigned points (0–10) with the corresponding TIRADS categories and found that as the point tally increased, risk of malignancy also increased, from 0.3% for 1 point to 68.4% for 10 or greater points. The risk of malignancy similarly correlated with TIRADS categories: TR1 0.3%, TR2 1.5%, TR3 4.8%, TR4 9.1%, and TR5 35%.

Other categorization systems proposed by the American Thyroid Association (ATA),[21] the American College of Endocrinology (ACE),[84] and the Korean Society for Thyroid Radiology (K-TIRADS)[81] comprise pattern-based classification without a quantitative point system. K-TIRADS consists of 4 patterns based on grayscale sonographic features: benign, low, intermediate, and high suspicion. The system was validated in a prospective study of 902 nodules, which reported malignancy risks of 0, 7.8, 25.4, and 79.3%, respectively.[85]

The ATA risk stratification system consists of 5 categories, based on various combinations of grayscale sonographic features: benign, very low suspicion, low suspicion, intermediate suspicion, and high suspicion, with estimated malignancy risks of less than 1%, less than 3%, 5% to 10%, 10% to 20%, and 70% to 90%, respectively.[21] These estimated malignancy risks were validated in a prospective study of 206 nodules, with reported malignancy rates of 2% for very low, 8% for low, 11% for intermediate, and 100% for high suspicion sonographic pattern.[92] Other studies have found lower malignancy rates, 55% to 58%, in nodules classified as ATA high suspicion pattern.[93,94] A critique of the ATA system is that nodules that have a suspicious feature such as microcalcifications, but are not hypoechoic, are not categorizable and therefore malignancy risk cannot be quantified. In validation studies, the number of nodules that do not fall into an ATA category ranges from 0% to 14%,[86,92,94] with one study finding that 18% of these noncategorizable nodules were malignant.[94]

Few studies have compared the performance of various stratification systems. Middleton and colleagues[86] used their dataset of 3422 nodules to compare ACR-TIRADS to ATA and K-TIRADS and concluded that fewer benign nodules would be subject to biopsy with ACR TIRADS than with either of the other systems. An Italian study of 987 nodules found similar accuracy when comparing the 5-tiered ATA system to 3- and 4-tiered systems recommended by the ACE[84] and the British Thyroid Association, respectively[93](Table 4).

MANAGEMENT
Indication for Fine-Needle Aspiration

Risk stratification systems inform two fundamental questions regarding thyroid nodule management: which nodules should be biopsied and how often should surveillance scans be performed for those which are not aspirated? Size is the most commonly used determinant for biopsy, but it is important to note that this tendency is based on its predictive value for clinically meaningful malignancy, not for the presence of malignancy alone.[95] Indeed, several observational studies of small (<1 cm) biopsy-proven carcinomas have revealed that small papillary thyroid cancers rarely grow or metastasize beyond the thyroid, and when these events do occur, delayed time to surgery does not affect overall survival.[96] These data, combined with risk of surgical complications, prompt most of the thyroid nodule management guidelines to recommend sampling of nodules only greater than or equal to 1 cm in maximal dimension.[21]

Although prior recommendations used an indiscriminant 1 cm threshold to recommend biopsy for all solid nodules, more recent guidelines have incorporated sonographic appearance to tailor the size criteria for biopsy. Specific size thresholds vary based on the stratification system (see **Table 4**), but in general

Table 4
Comparison of management recommendations in stratification systems of the ATA

Categorization	Description	FNA Size Threshold	Surveillance Interval if Benign Cytology
ATA			
Benign	Anechoic cyst	Not recommended	Not recommended
Very Low	Complex; spongiform	≥2 cm	≥24 mo or clinical surveillance
Low	Complex or solid hyper/isoechoic	≥1.5 cm	12–24 mo
Intermediate	Solid hypoechoic	≥1 cm	12–24 mo
High	Hypoechoic with suspicious feature	≥1 cm	Repeat FNA and US within 12 mo
ACR-TIRADS			
0 Benign	0 points (see **Table 2**)	Not recommended	
2 Not Suspicious	2 points (see **Table 2**)	Not recommended	
3 Mildly Suspicious	3 points (see **Table 2**)	FNA ≥2.5 cm Follow ≥1.5 cm	At 1, 3, and 5 y
4 Moderately Suspicious	4–6 points (see **Table 2**)	FNA ≥1.5 cm Follow ≥1.0 cm	At 1, 2, 3, and 5 y
5 Highly suspicious	≥7 points (see **Table 2**)	FNA ≥1.0 cm Follow ≥0.5 cm	Annually for 5 y
K-TIRADS			
2 Benign	Cystic, spongiform, complex with colloid inclusions	≥2 cm	Not stated
3 Low	Complex or solid hyper/isoechoic	≥1.5 cm	12–24 mo
4 Intermediate	Solid hypoechoic without suspicious features or hyper/isoechoic with suspicious features	≥1 cm	12–24 mo
5 High	Solid hypoechoic with suspicious features	≥0.5–1 cm	Repeat FNA and US within 6–12 mo
ACE			
Low	Cystic, spongiform, complex with colloid inclusions	≥2 cm and increasing in size or other clinical risk factor	≥12 mo or clinical surveillance
Intermediate	Solid or complex without suspicious features	≥2 cm	≥12 mo or clinical surveillance
High	Markedly hypoechoic or other suspicious features	≥0.5–1 cm	Repeat FNA

Data from Refs.[21,37,81,84].

recommend FNA of solid nodules greater than 1 cm with suspicious features and greater than 2 to 2.5 cm for nodules with a more reassuring pattern or cystic predominance. Nodules with intermediate to low suspicion features, when malignant, have a higher likelihood of being FTC rather than PTC.[90] A larger size threshold for aspiration of nodules with this pattern is based on data demonstrating that follicular carcinomas measuring less than 2 cm were not associated with distant metastases or mortality.[21,64]

Individualized factors that may affect clinical decision-making include history of head and neck irradiation, family history of thyroid cancer, or personal history of syndromes associated with thyroid cancer such as multiple endocrine neoplasia, Cowden syndrome, familial adenomatous polyposis, or Carney complex. Nodules found incidentally on PET scanning with ^{18}FDG avidity prove to be malignant in approximately 35% of cases[97]; however, recommended biopsy threshold for these nodules remains greater than or equal to 1 cm.[21] In addition, the patient's age, medical comorbidities, and life expectancy should be taken into consideration. Indeed, a recent retrospective study of 1129 patients older than 70 years with thyroid nodules found that 14.4% of the cohort died during a mean follow-up of 4 years. Only 0.9% (n = 10 patients) of the cohort died due to thyroid cancer; all were preoperatively identified as clinically significant thyroid cancers by imaging and/or cytology. A separate nonthyroidal malignancy or coronary artery disease at the time of nodule evaluation was associated with a more than 2-fold increased mortality compared with those without these diagnoses, validating a judicious approach to elderly patients with coexisting medical conditions during the workup of thyroid nodules.[98]

How to Perform Fine-Needle Aspiration

Biopsy of the thyroid is a safe, accurate, and rapid tool to assess the malignancy risk of a thyroid nodule. There are many variables to consider when attempting to obtain cytologic material from thyroid nodules including use of image guidance, needle size, use of anesthetic, and sampling technique.

Before widespread use of office-based sonography, most of the biopsies were palpation-guided. The limitation of this approach is the lack of direct needle visualization in the area of interest. For large, solid nodules, palpation-guided biopsy provides an adequate sample in most of the cases. However, nodules that have a cystic component, are not readily palpated, have a prior nondiagnostic FNA, or are posteriorly located are best sampled with US guidance of the needle.[21]

Most clinicians prefer to use a small bore needle (23–27 gauge), referred to as FNA, as the initial approach to thyroid sampling. In contrast, a large (21 gauge or bigger) needle is used by some to provide a core of thyroid tissue for histopathologic analysis or to provide more cellular material in the case of a prior nondiagnostic FNA.[99] This large needle biopsy is unnecessary in most cases, however, and exposes the patient to increased risk for bleeding and significant discomfort.

Although anesthetic is not essential, some prefer to use either injectable or topical lidocaine. Others argue that when using a fine needle (25 or 27 gauge), the procedure is associated with only minimal discomfort and the injection to administer lidocaine is a needless source of additional pain. Alternatively, topical lidocaine may be used to avoid an extra needle stick but it increases the length of the procedure while awaiting the anesthetic effect.

There are two approaches to guide the needle sonographically into the nodule: parallel and perpendicular. Physician preference determines the approach used in most cases but there are distinct advantages to each method. The parallel technique places the needle along the lateral edge of the probe parallel to the plane of the US waves, providing visualization of the needle along its entire path to the nodule. This method requires more exact maneuvering of the needle to find the plane of the US beam. The alternative approach, perpendicular to and in the center of the US probe, is a quicker and more direct path into the nodule. With this method, the needle tip alone is visualized as it traverses the plane of the US beam.

Once the nodule is punctured with the needle, the technique to obtain cellular material may include use of suction (aspiration) with a syringe or by capillary action with repetitive movement of the needle in the nodule without a syringe. Both techniques have demonstrated similar efficacy in obtaining an adequate sample.[100]

CYTOLOGY FINDINGS AND MANAGEMENT

The 2008 introduction of the Bethesda System for Reporting Thyroid Cytopathology[101] brought a much-needed, standardized method of reporting cytopathologic findings in a risk-stratified manner, allowing for a common language and providing practice standards amongst clinicians. Widely adopted since its publication, the Bethesda System was revised in 2017[102] to reflect new developments, such as the introduction of the NIFTP classification, as well as the use of molecular markers in nodules with indeterminate cytology.

The 2017 Bethesda System[102] retains the original 6 cytologic categories as outlined in **Table 5**. Category I, Nondiagnostic (ND) or Unsatisfactory, describes aspirates containing only blood, or an insufficient number of follicular cells, with the requirement being at least 6 groups composed of at least 10 follicular cells each. An exception is a sample with insufficient number of follicular cells, but abundant colloid, which can be classified as benign. It is difficult to accurately assess malignancy risk amongst Category I nodules, because many are reclassified on repeat biopsy, and malignancy rates among those that are resected are likely an overestimate of malignancy of all ND nodules due to selection bias. When an ND result is received, sonographic features may help guide the decision to monitor the nodule (eg, a mostly cystic, sonographically reassuring nodule) versus repeat the aspiration.[103]

Table 5
Bethesda System for cytologic diagnosis of thyroid nodules

Category	Category Name	Cytologic Features	Malignancy Risk (%)
I	Nondiagnostic or Unsatisfactory (ND)	Insufficient cellularity, obscuring blood	5–10
II	Benign	Normal-appearing follicular cells arranged in sheets or macrofollicles, abundant colloid	0–3
III	Atypical of Undetermined Significance or Follicular Lesion of Undetermined Significance (AUS/FLUS)	Sparsely cellular, microfollicles, mild nuclear changes	10–30
IV	Follicular Lesion/Suspicious for Follicular Lesion (FN/SFN)	Hypercellular, crowding, microfollicles, scant colloid	25–40
V	Suspicious for Malignancy (SFM)	Some features that suggest but not definitive for malignancy	50–75
VI	Malignant	Papillary architecture, definitive nuclear changes	97–99

Data from Cibas ES, Ali SZ. The 2017 Bethesda System for Reporting Thyroid Cytopathology. Thyroid 2017;27(11):1341–6.

Category II, Benign, is the most commonly assigned category (60%–70%)[101] and represents a less than 3% risk of malignancy. Category II nodules feature an adequate number of uniform, well-spaced follicular cells, arranged as macrofollicles or in sheets, and contain colloid. Category II also comprises aspirates featuring lymphocytic thyroiditis, and granulomatous (subacute) thyroiditis.

Categories III (Atypia of Undetermined Significance/Follicular Lesion of Undetermined Significance [AUS/FLUS]) and IV (Follicular Neoplasm or Suspicious for Follicular Neoplasm [FN/SFN]) feature cellular abnormalities that increase the risk, but are not definitive for malignancy. It is in this area where management decisions are often nuanced and in which there is much interest in developing tools to further risk stratify findings. Included in the AUS/FLUS category are sparsely cellular samples arranged in microfollicules, cells featuring mild nuclear changes, or an abundance of Hurthle cells.

The AUS/FLUS categorization has a wide range of risk of malignancy, between 5% and 48%,[102–105] but the rate will vary according to specific cytologic findings, the interpreting pathologist, and the community population. The introduction of the NIFTP classification further complicates the estimation of malignancy risk with this diagnosis because many NIFTP tumors were initially categorized as AUS on FNA. If NIFTP is not considered a cancer, overall malignancy rates in the category decline, with one analysis reporting a 6% to 18% risk of malignancy if NIFTP is not a cancer versus 10% to 30% if NIFTP is considered a cancer.[103,106] Although NIFTP is not technically a cancer by definition, it does require surgical removal, and so the higher estimates may be more relevant when it comes to surgical planning.[103]

Category IV, FN/SFN, consists of cytologic findings that are hypercellular and are arranged in a microfollicular or trabecular pattern. Crowding may be seen, and colloid is often scant. When malignancy is found in these nodules (10%–40%), it is typically follicular carcinoma or the follicular variant of papillary carcinoma, both of which are defined by capsular invasion and therefore cannot be diagnosed on FNA. Malignancy rates are similarly decreased when NIFTP is reclassified as nonmalignant (10%–40% vs 25%–40%).[103]

Molecular testing, to further risk stratify indeterminate nodules, has become common-place and is addressed in Sarah E. Mayson and Bryan R. Haugen's article, "Molecular Diagnostic Evaluation of Thyroid Nodules," in this issue. Recent data suggests sonographic features may also assist in risk stratification and subsequent decision-making in indeterminate nodules.[107]

The final 2 categories, V (Suspicious for Malignancy [SFN]) and VI (Malignant), have high rates of malignancy (60%–75% and 97%–99%, respectively) and are nearly always recommended to undergo resection. Cytologic findings here include typical nuclear and architectural features of papillary thyroid cancer: large cells, prominent nucleoli, nuclear grooves and inclusions, psammoma bodies, and cells that are arranged in papillae.[101]

SURVEILLANCE

Appropriate surveillance of nodules with benign cytology depends on sonographic features. In nodules with multiple suspicious sonographic features but benign cytology, most of the guidelines recommend repeat FNA within 6 to 12 months out of concern for a false-negative cytology result[21,81,84] (see **Table 4**). Several studies have determined that the rate of false-negative cytology is related to the sonographic pattern of nodules. Cytologically benign nodules with a reassuring US pattern have a risk of malignancy less than 2%, whereas those that are sonographically suspicious have a risk of malignancy of 17% to 20%.[108,109] For nodules with a benign FNA that have a reassuring sonographic pattern, the recommended follow-up interval is 12 to 24 months. The ATA further advises that nodules with a very low suspicion pattern and benign cytology may not require any subsequent imaging.[21] The long-term surveillance for sonographically stable nodules should be lengthened but the ideal monitoring intervals are unclear and the need for evaluation beyond 5 years is unknown due to limited evidence-based guidance.

The definition of nodule stability has traditionally focused on size, defined as a 20% increase in at least 2 nodule dimensions with a minimal increase of 2 mm or more or greater than 50% increase in volume.[21] More recently, however, the emergence of suspicious sonographic features has garnered more concern for the presence of an unrecognized malignancy. Several studies have established that many benign nodules exhibit growth and that the likelihood of malignancy does not increase with growth after initial benign FNA.[108–110] However, a recent study examined rates of growth in cytologically benign versus malignant nodules greater than 1 cm that did not undergo immediate resection and found that malignant nodules were more likely to grow, with a growth of more than 2 mm/y that predicts malignancy. Moreover, faster growth rate was associated with more aggressive carcinoma subtypes.[111] It is reasonable, therefore, to incorporate both sonographic features and significant growth into the decision to repeat an FNA.

A nodule that has had 2 benign biopsy results has a likelihood of malignancy that is virtually zero and no longer requires sonographic surveillance.[21,108] From a practical standpoint, this is helpful for a solitary nodule, but in a multinodular thyroid, continued surveillance will often be needed. In addition, long-term clinical, if not sonographic, follow-up is important because benign nodules that are large or medially located have the potential to cause compressive symptoms as they grow and may eventually require resection or nonsurgical ablation.

Nodules that do not undergo biopsy generally require continued sonographic surveillance, the recommended interval of which ranges from 6 to 24 months, again based on sonographic features (see **Table 4**). Of note, the ATA advises subcentimeter nodules with a very low suspicion pattern do not require subsequent sonographic follow-up.[21]

REFERENCES

1. Mazzaferri EL. Management of a solitary thyroid nodule. N Engl J Med 1993; 328(8):553–9.

2. Yang J, Schnadig V, Logrono R, et al. Fine-needle aspiration of thyroid nodules: a study of 4703 patients with histologic and clinical correlations. Cancer 2007; 111(5):306–15.

3. Yassa L, Cibas ES, Benson CB, et al. Long-term assessment of a multidisciplinary approach to thyroid nodule diagnostic evaluation. Cancer 2007;111(6): 508–16.

4. Ito Y, Miyauchi A, Kihara M, et al. Patient age is significantly related to the progression of papillary microcarcinoma of the thyroid under observation. Thyroid 2014;24(1):27–34.

5. SEER database. Available at: https://seer.cancer.gov/statfacts/html/thyro.html. Accessed March 20, 2018.

6. Hundahl SA, Fleming ID, Fremgen AM, et al. A national cancer data base report on 53,856 cases of thyroid carcinoma treated in the U.S., 1985-1995 [see commetns]. Cancer 1998;83(12):2638–48.

7. Moon JH, Hyun MK, Lee JY, et al. Prevalence of thyroid nodules and their associated clinical parameters: a large-scale, multicenter-based health checkup study. Korean J Intern Med 2018;33(4):753–62.

8. Acar T, Ozbek SS, Acar S. Incidentally discovered thyroid nodules: frequency in an adult population during Doppler ultrasonographic evaluation of cervical vessels. Endocrine 2014;45(1):73–8.

9. Liu Y, Lin Z, Sheng C, et al. The prevalence of thyroid nodules in northwest China and its correlation with metabolic parameters and uric acid. Oncotarget 2017; 8(25):41555–62.

10. Libutti SK. Understanding the role of gender in the incidence of thyroid cancer. Cancer J 2005;11(2):104–5.

11. Germano A, Schmitt W, Almeida P, et al. Ultrasound requested by general practitioners or for symptoms unrelated to the thyroid gland may explain higher prevalence of thyroid nodules in females. Clin Imaging 2018;50:289–93.

12. Ding X, Xu Y, Wang Y, et al. Gender disparity in the relationship between prevalence of thyroid nodules and metabolic syndrome components: the SHDC-CDPC community-based study. Mediators Inflamm 2017;2017:8481049.

13. Manole D, Schildknecht B, Gosnell B, et al. Estrogen promotes growth of human thyroid tumor cells by different molecular mechanisms. J Clin Endocrinol Metab 2001;86(3):1072–7.

14. Xu S, Chen G, Peng W, et al. Oestrogen action on thyroid progenitor cells: relevant for the pathogenesis of thyroid nodules? J Endocrinol 2013;218(1):125–33.

15. Zhao W, Han C, Shi X, et al. Prevalence of goiter and thyroid nodules before and after implementation of the universal salt iodization program in mainland China from 1985 to 2014: a systematic review and meta-analysis. PLoS One 2014; 9(10):e109549.

16. Ron E, Brenner A. Non-malignant thyroid diseases after a wide range of radiation exposures. Radiat Res 2010;174(6):877–88.

17. Schneider AB, Ron E, Lubin J, et al. Dose-response relationships for radiation-induced thyroid cancer and thyroid nodules: evidence for the prolonged effects of radiation on the thyroid. J Clin Endocrinol Metab 1993;77(2):362–9.

18. Sklar C, Whitton J, Mertens A, et al. Abnormalities of the thyroid in survivors of Hodgkin's disease: data from the Childhood Cancer Survivor Study. J Clin Endocrinol Metab 2000;85(9):3227–32.

19. Agrawal C, Guthrie L, Sturm MS, et al. Comparison of thyroid nodule prevalence by ultrasound in childhood cancer survivors with and without thyroid radiation exposure. J Pediatr Hematol Oncol 2016;38(1):43–8.

20. Hamming JF, Goslings BM, van Steenis GJ, et al. The value of fine-needle aspiration biopsy in patients with nodular thyroid disease divided into groups of suspicion of malignant neoplasms on clinical grounds. Arch Intern Med 1990; 150(1):113–6.

21. Haugen BR, Alexander EK, Bible KC, et al. 2015 American Thyroid Association Management guidelines for adult patients with thyroid nodules and differentiated thyroid cancer: the American Thyroid Association guidelines task force on thyroid nodules and differentiated thyroid cancer. Thyroid 2016;26(1):1–133.

22. Ross DS, Burch HB, Cooper DS, et al. 2016 American Thyroid Association guidelines for diagnosis and management of hyperthyroidism and other causes of thyrotoxicosis. Thyroid 2016;26(10):1343–421.

23. Jonklaas J, Sarlis NJ, Litofsky D, et al. Outcomes of patients with differentiated thyroid carcinoma following initial therapy. Thyroid 2006;16(12):1229–42.

24. Boelaert K, Horacek J, Holder RL, et al. Serum thyrotropin concentration as a novel predictor of malignancy in thyroid nodules investigated by fine-needle aspiration. J Clin Endocrinol Metab 2006;91(11):4295–301.

25. Golbert L, de Cristo AP, Faccin CS, et al. Serum TSH levels as a predictor of malignancy in thyroid nodules: a prospective study. PLoS One 2017;12(11): e0188123.

26. Haymart MR, Repplinger DJ, Leverson GE, et al. Higher serum thyroid stimulating hormone level in thyroid nodule patients is associated with greater risks of differentiated thyroid cancer and advanced tumor stage. J Clin Endocrinol Metab 2008;93(3):809–14.

27. McLeod DS, Cooper DS, Ladenson PW, et al. Prognosis of differentiated thyroid cancer in relation to serum thyrotropin and thyroglobulin antibody status at time of diagnosis. Thyroid 2014;24(1):35–42.

28. Elisei R, Bottici V, Luchetti F, et al. Impact of routine measurement of serum calcitonin on the diagnosis and outcome of medullary thyroid cancer: experience in 10,864 patients with nodular thyroid disorders. J Clin Endocrinol Metab 2004; 89(1):163–8.

29. Daniels GH. Screening for medullary thyroid carcinoma with serum calcitonin measurements in patients with thyroid nodules in the United States and Canada. Thyroid 2011;21(11):1199–207.

30. Suh I, Vriens MR, Guerrero MA, et al. Serum thyroglobulin is a poor diagnostic biomarker of malignancy in follicular and Hurthle-cell neoplasms of the thyroid. Am J Surg 2010;200(1):41–6.

31. Marqusee E, Benson CB, Frates MC, et al. Usefulness of ultrasonography in the management of nodular thyroid disease. Ann Intern Med 2000;133(9):696–700.

32. Kouvaraki MA, Shapiro SE, Fornage BD, et al. Role of preoperative ultrasonography in the surgical management of patients with thyroid cancer. Surgery 2003; 134(6):946–54 [discussion: 954–5].

33. Stulak JM, Grant CS, Farley DR, et al. Value of preoperative ultrasonography in the surgical management of initial and reoperative papillary thyroid cancer. Arch Surg 2006;141(5):489–94 [discussion: 494–6].

34. Moon HJ, Kim EK, Yoon JH, et al. Differences in the diagnostic performances of staging US for thyroid malignancy according to experience. Ultrasound Med Biol 2012;38(4):568–73.

35. Shimamoto K, Satake H, Sawaki A, et al. Preoperative staging of thyroid papillary carcinoma with ultrasonography. Eur J Radiol 1998;29(1):4–10.

36. Kwak JY, Han KH, Yoon JH, et al. Thyroid imaging reporting and data system for US features of nodules: a step in establishing better stratification of cancer risk. Radiology 2011;260(3):892–9.

37. Tessler FN, Middleton WD, Grant EG, et al. ACR thyroid imaging, reporting and data system (TI-RADS): white paper of the ACR TI-RADS committee. J Am Coll Radiol 2017;14(5):587–95.

38. Henrichsen TL, Reading CC, Charboneau JW, et al. Cystic change in thyroid carcinoma: prevalence and estimated volume in 360 carcinomas. J Clin Ultrasound 2010;38(7):361–6.

39. Brito JP, Gionfriddo MR, Al Nofal A, et al. The accuracy of thyroid nodule ultrasound to predict thyroid cancer: systematic review and meta-analysis. J Clin Endocrinol Metab 2014;99(4):1253–63.

40. Li W, Zhu Q, Jiang Y, et al. Partially cystic thyroid nodules in ultrasound-guided fine needle aspiration: prevalence of thyroid carcinoma and ultrasound features. Medicine 2017;96(46):e8689.

41. Moon WJ, Jung SL, Lee JH, et al. Benign and malignant thyroid nodules: US differentiation–multicenter retrospective study. Radiology 2008;247(3):762–70.
42. Bonavita JA, Mayo J, Babb J, et al. Pattern recognition of benign nodules at ultrasound of the thyroid: which nodules can be left alone? AJR Am J Roentgenol 2009;193(1):207–13.
43. Kim DW, Lee EJ, In HS, et al. Sonographic differentiation of partially cystic thyroid nodules: a prospective study. AJNR Am J Neuroradiol 2010;31(10):1961–6.
44. Jeh SK, Jung SL, Kim BS, et al. Evaluating the degree of conformity of papillary carcinoma and follicular carcinoma to the reported ultrasonographic findings of malignant thyroid tumor. Korean J Radiol 2007;8(3):192–7.
45. Kim DS, Kim JH, Na DG, et al. Sonographic features of follicular variant papillary thyroid carcinomas in comparison with conventional papillary thyroid carcinomas. J Ultrasound Med 2009;28(12):1685–92.
46. Ren J, Liu B, Zhang LL, et al. A taller-than-wide shape is a good predictor of papillary thyroid carcinoma in small solid nodules. J Ultrasound Med 2015; 34(1):19–26.
47. Chen SP, Hu YP, Chen B. Taller-than-wide sign for predicting thyroid microcarcinoma: comparison and combination of two ultrasonographic planes. Ultrasound Med Biol 2014;40(9):2004–11.
48. Moon HJ, Kwak JY, Kim EK, et al. A taller-than-wide shape in thyroid nodules in transverse and longitudinal ultrasonographic planes and the prediction of malignancy. Thyroid 2011;21(11):1249–53.
49. Grant EG, Tessler FN, Hoang JK, et al. Thyroid ultrasound reporting lexicon: white paper of the ACR thyroid imaging, reporting and data system (TIRADS) committee. J Am Coll Radiol 2015;12(12 Pt A):1272–9.
50. Kuo EJ, Thi WJ, Zheng F, et al. Individualizing surgery in papillary thyroid carcinoma based on a detailed sonographic assessment of extrathyroidal extension. Thyroid 2017;27(12):1544–9.
51. Lee CY, Kim SJ, Ko KR, et al. Predictive factors for extrathyroidal extension of papillary thyroid carcinoma based on preoperative sonography. J Ultrasound Med 2014;33(2):231–8.
52. Taki S, Terahata S, Yamashita R, et al. Thyroid calcifications: sonographic patterns and incidence of cancer. Clin Imaging 2004;28(5):368–71.
53. Arpaci D, Ozdemir D, Cuhaci N, et al. Evaluation of cytopathological findings in thyroid nodules with macrocalcification: macrocalcification is not innocent as it seems. Arq Bras Endocrinol Metabol 2014;58(9):939–45.
54. Kim MJ, Kim EK, Kwak JY, et al. Differentiation of thyroid nodules with macrocalcifications: role of suspicious sonographic findings. J Ultrasound Med 2008; 27(8):1179–84.
55. Lee J, Lee SY, Cha SH, et al. Fine-needle aspiration of thyroid nodules with macrocalcification. Thyroid 2013;23(9):1106–12.
56. Park YJ, Kim JA, Son EJ, et al. Thyroid nodules with macrocalcification: sonographic findings predictive of malignancy. Yonsei Med J 2014;55(2):339–44.
57. American Thyroid Association (ATA) Guidelines Taskforce on Thyroid Nodules and Differentiated Thyroid Cancer, Cooper DS, Doherty GM, et al. Revised American Thyroid Association management guidelines for patients with thyroid nodules and differentiated thyroid cancer. Thyroid 2009;19(11):1167–214.
58. Papini E, Guglielmi R, Bianchini A, et al. Risk of malignancy in nonpalpable thyroid nodules: predictive value of ultrasound and color-Doppler features. J Clin Endocrinol Metab 2002;87(5):1941–6.

59. Moon HJ, Kwak JY, Kim MJ, et al. Can vascularity at power Doppler US help predict thyroid malignancy? Radiology 2010;255(1):260–9.
60. Yang GCH, Fried KO. Most thyroid cancers detected by sonography lack intranodular vascularity on color Doppler imaging: review of the literature and sonographic-pathologic correlations for 698 thyroid neoplasms. J Ultrasound Med 2017;36(1):89–94.
61. Cappelli C, Castellano M, Pirola I, et al. The predictive value of ultrasound findings in the management of thyroid nodules. QJM 2007;100(1):29–35.
62. Lai X, Liu M, Xia Y, et al. Hypervascularity is more frequent in medullary thyroid carcinoma: compared with papillary thyroid carcinoma. Medicine 2016;95(49): e5502.
63. Hong MJ, Na DG, Baek JH, et al. Impact of nodule size on malignancy risk differs according to the ultrasonography pattern of thyroid nodules. Korean J Radiol 2018;19(3):534–41.
64. Machens A, Holzhausen HJ, Dralle H. The prognostic value of primary tumor size in papillary and follicular thyroid carcinoma. Cancer 2005;103(11):2269–73.
65. Lee S, Shin JH, Han BK, et al. Medullary thyroid carcinoma: comparison with papillary thyroid carcinoma and application of current sonographic criteria. AJR Am J Roentgenol 2010;194(4):1090–4.
66. Kim SH, Kim BS, Jung SL, et al. Ultrasonographic findings of medullary thyroid carcinoma: a comparison with papillary thyroid carcinoma. Korean J Radiol 2009;10(2):101–5.
67. Liu MJ, Liu ZF, Hou YY, et al. Ultrasonographic characteristics of medullary thyroid carcinoma: a comparison with papillary thyroid carcinoma. Oncotarget 2017;8(16):27520–8.
68. Zhou L, Chen B, Zhao M, et al. Sonographic features of medullary thyroid carcinomas according to tumor size: comparison with papillary thyroid carcinomas. J Ultrasound Med 2015;34(6):1003–9.
69. Langer JE, Mandel SJ. Sonographic imaging of cervical lymph nodes in patients with thyroid cancer. Neuroimaging Clin N Am 2008;18(3):479–89, vii-viii.
70. Kuna SK, Bracic I, Tesic V, et al. Ultrasonographic differentiation of benign from malignant neck lymphadenopathy in thyroid cancer. J Ultrasound Med 2006; 25(12):1531–7 [quiz: 1538–40].
71. Leboulleux S, Girard E, Rose M, et al. Ultrasound criteria of malignancy for cervical lymph nodes in patients followed up for differentiated thyroid cancer. J Clin Endocrinol Metab 2007;92(9):3590–4.
72. Sohn YM, Kwak JY, Kim EK, et al. Diagnostic approach for evaluation of lymph node metastasis from thyroid cancer using ultrasound and fine-needle aspiration biopsy. AJR Am J Roentgenol 2010;194(1):38–43.
73. Park JS, Son KR, Na DG, et al. Performance of preoperative sonographic staging of papillary thyroid carcinoma based on the sixth edition of the AJCC/UICC TNM classification system. AJR Am J Roentgenol 2009;192(1):66–72.
74. Leenhardt L, Erdogan MF, Hegedus L, et al. 2013 European thyroid association guidelines for cervical ultrasound scan and ultrasound-guided techniques in the postoperative management of patients with thyroid cancer. Eur Thyroid J 2013; 2(3):147–59.
75. Solbiati L, Osti V, Cova L, et al. Ultrasound of thyroid, parathyroid glands and neck lymph nodes. Eur Radiol 2001;11(12):2411–24.
76. Rosario PW, de Faria S, Bicalho L, et al. Ultrasonographic differentiation between metastatic and benign lymph nodes in patients with papillary thyroid carcinoma. J Ultrasound Med 2005;24(10):1385–9.

77. Ahuja AT, Ying M, Ho SS, et al. Distribution of intranodal vessels in differentiating benign from metastatic neck nodes. Clin Radiol 2001;56(3):197–201.

78. Ahuja A, Ying M. Sonography of neck lymph nodes. Part II: abnormal lymph nodes. Clin Radiol 2003;58(5):359–66.

79. Kim EK, Park CS, Chung WY, et al. New sonographic criteria for recommending fine-needle aspiration biopsy of nonpalpable solid nodules of the thyroid. AJR Am J Roentgenol 2002;178(3):687–91.

80. Frates MC, Benson CB, Charboneau JW, et al. Management of thyroid nodules detected at US: Society of Radiologists in Ultrasound consensus conference statement. Radiology 2005;237(3):794–800.

81. Shin JH, Baek JH, Chung J, et al. Ultrasonography diagnosis and imaging-based management of thyroid nodules: revised Korean Society of Thyroid Radiology consensus statement and recommendations. Korean J Radiol 2016;17(3): 370–95.

82. Horvath E, Majlis S, Rossi R, et al. An ultrasonogram reporting system for thyroid nodules stratifying cancer risk for clinical management. J Clin Endocrinol Metab 2009;94(5):1748–51.

83. Park JY, Lee HJ, Jang HW, et al. A proposal for a thyroid imaging reporting and data system for ultrasound features of thyroid carcinoma. Thyroid 2009;19(11): 1257–64.

84. Gharib H, Papini E, Garber JR, et al. American Association of Clinical Endocrinologists, American College of Endocrinology, and Associazione Medici Endocrinologi Medical guidelines for clinical practice for the diagnosis and management of thyroid nodules–2016 update. Endocr Pract 2016;22(5):622–39.

85. Na DG, Baek JH, Sung JY, et al. Thyroid imaging reporting and data system risk stratification of thyroid nodules: categorization based on solidity and echogenicity. Thyroid 2016;26(4):562–72.

86. Middleton WD, Teefey SA, Reading CC, et al. Multiinstitutional analysis of thyroid nodule risk stratification using the American College of Radiology thyroid imaging reporting and data system. AJR Am J Roentgenol 2017;208(6):1331–41.

87. Park CS, Kim SH, Jung SL, et al. Observer variability in the sonographic evaluation of thyroid nodules. J Clin Ultrasound 2010;38(6):287–93.

88. Russ G, Royer B, Bigorgne C, et al. Prospective evaluation of thyroid imaging reporting and data system on 4550 nodules with and without elastography. Eur J Endocrinol 2013;168(5):649–55.

89. Grani G, Lamartina L, Cantisani V, et al. Interobserver agreement of various thyroid imaging reporting and data systems. Endocr Connect 2018;7(1):1–7.

90. Ha EJ, Baek JH, Na DG. Risk stratification of thyroid nodules on ultrasonography: current status and perspectives. Thyroid 2017;27(12):1463–8.

91. Horvath E, Silva CF, Majlis S, et al. Prospective validation of the ultrasound based TIRADS (thyroid imaging reporting and data system) classification: results in surgically resected thyroid nodules. Eur Radiol 2017;27(6):2619–28.

92. Tang AL, Falciglia M, Yang H, et al. Validation of American Thyroid Association ultrasound risk assessment of thyroid nodules selected for ultrasound fine-needle aspiration. Thyroid 2017;27(8):1077–82.

93. Persichetti A, Di Stasio E, Guglielmi R, et al. Predictive value of malignancy of thyroid nodule ultrasound classification systems: a prospective study. J Clin Endocrinol Metab 2018;103(4):1359–68.

94. Yoon JH, Lee HS, Kim EK, et al. Malignancy risk stratification of thyroid nodules: comparison between the thyroid imaging reporting and data system and the

2014 American Thyroid Association management guidelines. Radiology 2016; 278(3):917–24.

95. Frates MC, Benson CB, Doubilet PM, et al. Prevalence and distribution of carcinoma in patients with solitary and multiple thyroid nodules on sonography. J Clin Endocrinol Metab 2006;91(9):3411–7.

96. Ito Y, Miyauchi A, Inoue H, et al. An observational trial for papillary thyroid microcarcinoma in Japanese patients. World J Surg 2010;34(1):28–35.

97. Soelberg KK, Bonnema SJ, Brix TH, et al. Risk of malignancy in thyroid incidentalomas detected by 18F-fluorodeoxyglucose positron emission tomography: a systematic review. Thyroid 2012;22(9):918–25.

98. Wang Z, Vyas CM, Van Benschoten O, et al. Quantitative analysis of the benefits and risk of thyroid nodule evaluation in patients >/=70 years old. Thyroid 2018; 28(4):465–71.

99. Carpi A, Nicolini A, Sagripanti A, et al. Large-needle aspiration biopsy for the preoperative selection of palpable thyroid nodules diagnosed by fine-needle aspiration as a microfollicular nodule or suspected cancer. Am J Clin Pathol 2000;113(6):872–7.

100. Tublin ME, Martin JA, Rollin LJ, et al. Ultrasound-guided fine-needle aspiration versus fine-needle capillary sampling biopsy of thyroid nodules: does technique matter? J Ultrasound Med 2007;26(12):1697–701.

101. Baloch ZW, Cibas ES, Clark DP, et al. The National Cancer Institute Thyroid fine needle aspiration state of the science conference: a summation. Cytojournal 2008;5:6.

102. Pusztaszeri M, Rossi ED, Auger M, et al. The Bethesda system for reporting thyroid cytopathology: proposed modifications and updates for the second edition from an international panel. Acta Cytol 2016;60(5):399–405.

103. Cibas ES, Ali SZ. The 2017 Bethesda system for reporting thyroid cytopathology. Thyroid 2017;27(11):1341–6.

104. Wang CC, Friedman L, Kennedy GC, et al. A large multicenter correlation study of thyroid nodule cytopathology and histopathology. Thyroid 2011;21(3):243–51.

105. Olson MT, Clark DP, Erozan YS, et al. Spectrum of risk of malignancy in subcategories of 'atypia of undetermined significance. Acta Cytol 2011;55(6):518–25.

106. Faquin WC, Wong LQ, Afrogheh AH, et al. Impact of reclassifying noninvasive follicular variant of papillary thyroid carcinoma on the risk of malignancy in The Bethesda system for reporting thyroid cytopathology. Cancer Cytopathol 2016;124(3):181–7.

107. Valderrabano P, McGettigan MJ, Lam CA, et al. Thyroid nodules with indeterminate cytology: utility of the American Thyroid Association sonographic patterns for cancer risk stratification. Thyroid 2018;28(8):1004–12.

108. Kwak JY, Koo H, Youk JH, et al. Value of US correlation of a thyroid nodule with initially benign cytologic results. Radiology 2010;254(1):292–300.

109. Rosario PW, Purisch S. Ultrasonographic characteristics as a criterion for repeat cytology in benign thyroid nodules. Arq Bras Endocrinol Metabol 2010;54(1): 52–5.

110. Durante C, Costante G, Lucisano G, et al. The natural history of benign thyroid nodules. JAMA 2015;313(9):926–35.

111. Angell TE, Vyas CM, Medici M, et al. Differential growth rates of benign vs. malignant thyroid nodules. J Clin Endocrinol Metab 2017;102(12):4642–7.

Molecular Diagnostic Evaluation of Thyroid Nodules

Sarah E. Mayson, MD*, Bryan R. Haugen, MD

KEYWORDS

- Thyroid nodule • Indeterminate cytology • Molecular testing • ThyroSeq • Afirma

KEY POINTS

- Sensitivity and specificity are inherent test characteristics, whereas positive predictive value and negative predictive value depend on the population prevalence of a given disease.
- Molecular diagnostic tests with high sensitivity and negative predicative value are used as rule-out tests for thyroid cancer, whereas those with high specificity and positive predictive value are used as rule-in tests.
- The next-generation molecular tests, Afirma GSC RNAseq panel and ThyroSeqv3 112-gene panel, have high sensitivity and sufficiently high enough specificity to function as rule-out and rule-in tests.
- Optimal molecular tests should have proven analytical validation, clinical validation and clinical usefulness, and should be performed in a Clinical Laboratory Improvements Amendments-approved laboratory.

INTRODUCTION

The historical management of thyroid nodules with indeterminate cytology has often been with diagnostic lobectomy or thyroidectomy. There is a substantial downside to this approach, in that many patients are subjected to operative risk, surgical complications, cost, and time off work for what is ultimately proven to be a benign thyroid nodule. Molecular diagnostic testing has been used over the last decade to help guide the management of thyroid nodules with indeterminate cytology and ultimately decrease the number of thyroid surgeries done for diagnostic purposes.

Disclosure Statement: Dr S.E. Mayson previously received research support from Rosetta genomics. Dr S.E. Mayson and Dr B.R. Haugen participated as investigators in the ThyroSeq v3 clinical validation study.
Division of Endocrinology, Metabolism and Diabetes, University of Colorado School of Medicine, MS 8106, 12801 East 17th Avenue, Aurora, CO 80045, USA
* Corresponding author.
E-mail address: Sarah.Mayson@ucdenver.edu

Endocrinol Metab Clin N Am 48 (2019) 85–97
https://doi.org/10.1016/j.ecl.2018.10.004
0889-8529/19/© 2018 Elsevier Inc. All rights reserved.
endo.theclinics.com

DISCUSSION

Bethesda Cytology/Indeterminate Fine Needle Aspiration

Clinical evaluation of patients with thyroid nodules, including the Bethesda System for Reporting Thyroid Cytopathology (TBSRTC), is reviewed in Carolyn Maxwell and Jennifer A. Sipos' article, "Diagnostic Evaluation of Thyroid Nodules," elsewhere in this issue. TBSRTC was first proposed in 2007, then revised more recently to include updated studies and the noninvasive follicular thyroid neoplasm with papillary-like nuclear features (NIFTP) category of surgical pathology.[1–3] TBSRTC is widely accepted as a standard reporting system for thyroid cytopathology. Whether NIFTP is considered in the benign or malignant surgical pathology category, benign and malignant cytopathology using TBSRTC are highly accurate, with a 0% to 3% risk of malignancy in the benign cytopathology category and 94% to 99% risk of malignancy in the malignant cytopathology category.[1]

The risk of malignancy in the atypia (or follicular lesion) of undetermined significance (AUS/FLUS; Bethesda III) and follicular neoplasm/suspicious for follicular neoplasm (FN/SFN; Bethesda IV) categories remains low enough to not justify surgical resection for all patients, yet high enough to not justify monitoring for all patients. Cibas and Ali[1] in the 2017 TBSRTC propose that the risk for malignancy for AUS/FLUS cytology is 6% to 18% when NIFTP is considered benign and 10% to 30% when NIFTP is considered malignant. Furthermore, they propose that the risk for malignancy for FN/SFN cytology is 10% to 40% when NIFTP is considered benign and 25% to 40% when NIFTP is considered malignant. These stated risks of malignancy are known to have case selection, partial verification, and publication biases that can overestimate and underestimate the true risk of malignancy in any given patient with an indeterminate cytology.[2]

The historical approach to patients with indeterminate cytology, especially before the introduction of TBSRTC, has been a diagnostic lobectomy or thyroidectomy. This approach led to unnecessary surgery in 60% to 94% of patients with indeterminate cytology. The 2015 American Thyroid Association (ATA) Guidelines for Patients with Thyroid Nodules and Differentiated Thyroid Cancer proposed a menu of options for patients with AUS/FLUS and FN/SFN.[4] The proposed primary approaches to patients with an AUS/FLUS cytology are repeat fine needle aspiration (FNA) or molecular testing, whereas patients with FN/SFN are recommended to undergo a diagnostic lobectomy or molecular testing. Both approaches recommend considering clinical and sonographic features as well as informed patient preference in decision making. The ATA guidelines also recommend considering a second opinion cytopathology review, especially for patients with AUS/FLUS cytology. The 2017 TBSRTC recommends repeat FNA, molecular testing, or diagnostic lobectomy for patients with AUS/FLUS cytology, and molecular testing or diagnostic lobectomy for patients with FN/SFN cytology. Consequently, molecular testing is a core diagnostic tool for many patients with Bethesda III and IV cytology. An algorithm illustrating how molecular diagnostic testing can be used in the management of thyroid nodules with indeterminate cytology is shown in **Fig. 1**.

Principles of Molecular Diagnostic Evaluation of Thyroid Nodules

There are 3 important concepts to consider when evaluating molecular diagnostic tests for patients with thyroid nodules: analytical validation, clinical validation, and clinical usefulness. We review analytical and clinical validation in detail in the following sections. Clinical usefulness refers to the psychological, social, and economic consequences of testing and impact on health outcomes in the context of the individual, family, and society.

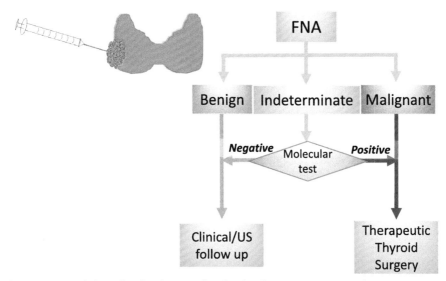

Fig. 1. Suggested algorithm for the use of molecular diagnostic testing in the management of thyroid nodules with indeterminate cytology. FNA, fine needle aspiration; US, ultrasound examination.

Analytical validation

Analytical validation refers to the ability of a test to perform in the context of limited input material, potentially interfering nontumor cell or blood contamination, as well as the reproducibility of the test across technical replicates and different processing or storage methods.[5] The 112-gene sequencing panel (ThyroSeqv3) underwent analytical validation on 238 surgical specimens and 175 FNA specimens.[6] The quality control first screens for acellular specimens, then nonthyroid specimens, then performs next-generation sequencing on specimens that pass the screen. This assay accurately detected genetic alterations down to 2.5 ng of input, accurately classified 10 samples with 12% tumor in 88% normal thyroid cells, and was accurate in 3 samples diluted to 12% in blood. This assay also made the same calls from 12 specimens in triplicate in the same run (precision) and in 3 different runs by different operators (reproducibility). The collected samples were shown to be stable at room temperature for 2 hours followed by storage at −20°C or 4°C for up to 72 hours. The genomic sequencing classifier (GSC) has undergone analytical validation, which has been submitted for publication, but this has not yet been published (Kennedy GC, personal communication). The 167 Gene Expression Classifier (Afirma GEC) underwent analytical validation using standard FNA collection into preservative, generating preanalytical, analytical, and reproducibility studies.[7] This assay accurately called benign or suspicious samples down to 10 ng input RNA, although the standard input for the assay is 15 ng. The assay was accurate down to 20% FNA content mixed with normal tissue and 17% FNA content mixed with whole blood. This assay also demonstrated 94% precision (intraassay) and 100% reproducibility (interlaboratory). The collected samples in preservative were stable for up to 6 days at room temperature.

Congress passed the Clinical Laboratory Improvements Amendments in 1988 establishing quality standards for laboratory testing. To ensure quality laboratory testing, all molecular tests should be performed in a Clinical Laboratory Improvements Amendments-certified laboratory.

Clinical validation
Clinical validation tests the ability of a diagnostic test to rule out disease (sensitivity, negative predictive value [NPV]) and rule in disease (specificity, positive predictive value [PPV]). Sensitivity and specificity evaluate the test characteristics and are independent of the disease prevalence in a population, whereas the NPV and PPV depend on the disease prevalence in a population. Sensitivity and specificity can be directly compared between different studies in different populations, whereas NPV and PPV cannot be directly compared (**Fig. 2**). To adequately evaluate NPV and PPV for a given molecular test, one needs to know the prevalence of malignancy for each Bethesda cytology category for a given institution or region, preferably over a 3- to 5-year period of time.[8] The most robust design of a clinical validation trial for molecular markers in patients with thyroid nodules is a prospective, blinded trial in consecutive patients collecting the test and all patients going to surgery for histopathologic confirmation.[9,10] A recently developed GSC underwent clinical validation using existing specimens from a previous prospective, blinded study.[9,11] Another large study of a 7-gene mutation panel underwent a large clinical validation study that was prospective, but not blinded.[12] The sensitivity and specificity of this 7-gene mutation panel was confirmed in many other independent studies,[13–15] which is another form of clinical validation. The 2 most recently published and most commonly used molecular tests have not undergone confirmation in independent studies.[10,11]

Types of Molecular Diagnostic Tests

A summary of the clinical validation of first-, second-, and next-generation molecular tests for indeterminate cytology thyroid nodules is outlined in **Table 1**.

First-generation molecular tests
In 2011, the Afirma GEC (Veracyte, South San Francisco, CA) for the diagnostic evaluation of thyroid nodules with indeterminate cytology became available for clinical use. This microarray based test uses a proprietary algorithm to differentiate benign from malignant nodules based on messenger RNA expression pattern. The GEC designates thyroid nodules as "benign" (negative test) or "suspicious" (positive test) according to the probability of malignancy derived from the expression pattern.[16] The

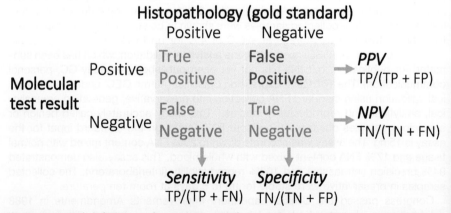

Fig. 2. Statistical definitions of sensitivity, specificity, negative predictive value (NPV), and positive predictive value (PPV). FN, false negative; FP, false positive; TN, true negative; TP, true positive.

Table 1
Paired sensitivity, specificity, negative predictive value (NPV), and positive predictive value (PPV) of clinical validation studies of molecular diagnostic tests

Generation	Test	Number of Nodules	Bethesda Category	Sensitivity (%)	Specificity (%)	Cancer Rate (%)	NPV (%)	PPV (%)
First	Afirma-GEC 167 RNA GEC	265	III-V	92	52	32	93	47
	7-gene panel	513	III-V	61	98	24	89	90
Second	ThyroSeq v2 19-gene panel	95	III	91	92	23	97	77
		143	IV	90	93	27	96	83
	ThyGenX/ThyraMIR 8-gene panel/microRNA GEC	109	III-IV	89	85	32	94	74
Third	Afirma-GSC RNAseq panel	191	III-IV	91	68	24	96	47
	ThyroSeq v3 112-gene panel	286	III-IV	94	82	28[a]	97	66

[a] Combined cancer/noninvasive follicular thyroid neoplasm with papillary-like nuclear features (NIFTP) prevalence. Prevalence of NIFTP not determined in other studies.

manufacturer recommends 2 dedicated FNA passes collected in a nucleic acid preservative for sample acquisition.

A prospective, double-blinded, multicenter clinical validation study included 4812 FNA samples, 577 (12%) of which had indeterminate cytology, with 265 samples subsequently analyzed. The sensitivity and specificity were 92% and 52% for all thyroid nodules with indeterminate cytology (Bethesda III/IV/V), 90% and 53% for AUS/FLUS (Bethesda III), and 90% and 49% for FN/SFN (Bethesda IV). Given the prevalence of malignancy of 24% for Bethesda III nodules and 25% for Bethesda IV in this study, the NPV and PPV were 95% and 38% and 94% and 37%, respectively.[9] A recent metaanalysis of 18 postvalidation studies (4 prospective and 14 retrospective) calculated the test characteristics of the GEC using only indeterminate nodules that were surgically excised. This confirmed a sensitivity of approximately 90%, which is consistent with the clinical validation study; however, the specificity was considerably lower at 27% (vs 52%).[9,17] Veracyte offers add-on *BRAF* V600 E mutational testing; however, there is a negligible impact on test performance given the low prevalence of this mutation in Bethesda III/IV nodules.[18]

A follow-up multicenter study that included 5 academic centers from the original validation cohort evaluated 346 consecutive patients with indeterminate thyroid nodules who underwent GEC testing.[19] Overall, 51% of nodules were GEC benign, 44% were GEC suspicious, and the results of testing affected clinical care recommendations in one-half of the patients.[19] This study and others have demonstrated significant site to site variability in the benign call rate (range, 27%–53%) and in the malignancy rate of GEC suspicious nodules (range, 15.6%–70.0%).[19–26] This parallels the site-to-site variability in the malignancy rates of Bethesda III and VI nodules.[27]

Architectural versus cytologic atypia in the AUS/FLUS (Bethesda III) category impacts the GEC benign call rate and malignancy rate of resected GEC suspicious nodules. Baca and colleagues[28] evaluated 227 nodules with AUS cytology and GEC testing and demonstrated a higher GEC benign call rate for AUS nodules with architectural atypia (65%) versus those with cytologic atypia (59%) or both (38%). Furthermore, the malignancy rate of resected GEC suspicious nodules was 19% in the setting of architectural atypia versus 45% for cytologic atypia or 57% for both. Importantly, the specificity of the GEC in Hurthle cell nodules has been shown to be very low (approximately 12%), such that a positive result has a negligible impact on the posttest probability of malignancy.[29]

The high sensitivity of the GEC supports its use as a rule-out test for thyroid cancer in Bethesda III/IV nodules when the population prevalence of malignancy is similar to or lower than that of the validation cohort. In this context, the NPV is high and negative testing provides patients with the option to pursue clinical surveillance instead of immediate diagnostic surgery. The low specificity and PPV of the GEC means that a positive test is insufficient to predict that a nodule is malignant and subsequent clinical decision making must integrate cytology results, ultrasound findings, and clinical risk factors. The clinical usefulness of testing is low in Bethesda V nodules given the relatively high pretest probability of malignancy in this population and therefore use of the GEC in this context is not recommended. The routine use of this test does not seem to be cost-effective unless the population prevalence of malignancy is especially low (<10%).[30]

Longer term follow-up studies evaluating the clinical behavior of GEC benign nodules have been reassuring. Low surgical excision rates of GEC benign nodules have been demonstrated in several studies.[8,31–34] Angell and colleagues[32] found that only 5 of 90 (5.5%) indeterminate GEC benign nodules in their cohort ultimately underwent surgical excision with 1 malignancy identified. The GEC benign nodules demonstrated comparable growth to nodules with benign cytology after a median follow-up of 13 months. Deaver and colleagues[8] found that only 5 of 73 (6.8%) GEC benign nodules in their cohort underwent surgery with only 1 nodule harboring an incidental focus of papillary microcarcinoma that was not targeted during FNA. Size remained stable in the majority (>70%) of GEC benign nodules over a median follow-up of 46 months for Bethesda III and 62 months for Bethesda IV.

The Afirma GEC test has been replaced by the Afirma GSC test, which is described in the next-generation testing section.

Genetic alterations affecting the mitogen-activated protein kinase and phosphoinositide 3-kinase signaling pathways are common in thyroid cancer.[35–37] The miRInform Thyroid (Asuragen, Austin, TX) test, rebranded as ThyGenX Thyroid Oncogene Panel (Interpace Diagnostics, Parsippany, NJ), evaluates for common genetic alterations in 7 genes (BRAF V600 E, NRAS codon 61, HRAS codon 61, and KRAS codons 12/13 point mutations and RET/PTC1, RET/PTC3, and PAX8/PPAR rearrangements) that are found in approximately 70% of thyroid cancers.[12] One dedicated FNA pass collected in a nucleic acid preservative is recommended for sample acquisition. The use of DNA-based mutational panels on ThinPrep material and air-dried smears has also been successfully demonstrated.[38,39]

The largest study to evaluate the performance of the 7-gene panel was a single-center, nonblinded prospective study, in which 1056 indeterminate nodules had molecular testing and 513 nodules with surgical pathology were analyzed. In total, 247 Bethesda III, 214 Bethesda IV, and 52 Bethesda V nodules were included and the prevalence of malignancy was 14%, 27%, and 54%, respectively. The sensitivity and specificity of the 7-gene panel were, respectively, 61% and 98% for the entire cohort, 63% and 99% for Bethesda III nodules, 57% and 97% for Bethesda IV, and 68% and 96% for Bethesda V.[12] The posttest probability of malignancy is affected by the mutation detected; for example, the risk of malignancy is 100% with BRAF V600 E mutations, whereas RAS mutations are known to occur in both benign and malignant thyroid neoplasms.

Before publication of the 2015 ATA Guidelines for Patients with Thyroid Nodules and Differentiated Thyroid Cancer, the clinical implication of a positive 7-gene panel was to direct patients to thyroidectomy rather than lobectomy, allowing for a 2-step surgical procedure to be avoided in cases when the nodule was proven to be malignant after diagnostic lobectomy. Unlike prior guidelines on this topic, the 2015 ATA Guidelines endorse either a lobectomy or a thyroidectomy as an appropriate surgical procedure for many thyroid cancers less than 4 cm in size, such that 2-step surgical procedures are no longer routinely required.[4] Consequently, the 7-gene mutation panel has a diminished role in surgical decision making in current clinical practice, primarily owing to the low sensitivity of this test.

Second-generation tests

The first molecular tests developed for the diagnostic evaluation of indeterminate thyroid nodules either had high sensitivity or specificity, but not both. The goal of subsequent test development has been to improve test characteristics such that a single test could serve the dual purposes of rule-in and rule-out. ThyroSeq uses next-generation sequencing and an expanded list of genetic alterations beyond the 7-gene panel, whereas ThyrGenX/ThyraMIR combines the 7-gene mutation panel with a classifier that analyzes the expression of small noncoding microRNAs (miRNAs). Another miRNA classifier test, the RosettaGX Reveal (Rosetta Genomics, Jersey City, NJ), was unique in that it could be performed on existing cytology smears; however, it is no longer available for clinical use.[40]

The ThyroSeq test (CBL Path Inc, North Haven, CT) is a custom panel of 284 mutational hot spots in 12 genes associated with thyroid cancer. Either 1 or 2 drops from the first FNA pass or 1 dedicated pass are sufficient for sample acquisition. To validate the analytical performance of this test, Nikiforova and colleagues[41] sequenced 228 DNA samples from thyroid neoplasms and benign nonneoplastic lesions, including frozen, formalin-fixed, and thyroid FNA specimens, and identified mutations in 110 of 145 thyroid cancers (76%) and 5 of 83 benign specimens (6%). The subsequent ThyroSeq v2 test is an expanded panel that adds telomerase reverse transcriptase (*TERT*) gene promoter mutations, testing for 38 types of RET fusion genes, and expression analysis of 8 genes to confirm follicular cell sample adequacy and identify nonthyroidal lesions (eg, parathyroid). A single-center study of 143 consecutive Bethesda IV nodule FNA samples with known surgical outcomes were analyzed using the ThyroSeq v2 (91 retrospective and 52 prospective samples) to yield a 90% sensitivity and 93% specificity.[42] A separate study of 462 Bethesda III nodules demonstrated a sensitivity of 91% and specificity of 92% for an updated version of ThyroSeq v2 (14 gene mutations and 42 gene fusions) based on histopathology from 95 patients who underwent surgery.[43] The largest postvalidation study to independently evaluate ThyroSeq v2 included 190 consecutive indeterminate (Bethesda III/IV) thyroid nodules. The test characteristics were calculated based on the 102 nodules with surgical histology yielding an overall sensitivity of 70%, specificity 77%, NPV 91%, and PPV 42% with a prevalence of cancer/NIFTP of 20%. The authors found that the test performance was significantly better for Bethesda IV than III nodules.[44]

ThyGenX/ThyraMIR (Interpace Diagnostics) combines targeted sequencing for 5 gene mutations and 3 gene fusion transcripts with a proprietary 10-miRNA GEC that classifies nodules as having a low-risk or high-risk miRNA profile. ThyraMIR testing is reflexively triggered when ThyGenX is negative for genetic alterations or if a mutation with a lower specificity for malignancy is detected. Recommended sample acquisition is with 1 dedicated FNA pass collected in a nucleic acid preservative. The clinical validation study included a cross-sectional cohort of 109 Bethesda III/IV thyroid nodules from 12 clinical sites. The sensitivity was 89%, specificity 85%, NPV 94%, and PPV 74% with a population prevalence of malignancy of 32%. A negative ThyGenX plus a low-risk ThyraMIR is associated with a residual risk of malignancy of 6%.[45] There have been no postvalidation studies of ThyGenX/ThyraMIR.

Third-generation tests
The ThyroSeq v3 Genomic Classifier (GC) and Afirma GSC are the newest tests available for the molecular evaluation of thyroid nodules with indeterminate cytology, both with improved sensitivity and specificity compared with prior iterations of testing.

The ThyroSeq v3 GC is a targeted next-generation sequencing test that evaluates for point mutations, gene fusions, copy number alterations, and abnormal gene expression in 112 thyroid cancer-related genes. Each genetic alteration that is detected is assigned a score between 0 and 2 and the total score is calculated for the sample. A total score of 0 or 1 is considered negative, and a score of 2 or more is positive. In addition to providing a binary positive/negative result, ThyroSeq v3 also reports mutations and other genetic alterations that are identified and the associated risk of malignancy.

The analytical performance of the GC was recently evaluated in a study that included a training set of 238 tissue samples (205 thyroid samples) and validation set of 175 indeterminate (Bethesda III–V) FNA samples with known histology (52.6% malignant). Oncocytic lesions were included in both the training set (n = 68) and validation set (n = 14). The achieved sensitivity, specificity, and accuracy were, respectively, 94%, 89.4%, and 92.1% in the training set and 98%, 81.8%, and 90.9% in the validation set. Although only a 2.5-ng nucleic acid sample was needed in the analytical validation study, the manufacturer recommends that a dedicated pass be performed (the second pass into the nodule) for sample acquisition, and for larger nodules the needles from all other passes should be washed into the same vial.

A prospective, double-blinded, clinical validation study of 286 indeterminate (Bethesda III–V) thyroid nodules at 10 clinical sites using ThyroSeq v3 GC was recently published.[10] Twenty samples (7%) failed a presequencing step owing to low nucleic acid quantity and 9 samples (3%) had inadequate samples owing to low expression of thyroid cell markers, leaving 257 samples for informative molecular analysis. The sensitivity and specificity were 91.4% and 84.9% for Bethesda III (154 nodules) and 97% and 75% for Bethesda IV (93 nodules), respectively. The NPV and PPV were, respectively, 97.1% and 64% for Bethesda III (cancer/NIFTP prevalence 23%) and 98% and 68% for Bethesda IV (cancer/NIFTP prevalence 35%). There were 11 NIFTP nodules (4%) in the study cohort, all of which were classified as positive. In addition, all 10 Hurthle cell carcinomas were correctly classified and the negative call rate for oncocytic lesions was 53% (vs 61% for Bethesda III/IV nodules overall). Further research is needed to clarify the clinical significance of detecting mutant alleles at very low levels (<10%) within a sample using next-generation sequencing, which is a highly sensitive technique. Furthermore, the long-term outcomes of nodules harboring low risk genetic alterations (GC score 1), which are reported clinically as currently negative, have yet to be determined. Fortunately, only 21 of 257 samples (8.2%) were assigned a GC score of 1 in this cohort.

The Afirma GSC is an RNA sequencing-based test that includes 12 classifiers composed of 10,196 genes (1115 core genes) plus 7 additional components to identify parathyroid lesions, MTC, *BRAF* V600 E mutations, *RET/PTC1* or *RET/PTC3* fusions, and Hurthle cell lesions. No studies assessing the analytical performance of the GSC have been published to date; however, a blinded clinical validation study that used the same cohort as the GEC validation study assessed the GSC performance in 191 indeterminate (Bethesda III/IV) thyroid nodules from 49 sites. This study demonstrated a high sensitivity of 91%, moderate specificity of 68%, NPV of 96%, and PPV of 47% with a cancer prevalence of 24% (NIFTP prevalence unknown). The sensitivity and specificity were, respectively, 92.9% and 70.9% for Bethesda III (114 nodules) and 88.2% and 64.4% for Bethesda IV (76 nodules). The NPV and PPV were, respectively, 96.8% and 51% for Bethesda III and 95% and 41.7% for Bethesda IV. To address the poor specificity of the GEC with Hurthle cell lesions, the GSC has 2 dedicated Hurthle cell classifiers. A subanalysis of 26 Hurthle cell neoplasms in this study yielded a sensitivity and specificity of 88.9% and 58.8%, respectively (vs 88.9% and 11.8% with the GEC, respectively).[11] Although the classifier has been trained to identify NIFTP lesions as suspicious, the performance of the GSC in NIFTP is unknown, because the validation cohort existed before NIFTP was described. The manufacturer recommends 2 dedicated FNA passes collected in a nucleic acid preservative for sample acquisition.

OUR EXPERIENCE

At the University of Colorado Hospital, many factors impact our decision to recommend molecular diagnostic testing to our patients with indeterminate thyroid nodules. The most common indication for molecular testing in our clinical practice is to help guide the selection of patients with Bethesda III/IV cytology results who can be managed with clinical follow-up instead of immediate diagnostic thyroid surgery. With this goal in mind, we select a test with a high sensitivity (>90%) that translates to a high NPV in our patient population. A recent review of 2019 thyroid nodule FNAs between 2011 and 2015 at our institution found that the malignancy rate varied significantly from year to year ranging from 8% to 38% for Bethesda III nodules (3-year average of 21%–30%) and from 0% to 42% for Bethesda IV (3-year average of 24%–34%).[8] Because the NPV and PPV of molecular diagnostic tests depend on the prevalence of malignancy in the population being evaluated, it is critical to have an ongoing dialogue with your pathologist to help guide interpretation of molecular test results and clinical decision making. We do not recommend molecular testing for the purpose of ruling out thyroid cancer when the pretest probability of malignancy is high, such as when indeterminate cytology is documented in the presence of strong clinical risk factors for thyroid cancer (eg, history of head/neck ionizing radiation exposure), the ATA high suspicion sonographic pattern, or Bethesda V cytology.

Because we have on-site cytology review at our institution, we often have the opportunity to collect for molecular testing at the time of the initial biopsy procedure if the preliminary cytology results indicate that an indeterminate result is likely. Our practice is either to perform a dedicated pass for molecular testing or to wash the passes collected for cytology (generally 2–3) in the nucleic acid preservative solution in lieu of a dedicated pass. We generally store samples for molecular testing in the freezer while awaiting final pathology results. After molecular testing is completed, we interpret the results in the context of the patient's clinical risk factors for malignancy, ultrasound findings, and cytology results and use these in combination to guide clinical management. To our knowledge, no published studies have attempted to evaluate the impact of different ultrasound findings or patterns on the posttest probability of malignancy in the context of different cytology and molecular test results. This area warrants attention in future studies.

SUMMARY

Molecular diagnostic testing for indeterminate thyroid nodules was first introduced nearly a decade ago and has since undergone significant evolution as a result of advances in test methodology and in our understanding of the molecular basis of thyroid tumorigenesis. The most recent generation of molecular tests (eg, Afirma GSC and ThyroSeq v3) demonstrate substantial improvements in paired sensitivity and specificity. These tests have the potential to significantly impact the management of thyroid nodules with indeterminate cytology in current clinical practice. Long-term outcomes of patients with negative molecular testing and independent clinical validation of these next-generation molecular tests will help to shape how we use these tests in clinical practice.

REFERENCES

1. Cibas ES, Ali SZ. The 2017 Bethesda System for Reporting Thyroid Cytopathology. Thyroid 2017;27(11):1341–6.
2. Pusztaszeri M, Rossi ED, Auger M, et al. The Bethesda System for Reporting Thyroid Cytopathology: proposed modifications and updates for the second edition from an international panel. Acta Cytol 2016;60(5):399–405.
3. Ali SZ, Cibas ES, SpringerLink (Online service). The Bethesda System for Reporting Thyroid Cytopathology: definitions, criteria, and explanatory notes. New York: Springer; 2010.
4. Haugen BR, Alexander EK, Bible KC, et al. 2015 American Thyroid Association management guidelines for adult patients with thyroid nodules and differentiated

thyroid cancer: the American Thyroid Association guidelines task force on thyroid nodules and differentiated thyroid cancer. Thyroid 2016;26(1):1–133.

5. Pankratz DG, Hu Z, Kim SY, et al. Analytical performance of a gene expression classifier for medullary thyroid carcinoma. Thyroid 2016;26(11):1573–80.

6. Nikiforova MN, Mercurio S, Wald AI, et al. Analytical performance of the ThyroSeq v3 genomic classifier for cancer diagnosis in thyroid nodules. Cancer 2018; 124(8):1682–90.

7. Walsh PS, Wilde JI, Tom EY, et al. Analytical performance verification of a molecular diagnostic for cytology-indeterminate thyroid nodules. J Clin Endocrinol Metab 2012;97(12):E2297–306.

8. Deaver KE, Haugen BR, Pozdeyev N, et al. Outcomes of Bethesda categories III and IV thyroid nodules over 5 years and performance of the Afirma gene expression classifier: a single-institution study. Clin Endocrinol (Oxf) 2018. [Epub ahead of print].

9. Alexander EK, Kennedy GC, Baloch ZW, et al. Preoperative diagnosis of benign thyroid nodules with indeterminate cytology. N Engl J Med 2012;367(8):705–15.

10. Steward DL, Carty SE, Sippel RS, et al. Performance of a multigene genomic classifier in thyroid nodules with indeterminate cytology: a prospective blinded multicenter study. JAMA Oncol 2018. [Epub ahead of print].

11. Patel KN, Angell TE, Babiarz J, et al. Performance of a genomic sequencing classifier for the preoperative diagnosis of cytologically indeterminate thyroid nodules. JAMA Surg 2018;153(9):817–24.

12. Nikiforov YE, Ohori NP, Hodak SP, et al. Impact of mutational testing on the diagnosis and management of patients with cytologically indeterminate thyroid nodules: a prospective analysis of 1056 FNA samples. J Clin Endocrinol Metab 2011;96(11):3390–7.

13. Nikiforov YE, Steward DL, Robinson-Smith TM, et al. Molecular testing for mutations in improving the fine-needle aspiration diagnosis of thyroid nodules. J Clin Endocrinol Metab 2009;94(6):2092–8.

14. Cantara S, Capezzone M, Marchisotta S, et al. Impact of proto-oncogene mutation detection in cytological specimens from thyroid nodules improves the diagnostic accuracy of cytology. J Clin Endocrinol Metab 2010;95(3):1365–9.

15. Moses W, Weng J, Sansano I, et al. Molecular testing for somatic mutations improves the accuracy of thyroid fine-needle aspiration biopsy. World J Surg 2010;34(11):2589–94.

16. Chudova D, Wilde JI, Wang ET, et al. Molecular classification of thyroid nodules using high-dimensionality genomic data. J Clin Endocrinol Metab 2010;95(12): 5296–304.

17. Vargas-Salas S, Martinez JR, Urra S, et al. Genetic testing for indeterminate thyroid cytology: review and meta-analysis. Endocr Relat Cancer 2018;25(3): R163–77.

18. Kloos RT, Reynolds JD, Walsh PS, et al. Does addition of BRAF V600E mutation testing modify sensitivity or specificity of the Afirma Gene Expression Classifier in cytologically indeterminate thyroid nodules? J Clin Endocrinol Metab 2013;98(4): E761–8.

19. Alexander EK, Schorr M, Klopper J, et al. Multicenter clinical experience with the Afirma gene expression classifier. J Clin Endocrinol Metab 2014;99(1):119–25.

20. Harrell RM, Bimston DN. Surgical utility of Afirma: effects of high cancer prevalence and oncocytic cell types in patients with indeterminate thyroid cytology. Endocr Pract 2014;20(4):364–9.

21. McIver B, Castro MR, Morris JC, et al. An independent study of a gene expression classifier (Afirma) in the evaluation of cytologically indeterminate thyroid nodules. J Clin Endocrinol Metab 2014;99(11):4069–77.
22. Harrison G, Sosa JA, Jiang X. Evaluation of the Afirma gene expression classifier in repeat indeterminate thyroid nodules. Arch Pathol Lab Med 2017;141(7): 985–9.
23. Al-Qurayshi Z, Deniwar A, Thethi T, et al. Association of malignancy prevalence with test properties and performance of the gene expression classifier in indeterminate thyroid nodules. JAMA Otolaryngol Head Neck Surg 2017;143(4):403–8.
24. Jug R, Jiang X. Noninvasive follicular thyroid neoplasm with papillary-like nuclear features: an evidence-based nomenclature change. Patholog Res Int 2017;2017: 1057252.
25. Lastra RR, Pramick MR, Crammer CJ, et al. Implications of a suspicious Afirma test result in thyroid fine-needle aspiration cytology: an institutional experience. Cancer Cytopathol 2014;122(10):737–44.
26. Sacks WL, Bose S, Zumsteg ZS, et al. Impact of Afirma gene expression classifier on cytopathology diagnosis and rate of thyroidectomy. Cancer Cytopathol 2016; 124(10):722–8.
27. Bongiovanni M, Spitale A, Faquin WC, et al. The Bethesda System for Reporting Thyroid Cytopathology: a meta-analysis. Acta Cytol 2012;56(4):333–9.
28. Baca SC, Wong KS, Strickland KC, et al. Qualifiers of atypia in the cytologic diagnosis of thyroid nodules are associated with different Afirma gene expression classifier results and clinical outcomes. Cancer Cytopathol 2017;125(5):313–22.
29. Brauner E, Holmes BJ, Krane JF, et al. Performance of the Afirma gene expression classifier in Hurthle cell thyroid nodules differs from other indeterminate thyroid nodules. Thyroid 2015;25(7):789–96.
30. Wu JX, Lam R, Levin M, et al. Effect of malignancy rates on cost-effectiveness of routine gene expression classifier testing for indeterminate thyroid nodules. Surgery 2016;159(1):118–26.
31. Duick DS, Klopper JP, Diggans JC, et al. The impact of benign gene expression classifier test results on the endocrinologist-patient decision to operate on patients with thyroid nodules with indeterminate fine-needle aspiration cytopathology. Thyroid 2012;22(10):996–1001.
32. Angell TE, Frates MC, Medici M, et al. Afirma benign thyroid nodules show similar growth to cytologically benign nodules during follow-up. J Clin Endocrinol Metab 2015;100(11):E1477–83.
33. Sipos JA, Blevins TC, Shea HC, et al. Long-term nonoperative rate of thyroid nodules with benign results on the Afirma gene expression classifier. Endocr Pract 2016;22(6):666–72.
34. Witt RL. Outcome of thyroid gene expression classifier testing in clinical practice. Laryngoscope 2016;126(2):524–7.
35. Cancer Genome Atlas Research Network. Integrated genomic characterization of papillary thyroid carcinoma. Cell 2014;159(3):676–90.
36. Landa I, Ibrahimpasic T, Boucai L, et al. Genomic and transcriptomic hallmarks of poorly differentiated and anaplastic thyroid cancers. J Clin Invest 2016;126(3): 1052–66.
37. Pozdeyev N, Gay LM, Sokol ES, et al. Genetic analysis of 779 advanced differentiated and anaplastic thyroid cancers. Clin Cancer Res 2018;24(13):3059–68.
38. Eszlinger M, Krogdahl A, Munz S, et al. Impact of molecular screening for point mutations and rearrangements in routine air-dried fine-needle aspiration samples of thyroid nodules. Thyroid 2014;24(2):305–13.

39. Krane JF, Cibas ES, Alexander EK, et al. Molecular analysis of residual ThinPrep material from thyroid FNAs increases diagnostic sensitivity. Cancer Cytopathol 2015;123(6):356–61.
40. Lithwick-Yanai G, Dromi N, Shtabsky A, et al. Multicentre validation of a microRNA-based assay for diagnosing indeterminate thyroid nodules utilising fine needle aspirate smears. J Clin Pathol 2017;70(6):500–7.
41. Nikiforova MN, Wald AI, Roy S, et al. Targeted next-generation sequencing panel (ThyroSeq) for detection of mutations in thyroid cancer. J Clin Endocrinol Metab 2013;98(11):E1852–60.
42. Nikiforov YE, Carty SE, Chiosea SI, et al. Highly accurate diagnosis of cancer in thyroid nodules with follicular neoplasm/suspicious for a follicular neoplasm cytology by ThyroSeq v2 next-generation sequencing assay. Cancer 2014; 120(23):3627–34.
43. Nikiforov YE, Carty SE, Chiosea SI, et al. Impact of the multi-gene ThyroSeq next-generation sequencing assay on cancer diagnosis in thyroid nodules with atypia of undetermined significance/follicular lesion of undetermined significance cytology. Thyroid 2015;25(11):1217–23.
44. Valderrabano P, Khazai L, Leon ME, et al. Evaluation of ThyroSeq v2 performance in thyroid nodules with indeterminate cytology. Endocr Relat Cancer 2017;24(3): 127–36.
45. Labourier E, Shifrin A, Busseniers AE, et al. Molecular testing for miRNA, mRNA, and DNA on fine-needle aspiration improves the preoperative diagnosis of thyroid nodules with indeterminate cytology. J Clin Endocrinol Metab 2015;100(7): 2743–50.

Clinical Assessment and Risk Stratification in Differentiated Thyroid Cancer

Fernanda Vaisman, MD, PhD[a],*, R. Michael Tuttle, MD[b]

KEYWORDS

- Risk stratification • Thyroid cancer • Mortality • Recurrence • Response to therapy

KEY POINTS

- Initial risk stratification provides valuable information to guide initial staging, therapy, and follow-up recommendations.
- Dynamic risk stratification is used to modify initial risk estimates so that additional therapy and follow-up can be tailored to real-time risk estimates.
- The eighth edition of the American Joint Committee on Cancer/TNM (tumor, node, and metastases) staging system downstages a substantial number of patients and improves prediction of outcomes across the 4 stage groups.

INTRODUCTION

In the last decade, there has been a shift in paradigm regarding differentiated thyroid cancer staging and management from a standardized approach to an individualized way of assessing and treating these patients. These changes were mostly due to the development of risk assessment tools, which made it possible, in an early time in follow-up, to predict major outcomes such as disease-specific mortality, risk of persistence/recurrence of structural disease, and also the chances of therapeutic failure.

One of the milestones for these changes was the 2009 revised American Thyroid Association guideline. It strongly endorsed a risk classification, taking into account not only the mortality risk but also the risk of recurrence and persistence of structural disease, which has a greater impact in thyroid cancer management, as the disease-specific mortality is usually low.[1] It emphasized the importance of factors such as histology, quality of the first surgery, and postoperative thyroglobulin (Tg) into postoperative evaluation, and also into the decision-making process regarding adjuvant therapy with radioactive iodine (RAI).[2]

The authors have nothing to disclose.
[a] Endocrinology Service, Instituto Nacional do Cancer, Praça da Cruz Vermelha 23, 8° andar, centro, Rio de Janeiro, RJ 20230-130, Brazil; [b] Endocrinology Service, Department of Medicine, Memorial Sloan Kettering Cancer Center, 1275 York Avenue, New York, NY 10021, USA
* Corresponding author.
E-mail address: fevaisman@globo.com

Endocrinol Metab Clin N Am 48 (2019) 99–108
https://doi.org/10.1016/j.ecl.2018.11.002
0889-8529/19/© 2018 Elsevier Inc. All rights reserved.

endo.theclinics.com

However, after the first therapy, re-evaluation is needed to better predict long-term outcomes and to tailor follow-up. In 2010, Tuttle and colleagues[3] proposed a dynamic restratification based on response to therapy. This approach was also important to individualized differentiated thyroid cancer (DTC) management as it is practiced today.

Almost 10 years later, those tools had been refined, and some details have changed to better separate patients who are more likely to have bad outcomes from the majority who will have a good prognosis. This article aims to review those risk assessment tools and describe how they have been modified in recent years to improve prognostication.

DISCUSSION
Assessing Risk of Mortality

Mortality is usually the main concern cancer patients carry when they come to the office for the first time. Hence, it is crucial to have an accurate classification that can predict cancer-specific mortality that can be used in this first postoperative visit. As with other solid tumors, the American Joint Committee on Cancer (AJCC) staging, known as TNM (tumor, node, and metastases), is widely used. It takes into account tumor size and primary tumor local invasion, the presence of metastatic lymph nodes, and the presence of distant metastases, all of them divided by age group. When compared with other proposed staging systems, the AJCC/TNM system performs well and is the most commonly used system in tumor registries worldwide The age cut-off in this edition was 45 years of age at diagnosis.[4]

Recently, the eighth edition was published with a few changes that seem to enhance the accuracy of disease-specific mortality prediction.[5,6]

First, the age point for cut-off was increased to 55 years of age at diagnosis. An international multicenter study with almost 10,000 patients showed that this change in age groups was better to separate stage III from stage IV patients. In this study, using age 45 years as a cutoff, 10-year disease specific survival (DSS) rates for stage I–IV were 99.7%, 97.3%, 96.6%, and 76.3%, respectively. Using age 55 years as a cutoff, 10-yearDSS rates for stage I–IV were 99.5%, 94.7%, 94.1%, and 67.6%, respectively. This change resulted in a significant downstaging of many patients while retaining good separation of the stages.[7] Supporting the hypothesis that mutational status could play a role in the poor outcomes seen in older patients, in 2018, Kim and colleagues[8] were able to show that patients diagnosed at older than 55 years of age had 103 differently expressed genes when compared with younger patients and that those were related to pathways associated with aggressiveness of thyroid cancer, such as TGF-beta pathway, supporting, from a genetic perspective, this new age cut-off.

Second, there was a re-evaluation of the prognostic significance of minor extrathyroidal extension (mETE), defined as subclinical perithyroidal invasion that can only be detected on histologic examination (not apparent on clinical examination or imaging). In the seventh edition, any tumor with mETE was classified as T3. The prognostic impact of this microscopic extension has been analyzed, and studies showed that the presence of mETE alone does not influence disease-free survival or disease-specific survival, locoregional failure, and distant metastases failure. A recent study by Tam and colleagues[9] suggested that tumor size in fact is the independent predictor of those outcomes. With those considerations, the AJCC changed the T3 classification for T3a, tumors above 4 cm confined to the thyroid gland and T3b for tumors that show gross extrathyroidal extension (gETE) into strap muscles.

The third major change from the seventh to the eighth edition was regarding mediastinal metastatic lymph nodes, referred to as level VII lymph nodes. Previously, N1a was used only if the metastatic lymph nodes were found in level VI (ie, central compartment: pretracheal, paratracheal, or prelaryngeal). Now, those mediastinal lymph nodes are also called N1a, while N1b is used for metastatic lymph nodes found in the lateral neck (levels II-V).[5,10]

The fourth major change was that N1 disease no longer upstages older patients to stage III or IV disease. Although lymph node metastases in older patients does have a significant impact on disease-specific mortality, this effect is less important in younger patients and even in older patients does not convey a mortality risk that is usually associated with stage III/IV disease.[6] Thus, in patients younger than 55 years of age, N1 disease is classified as stage I disease while in patients older than 55 years, N1 disease is classified as stage II disease.

Multiple publications have now demonstrated that the eighth edition staging system does downstage a significant number of low-risk patients and also provides a better separation between the stage groups than the seventh edition.[6,10–13]

Patients younger than 55 years of age at diagnosis can only be stage I (no distant metastases) or stage II (distant metastases present). Patients at least 55 years old at diagnosis are classified as stage IVb if distant metastases are present. If not (M0/Mx), the presence or absence of gross extrathyroidal extension is the next major decision point. In the absence of gross extrathyroidal extension, tumors of no more than 4 cm confined to the thyroid (N0/Nx) are stage I, while tumors greater than 4 cm or with any cervical lymph node metastases are stage II. Conversely, patients with gross extrathyroidal extension can be stage II, III, or IVa depending on which surrounding structures are invaded by the tumor. It is important to note that any information obtained up to 4 months after initial surgery should be used to determine the AJCC stage. This includes any additional metastatic foci found on subsequent structural/functional imaging or physical examination up to 4 months after initial therapy.

Assessing Recurrence/Persistence

As already mentioned, the ATA 2009 guidelines for the management of thyroid nodules and thyroid cancer brought to light this new way of thinking about risk assessment based on the chances of recurrence and persistence of disease instead of only mortality. This approach seemed appropriate because of the low mortality rates and the paradox seen, especially in young patients, between recurrence/persistence and mortality. Studies such as Mazzaferri and colleagues in 2001 have demonstrated that although the risk of disease-specific mortality increases with age, the risk of recurrence versus age at diagnosis demonstrates a U-shaped curve, with higher risks of recurrence in younger and older patients.[14] To address that issue, in 2009, the ATA endorsed a stratification based on histopathology features, presence of lymph node and distant metastases, and some information from postoperative evaluation such as results of post-therapy iodine scan, when iodine is performed, thyroglobulin values, and cross-sectional images.

In 2010, Tuttle and colleagues[3] showed that this newly proposed risk stratification system was more accurate to predict recurrence/persistence than the AJCC, as this system accounts for a proportion of variance explained of 34%, being also better than the other commonly used staging systems such as MACIS and the former MSKCC system.[4,15,16]

In 2015, the revised ATA guidelines incorporated new data into that same classification and modified the risk of recurrence classification system by adding additional variables that relate to size and number of lymph node metastases, vascular invasion, specific histologies, and molecular profiling as additional risk factors that can be used to refine risk estimation. The prognostic significance of lymph node metastases in DTC is still controversial.[17,18] Most studies show that the presence of lymph node metastases has a small impact on overall survival, being more significant in older patients despite a great impact on recurrence/persistence rates and impairment of quality of life in all age groups.[4,5]

In the past, the presence of nodal metastasis and its location in the neck were the only factors analyzed to stratify node disease.[6] Recently, the number of affected lymph nodes, their size and location, and the presence of extranodal extension (ENE) have been shown to be important for estimating the risk of nodal disease recurrence/persistence.[7] In 2015, the ATA recommended that low-risk disease be defined as when there is no evidence of clinical nodal metastases (cN0) or when micrometastases (less than 2 mm) in 5 or fewer lymph nodes is present. Patients with clinically evident lymph nodes (cN1) and/or more than 5 lymph nodes, all less than 3 cm, should be classified as intermediate risk. High risk was attributed to patients with metastatic lymph nodes larger than 3 cm. The presence of ENE was not included as an independent factor, but the presence of more than 3 lymph nodes with ENE was considered a high-risk feature, with a 40% risk of recurrence/persistence.[18] The degree of vascular invasion is an important variable in follicular thyroid cancer (higher risk if there are more than 4 foci of vascular invasion). Although not required, mutational information can also be used to refine the risk stratification if available.

The clinical implication of this new stratification has also an impact in adjuvant radioiodine (RAI) therapy, as low nodal volume disease to be managed without adjuvant RAI therapy; for example,[3] minimally invasive FTC could now be treated as low risk, allowing the individualization of initial therapy.

Recently, Ghaznavi and colleagues[13] suggested merging the TNM eighth edition and the ATA stratification system to improve risk stratification for individual patients. They identified 6 cohorts based on AJCC stage, ATA risk, and age and showed the respective disease-free survival (DSS) rates after 6 years of follow-up:

Stage I/ATA low risk, younger and older, 100% DSS[2]
Stage I/ATA intermediate risk, younger and older, 98% DSS[3]
Stage I/ATA high risk, younger, 95% DSS[4]
Stage I/ATA high risk, older, 89% DSS[5]
Stage II/ATA high risk, younger, 78% DSS[6]
Stage II/ATA high risk, older, 61% DSS

Especially in the high-risk group, this approach has had a major difference and will probably allow even more individualization in the future.[13]

Different from mortality risk, age usually is not taken into account as a major predictive factor for recurrence/persistence of disease. However, it may be key in some specific groups. Recently, Shah and Boucai[19] showed that for ATA high-risk patients, those younger than 55 years had twice the chance of having excellent response than older patients, so that the authors considered age as a key predictor of response to therapy and disease-specific survival in ATA high-risk thyroid cancer patients.

Assessing Long-Term Risk of Persistence/Recurrence and Tailoring Long Term Follow-up

Although initial risk stratification provides important prognostic information that can allow individualized management recommendations, clinicians have long recognized that risk estimates need to be adjusted over time as a function of response to initial therapy and biological behavior of the disease. In 2010, the MSKCC thyroid cancer group proposed a nomenclature and dynamic risk stratification system that could be used to modify initial risk estimates based on clinical data obtained during follow-up.[3] In this system, patients are continually reclassified as having either an excellent, indeterminate, or incomplete response (biochemical and structural) to therapy based on the cumulative data obtained at any point during follow-up. The definitions were

Excellent response: no clinical, biochemical or structural evidence of disease
Biochemical incomplete response: abnormally elevated serum thyroglobulin (Tg) or rising antithyroglobulin antibody (TgAb) levels in the absence of localizable disease
Structural incomplete response: persistent or newly identified locoregional or distant metastases with or without abnormal Tg or TgAb
Indeterminate response: nonspecific biochemical or structural findings that cannot be confidently classified as either benign or malignant (**Table 1**)[3]

As expected, regardless of the initial risk estimates, patients achieving an excellent response to therapy within the first 2 years had a substantially lower risk of recurrence/persistent disease than those who demonstrated an incomplete response to therapy (less than 3%–5% in the excellent response group vs more than 85% in the structural incomplete group). These data were validated in several cohorts worldwide.[20–22] Vaisman and colleagues[23] showed similar results in Brazil, where 99% if patients with excellent response to therapy had no evidence of disease at the end of 10 years of follow-up, 81% with indeterminate response, 56% with biochemical incomplete response, and only 10% of patients with structural evidence of disease that remained after the first 2 years had no evidence of disease at 10 years.

In the subsequent years, the response to therapy stratification was already being used to guide and tailor long-term follow-up. The ATA 2015 guidelines had recommended that once one has an excellent response to therapy, it should lead to an early decrease in the intensity and frequency of follow-up and the degree of thyroid-stimulating hormone (TSH) suppression, as the chances of recurrence from that point on are low (1%–4%). If associated with stable or declining serum Tg values, a biochemical incomplete response should lead to continued observation with ongoing TSH suppression in most patients. Rising Tg or anti-Tg antibody values should prompt

Table 1
Response to therapy- TT + radioactive iodine (6-24 months after initial therapy)

Excellent Response	Indeterminate Response	Biochemical Incomplete Response	Structural Incomplete Response
All of the following: • Suppressed <0.2 and stimulated Tg <1 ng/mL • No evidence of disease on neck ultrasound, • Additional cross-sectional and/or nuclear medicine imaging negative (if performed)	Any of the following: • Suppressed Tg <1 ng/mL with stimulated Tg ≥1 and <10 nq/mL • Nonspecific imaging findings without definite evidence of disease	Any of the following in the absence of structurally identifiable disease: • Suppressed Tg ≥1 ng/mL • Stimulated Tg ≥10 ng/mL • Rising Tg values • Rising TgAb	Any of the following regardless of Tg values: • Persistent or newly identified disease on cross-sectional imaging and/or nuclear medicine imaging

additional investigations and potentially additional therapies; an indeterminate response should lead to continued observation with appropriate serial imaging of the nonspecific lesions and serum Tg monitoring. Nonspecific findings that become suspicious over time can be further evaluated with additional imaging or biopsy, and a structural incomplete response may lead to additional treatments or ongoing observation depending on multiple clinicopathologic factors including the size, location, rate of growth, RAI avidity, fluorodeoxyglucose (18FDG) avidity, and specific pathology of the structural lesions.[18] It is important to point out that patients with structural incomplete response to initial therapy will probably have less than 15% of chance of becoming free of disease despite additional therapy, meaning that most therapies will have a palliative purpose in those cases. Hence, it is crucial to weigh carefully risks and benefits from any additional therapy proposed.

On the other hand, the ATA also proposed a less aggressive initial approach for low- and intermediate-risk patients. However, those definitions were developed for patients who underwent total thyroidectomy followed by RAI, and this is not the standard treatment for every patient. Low-risk patients are not routinely treated with RAI, for example, and lobectomy can be an option for a small intrathyroidal tumor. Hence, some definition of the 4 possibilities on how patients responded to these different modalities of initial therapy had to be developed. To address this issue, Momesso and colleagues[24] published and validated those concepts for patients who were treated with less than total thyroidectomy and no RAI. As expected, an excellent response to therapy decreased dramatically the risk of recurrence/persistence structural disease based on the ATA risk, as it dropped from 2.5% and 9.5% in the low- and intermediate-risk groups, respectively, to 0%. Likewise, an indeterminate response to treatment without RAI reduced the risk of recurrence based on the initial ATA risk estimates (**Table 2**).

Table 2
Response to therapy- TT without radioactive iodine and lobectomy (6–24 months after initial therapy)

Excellent Response	Indeterminate Response	Biochemical Incomplete Response	Structural Incomplete Response
Total thyroidectomy: All of the following: • Nonstimulated <0.2 and stimulated Tg <1 ng/mL • No evidence of disease on neck ultrasound, Lobectomy: All of the following: • Nonstimulated <30 and stimulated Tg <1 ng/mL • No evidence of disease on neck US,	Total thyroidectomy: Any of the following: • Non stimulated Tg 0.2–5 ng/mL with stimulated Tg ≥2 and <10 ng/mL • Nonspecific imaging findings without definite evidence of disease Lobectomy: • Nonspecific imaging findings without definite evidence of disease	Total thyroidectomy: Any of the following in the absence of structurally identifiable disease: • Nonstimulated Tg ≥5 ng/mL • Stimulated Tg ≥10 ng/mL • Rising Tg values • Rising TgAb Lobectomy: • Nonstimulated Tg ≥30 ng/mL • Rising Tg levels over time with similar TSH levels • Rising TgAb	Total thyroidectomy: Any of the following regardless of Tg values: • Persistent or newly identified disease on cross-sectional imaging and/or nuclear medicine imaging Lobectomy: • Persistent or newly identified disease on cross-sectional imaging and/or nuclear medicine imaging

Assessing the Risk for Therapeutic Failure

When considering risk stratification schemes, it is also critical to be specific about what outcomes one trying to predict with risk stratification schemes. Clinicians have traditionally considered the risks of recurrence, distant metastases, and death from disease to be primary endpoints of interest. But from a practical clinical perspective, the real risk one is trying to predict is the risk of failure of initial therapy. It is the combination of both the aggressive tumor biology and the high likelihood of failure to respond to initial therapy that places older patients with gross extrathyroidal extension and non-RAI avid (FDG positron emission tomography [PET] positive) metastatic lesions at highest risk of dying from disease. The few older patients presenting with high-risk disease who respond well to initial treatments (tumor completely resected even if major neck structures need to be removed, RAI-avid metastatic lesions) have a much better prognosis than similar older patients with persistent disease that does not respond to therapy.

In that sense, some additional evaluation has been proposed to understand how likely it is that the tumor will respond to therapy and again try to individualize it for each case.

The guidelines suggest that the FDG-PET/computed tomography (CT) could be useful when patients, after initial therapy, remain with high serum levels of thyroglobulin or increasing thyroglobulin trend with all cross-sectional imaging being negative.[18] However, despite having a high sensitivity (ranging from 85% to 100%), the specificity is still low in this scenario (around 75%), and it depends on the tumor burden.[25]

More recently, FDG-PET/CT has been used as a prognostic tool. Wang and colleagues[26] showed that patients with positive lesions on FDG-PET/CT were less likely to respond to high doses of RAI. The same group also showed that FDG-PET/CT positive metastatic patients had worse prognosis than the negative ones, despite on the RAI avidity.[27]

The so called flip-flop phenomenon describes the condition when the tumor no longer is able to uptake iodine or this uptake is low and is FDG-avid because of intense glucose uptake and metabolism. These tumors tend to be larger and more invasive[28] and have aggressive histology[29] and more mutations compared with FDG-negative tumors.[30] Nowadays, FDG-PET/CT is a useful tool to predict RAI refractory tumors.

In order to individualize even more, risk stratification in thyroid cancer is heading to a genetic perspective, which will probably, in the near future, be combined with the clinical assessment and improved prognostic accuracy. Studies have suggested, for instance, that tumors that carry RAS mutations are more likely to be RAI avid[31] compared with those that carry BRAF + TERT mutations.[32–35]

SUMMARY

In conclusion, risk stratification is a multistep process in which the risk of disease-related death and initial risk of recurrence/persistence, estimated by AJCC and ATA risk systems respectively, are used to guide initial management recommendations. Ongoing response-to-therapy reassessments and dynamic risk stratification are then used to further tailor management recommendations as new data become available over time. This ongoing iterative process moves one closer to their goal of providing personalized oncology recommendations that maximize benefit while minimizing the risks of excessive treatment and follow-up.

REFERENCES

1. Cooper DS, Doherty GM, Haugen BR, et al. Revised American Thyroid Association management guidelines for patients with thyroid nodules and differentiated thyroid cancer. Thyroid 2009;19:1167–214.
2. Rondeau G, Tuttle RM. Similarities and differences in follicular cell-derived thyroid cancer management guidelines used in Europe and the United States. Semin Nucl Med 2011;41(2):89–95.
3. Tuttle RM, Tala H, Shah J, et al. Estimating risk of recurrence in differentiated thyroid cancer after total thyroidectomy and radioactive iodine remnant ablation: using response to therapy variables to modify the initial risk estimates predicted by the new American Thyroid Association staging system. Thyroid 2010;20(12):1341–9.
4. Brierley JD, Panzarella T, Tsang RW, et al. A comparison of different staging systems predictability of patient outcome. Thyroid carcinoma as an example. Cancer 1997;79(12):2414–23.
5. Perrier ND, Brierley JD, Tuttle RM. Differentiated and anaplastic thyroid carcinoma: major changes in the American Joint Committee on Cancer eighth edition cancer staging manual. CA Cancer J Clin 2018;68(1):55–63.
6. Tuttle RM, Haugen B, Perrier ND. Updated American Joint Committee on Cancer/tumor-node-metastasis staging system for differentiated and anaplastic thyroid cancer (eighth edition): what changed and why? Thyroid 2017;27(6):751–6.
7. Nixon IJ, Wang LY, Migliacci JC, et al. An international multi-institutional validation of age 55 years as a cutoff for risk stratification in the AJCC/UICC staging system for well-differentiated thyroid cancer. Thyroid 2016;26(3):373–80.
8. Kim K, Kim JH, Park IS, et al. The updated AJCC/TNM staging system for papillary thyroid cancer (8th Edition): from the perspective of genomic analysis. World J Surg 2018. [Epub ahead of print].
9. Tam S, Boonsripitayanon M, Amit M, et al. Survival in differentiated thyroid cancer: comparing the AJCC cancer staging 7th and 8th editions. Thyroid 2018;28(10):1301–10.
10. van Velsen EFS, Stegenga MT, van Kemenade FJ, et al. Comparing the prognostic value of the eighth edition of the American Joint Committee on Cancer/tumor node metastasis staging system between papillary and follicular thyroid cancer thyroid cancer. Thyroid 2018;28(8):976–81.
11. Kim TH, Kim YN, Kim HI, et al. Prognostic value of the eighth edition AJCC TNM classification for differentiated thyroid carcinoma. Oral Oncol 2017;71:81–6.
12. Pontius LN, Oyekunle TO, Thomas SM, et al. Projecting survival in papillary thyroid cancer: a comparison of the seventh and eighth editions of the American Joint Commission on Cancer/Union for International Cancer Control Staging Systems in two contemporary national patient cohorts. Thyroid 2017;27(11):1408–16.
13. Ghaznavi SA, Ganly I, Shaha AR, et al. Using the ATA risk stratification system to refine and individualize the AJCC 8th edition disease specific survival estimates in differentiated thyroid cancer. Thyroid 2018;28(10):1293–300.
14. Mazzaferri EL, Kloos RT. Clinical review 128: current approaches to primary therapy for papillary and follicular thyroid cancer. J Clin Endocrinol Metab 2001;86(4):1447–63.
15. Sherman SI, Brierley JD, Sperling M, et al. 3rd Prospective multicenter study of thyroid carcinoma treatment: initial analysis of staging and outcome. National Thyroid Cancer Treatment Cooperative Study Registry Group. Cancer 1998;83:1012–21.

16. Verburg FA, Mader U, Kruitwagen CL, et al. A comparison of prognostic classification systems for differentiated thyroid carcinoma. Clin Endocrinol (Oxf) 2010; 72:830–8.

17. Randolph GW, Duh Q, Heller KS, et al. The prognostic significance of nodal metastasis from papillary thyroid carcinoma can be stratified based on the size and number of metastatic lymph nodes, as well as the presence of extranodal extension. Thyroid 2012;22(11):1144–52.

18. Haugen BR, Alexander EK, Bible KC, et al. 2015 American Thyroid Association management guidelines for adult patients with thyroid nodules and differentiated thyroid cancer: the American Thyroid Association Guidelines Task Force on Thyroid Nodules and Differentiated Thyroid Cancer. Thyroid 2016;26(1):1–133.

19. Shah S, Boucai L. Effect of age on response to therapy and mortality in patients with thyroid cancer at high risk of recurrence. J Clin Endocrinol Metab 2018; 103(2):689–97.

20. Vaisman F, Tala H, Grewal R, et al. In differentiated thyroid cancer and incomplete structural response to therapy is associated with significantly worse clinical outcomes than only an incomplete thyroglobulin response. Thyroid 2011;21: 1317–22.

21. Castagna MG, Maino F, Cipri C, et al. Delayed risk stratification, to include the response to initial therapy (surgery and radioiodine ablation), has better outcome predictivity in differentiated thyroid cancer patients. Eur J Endocrinol 2011;165: 441–6.

22. Pitoia F, Bueno F, Urciuoli C, et al. Outcome of patients with differentiated thyroid cancer risk stratified according to the American thyroid association and Latin-American thyroid society risk of recurrence classification systems. Thyroid 2013;23:1401–7.

23. Vaisman F, Momesso D, Bulzico DA, et al. Spontaneous remission in thyroid cancer patients after biochemical incomplete response to initial therapy. Clin Endocrinol 2012;77:132–8.

24. Momesso DP, Vaisman F, Yang SP, et al. Dynamic risk stratification in patients with differentiated thyroid cancer treated without radioactive iodine. J Clin Endocrinol Metab 2016;101(7):2692–700.

25. Leboulleux S, Schroeder PR, Schlumberger M, et al. The role of PET in follow-up of patients treated for differentiated epithelial thyroid cancers. Thyroid 2001; 11(12):1169–75.

26. Wang W, Larson SM, Tuttle RM, et al. Resistance of [18f]-fluorodeoxyglucose-avid metastatic thyroid cancer lesions to treatment with high-dose radioactive iodine. Thyroid 2001;11(12):1169–75.

27. Richard RJ, Wan Q, Grewal RK, et al. Larson real- time prognosis for metastatic thyroid carcinoma based on 2-[18F]Fluoro-2-Deoxy-D-glucose positron emission tomography scanning. J Clin Endocrinol Metab 2006;91(2):498–505.

28. Esteva D, Muros MA, Llamas-Elvira JM, et al. Clinical and pathological factors related to 18F-FDG-PET positivity in the diagnosis of recurrence and/or metastasis in patients with differentiated thyroid cancer. Ann Surg Oncol 2009;16(7): 2006–13.

29. Rivera M, Ghossein RA, Schoder H, et al. Histopathologic characterization of radioactive iodine-refractory fluorodeoxyglucose-positron emission tomography-positive thyroid carcinoma. Cancer 2008;113(1):48–56.

30. Ricarte-Filho JC, Ryder M, Chitale DA, et al. Mutational profile of advanced primary and metastatic radioactive iodine-refractory thyroid cancers reveals distinct

pathogenetic roles for BRAF, PIK3CA, and AKT1. Cancer Res 2009;69(11): 4885–93.

31. Sabra MM, Dominguez JM, Grewal RK, et al. Clinical outcomes and molecular profile of differentiated thyroid cancers with radioiodine-avid distant metastases. J Clin Endocrinol Metab 2013;98(5):E829–36.

32. Yang X, Li J, Li X, et al. TERT Promoter mutation predicts radioiodine-refractory character in distant metastatic differentiated thyroid cancer. J Nucl Med 2017; 58(2):258–65.

33. Penna GC, Pestana A, Cameselle JM, et al. TERTp mutation is associated with a shorter progression free survival in patients with aggressive histology subtypes of follicular-cell derived thyroid carcinoma. Endocrine 2018;61(3):489–98.

34. Liu R, Bishop J, Zhu G, et al. Mortality risk stratification by combining BRAF V600E and TERT promoter mutations in papillary thyroid cancer: genetic duet of BRAF and TERT promoter mutations in thyroid cancer mortality. JAMA Oncol 2017;3(2):202–8.

35. Xing M, Liu R, Liu X, et al. BRAF V600E and TERT promoter mutations cooperatively identify the most aggressive papillary thyroid cancer with highest recurrence. J Clin Oncol 2014;32(25):2718–26.

Genetic-guided Risk Assessment and Management of Thyroid Cancer

Mingzhao Xing, MD, PhD

KEYWORDS

- Thyroid cancer • Genetic molecular marker • *BRAF* V600E mutation
- *TERT* promoter Mutation • *RAS* mutation • Risk stratification • Prognosis

KEY POINTS

- Controversies exist on how to optimally manage thyroid cancer because the prognosis is often uncertain based on clinical backgrounds.
- Prognostic genetic markers in thyroid cancer, exemplified by *BRAF* V600E and *TERT* promoter mutations, have been well characterized and widely appreciated.
- The genetic duet of *BRAF* V600E/*RAS* and *TERT* promoter mutations is a most robust prognostic genetic pattern for poor prognosis of differentiated thyroid cancer.
- The high negative predictive values of the prognostic genetic markers are equally valuable.
- The best prognostic value of genetic markers in thyroid cancer is achieved through a clinical risk level-based and genotype-individualized manner.

INTRODUCTION

Thyroid cancer is a common endocrine malignancy, which histologically includes follicular epithelial cell–derived thyroid cancer and parafollicular C-cell–derived medullary thyroid cancer (MTC).[1] The former consists of papillary thyroid cancer (PTC), follicular thyroid cancer (FTC), and anaplastic thyroid cancer (ATC). PTC and FTC are the most common thyroid cancers, accounting for 80% to 90% and 5% to 10% of all thyroid malignancies, respectively. ATC and MTC are uncommon, each accounting for 2% to 3% of thyroid malignancies. PTC is further classified into several variants,

Conflict of Interest Disclosure: M. Xing receives royalties as coholder of a licensed US patent related to *BRAF* V600E mutation in thyroid cancer.

Funding Support: This work was supported by US National Institutes of Health grants R01CA215142 and R01CA189224 to M. Xing.

Division of Endocrinology, Diabetes and Metabolism, Department of Medicine, Johns Hopkins University School of Medicine, 1830 East Monument Street, Suite 333, Baltimore, MD 21287, USA

E-mail address: mxing1@jhmi.edu

including most commonly conventional PTC (CPTC), followed by follicular-variant PTC (FVPTC), tall-cell PTC (TCPTC), and a few other rare variants.[1–3]

PTC and FTC are differentiated thyroid cancer (DTC), which are generally indolent clinically with a low overall mortality but significant recurrence rate with the current treatments. Disease recurrence of thyroid cancer is associated with increased risk of patient morbidity and mortality. ATC can develop from preexisting DTC or *de novo*. Although ATC is uncommon, it is the most aggressive type of thyroid cancer, with a rapid lethality. There is also poorly differentiated thyroid cancer (PDTC), which can develop from DTC and has an intermediate clinical aggressiveness between DTC and ATC. PTC of tumor ≤ 1.0 cm is uniquely defined as papillary thyroid microcarcinoma (PTMC),[4] which has an excellent clinical outcome in general but can be associated with poor prognosis and even mortality in some patients. The main goal in the clinical management of thyroid cancer is to prevent disease recurrence, patient morbidity, and mortality while minimizing treatment-associated adverse consequences. Achievement of the optimal balance between therapeutic benefits and treatment complications relies on accurate risk stratification of thyroid cancer. This is currently pursued primarily based on the assessment of clinicopathologic backgrounds, which has achieved considerably improved accuracy with comprehensive clinical approaches in recent years.[5] However, controversies on how to optimally manage patients with thyroid cancer are still commonly encountered in clinical practice and in academic forums. The main challenge is that classical clinicopathologic risk assessment is often inaccurate in thyroid cancer. An example is that clinically apparent low-risk thyroid cancer may turn out to be aggressive with poor outcomes, making clinical judgment and hence treatment decision making challenging. As a result, overtreatment of inherently low-risk thyroid cancer and undertreatment of potentially aggressive thyroid cancer are both common. Given the rapid increase in thyroid cancer incidence in recent decades and the currently large number of living patients with thyroid cancer,[2,6] better risk stratification for more accurate management of thyroid cancer has become an even more important task than ever.

Molecular-based risk stratification of thyroid cancer has become an attractive strategy in guiding precision management of thyroid cancer in recent years.[7] This is practically particularly important and promising for DTC given its high incidence[2,6] and well-known prognostic molecular markers,[1,7–14] which are the main focus of the present discussion.

MAJOR ONCOGENIC GENETIC ALTERATIONS IN THYROID CANCER

Among the many genetic alterations in thyroid cancer, the prognostically most promising are oncogenic mutations, most prominently *BRAF* V600E and *TERT* promoter mutations and a few others.[1,7–14] The occurrence of these mutations has an excellent concordance between the primary DTC and the matched metastatic tumor, consistent with their role in the progression of thyroid cancer.[15]

BRAF V600E Mutation in Thyroid Cancer

The *BRAF* V600E mutation was initially found to exist in thyroid cancer in 2003,[16–21] which occurred with a prevalence of about 45% to 50% in PTC, 25% to 30% in ATC, and none in FTC and benign thyroid neoplasm.[13] This is the most common activating point mutation in the *BRAF* gene, resulting in a valine-to-glutamic acid change in the BRAF protein, causing constitutive activation of the BRAF protein kinase and hence oncogenic activation of the microtubule-associated protein (MAP) kinase pathway.[22] Over the last 15 years, numerous studies have been devoted to the characterization of the prognostic value of this mutation.[1,7,9,10,12–14,23] In 2005, a Johns Hopkins study for the first time demonstrated the association of *BRAF* V600E with poor clinical outcomes of PTC, including increased disease recurrence and radioactive iodine (RAI) refractoriness of recurrent tumors, in addition to aggressive pathologic behaviors, such as extrathyroidal invasion and lymph node metastasis.[24] Subsequent studies widely confirmed these findings, although inconsistent studies were sometimes also reported.[14,25] A multicenter study on 2099 cases of PTC demonstrated that *BRAF* V600E had an independent prognostic value for the recurrence of PTC.[26] A multicenter study on 1849 patients with PTC showed a strong association between *BRAF* V600E and PTC-specific mortality.[27] Overall, these and other studies demonstrate an important oncogenic role of *BRAF* V600E in the progression and aggressiveness of PTC.

Telomerase Reverse Transcriptase Promoter Mutations in Thyroid Cancer

The telomerase reverse transcriptase (TERT) was initially identified and characterized with a fundamental function to maintain the integrity of chromosomes by adding telomeres to their ends in the early 1980s.[28,29] TERT is now widely known to also promote various cancer-hallmark cellular and molecular activities.[30] These functions of TERT drive cell immortality and oncogenesis. Two somatic mutations, chr5:1,295,228C>T and chr5:1,295,250C>T (termed here as C228T and C250T, respectively), in the promoter of the *TERT* gene, were found in melanoma[31,32] and other cancers, including thyroid cancer.[33] Both *TERT* promoter mutations are predicted to generate a consensus binding site for E-twenty-six (ETS) transcription factors and confer the *TERT* promoter increased transcriptional activities.[31,32] GABPA, an ETS transcriptional factor, was demonstrated to selectively bind the mutant promoter of the *TERT* gene and promote the expression of *TERT*.[34] Indeed, *TERT* promoter mutations were found to be associated with increased expression of messenger RNA and protein of TERT and telomere length.[35] *TERT* C228T is far more common than *TERT* C250T in thyroid cancer, and the 2 collectively occur in 10% to 15% DTC, 40% to 45% PDTC and ATC, and virtually none in benign thyroid neoplasm.[8,11] *TERT* promoter mutations have been widely found to be associated with aggressive tumor behaviors and poor clinical outcomes of thyroid cancer; it occurs particularly commonly in aggressive DTC, PDTC, and ATC and is associated with increased recurrence and mortality of DTC.[15,33,36–45] These studies suggest a strong oncogenic role of *TERT* promoter mutations in the development of aggressiveness of thyroid cancer.

Genetic Duet of BRAF V600E and Telomerase Reverse Transcriptase Promoter Mutations in Thyroid Cancer

The initial 2013 study reporting *TERT* promoter mutations in thyroid cancer also reported an interesting association between *BRAF* V600E and *TERT* promoter mutations in PTC.[33] This phenomenon has been widely confirmed in many other studies in both primary PTC and metastatic PTC.[8,11,15] The prevalence of the genetic duet of *BRAF* V600E and *TERT* promoter mutations in primary PTC was 7.7% (145/1892) on average.[11] Several studies also reported an association between *TERT* promoter mutations and the *BRAF* V600E mutation in melanoma,[31,46] suggesting that this is a general phenomenon in human cancer. Given the known oncogenic role of *BRAF* V600E and *TERT* promoter mutations each in thyroid cancer, it was speculated and demonstrated that this mutation duet was a robust genetic background for the most severe aggressiveness of PTC, hence predicting the worst clinicopathologic outcomes of PTC.[45] In this study, when the cohort was divided into 4 groups: no mutation, *BRAF* V600E, *TERT* promoter mutations, and the genetic duet of coexisting mutations, each mutation alone had a modest adverse effect, whereas the mutation duet had a robust effect on the poor clinicopathologic outcomes of PTC, including extrathyroidal invasion, lymph node metastasis, distant metastasis, and disease recurrence (**Fig. 1**).[45] This pattern of the effects of the genetic duet of *BRAF* V600E and *TERT* promoter mutations was similarly observed with PTC-related patient mortality,[44] which was fully confirmed in an expanded large study on 1051 patients with PTC, showing a robust synergistic adverse effect of the genetic duet on PTC-specific patient survival; the mortality was virtually zero in the absence of either mutation, slightly increased with either mutation alone, and robustly increased with the genetic duet (**Fig. 2**).[39] Many subsequent studies demonstrated a similarly robust synergistic adverse effect of the genetic duet of *BRAF* V600E and *TERT* promoter mutations on clinicopathologic outcomes of thyroid cancer.[15,37,42,47,48] This remarkable clinical finding of the genetic duet was beautifully explained by a novel molecular mechanism described recently.[49] In this mechanism, the BRAF V600E constitutively activates the MAP kinase pathway, causing the phosphorylation and activation of FOS, which, as a novel transcriptional factor for the *GABPB* gene, binds and activates the promoter of *GABPB* and upregulates its expression. GABPB, at elevated level, drives the formation of GABPA/GABPB complex, which in turn selectively binds and activates the mutant *TERT* promoter and robustly promotes the expression of *TERT*, conferring strong TERT oncogenicity. This represents a robust molecular mechanism underpinning the synergism between the *BRAF* V600E and *TERT* promoter mutations in driving the aggressiveness and poor clinical outcomes of thyroid cancer.

RAS Mutation and Its Genetic Duet with Telomerase Reverse Transcriptase Promoter Mutation in Thyroid Cancer

RAS mutations are common in follicular thyroid neoplasms, occurring in about 20% to 25% follicular thyroid adenoma, 30% to 45% FVPTC, 30% to 45% FTC, 20% to 40%

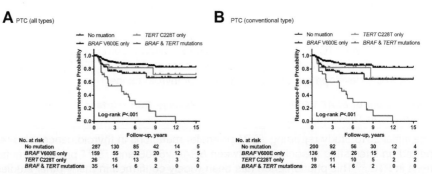

Fig. 1. Impacts of *BRAF* V600E or *TERT* promoter mutation alone or their coexistence on disease-free survival of patients with papillary thyroid cancer (PTC). Kaplan-Meier analyses of 507 patients with PTC were performed. (*A*) shows the analysis results of patients with PTC of all types and (*B*) shows the analysis results of patients with conventional-variant PTC only. Four groups of patients were included in each panel, including patients with neither mutation (*black line*), *TERT* mutation only (*green line*), *BRAF* V600E mutation only (*blue line*), and the genetic duet of the two coexisting mutations (*red line*). (*Adapted from* Xing M, Liu R, Liu X, et al. BRAF V600E and TERT promoter mutations cooperatively identify the most aggressive papillary thyroid cancer with highest recurrence. J Clin Oncol 2014;32(25):2718–26. Reprinted with permission. © 2014 American Society of Clinical Oncology. All rights reserved.)

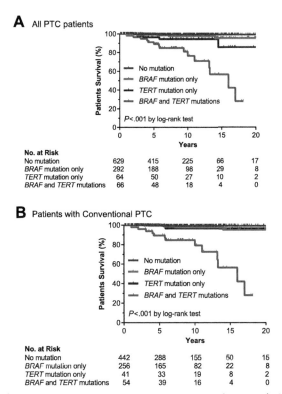

Fig. 2. Impacts of *BRAF* V600E or *TERT* promoter mutation alone or their coexistence on disease-specific survival of patients with PTC. Kaplan-Meier analyses of 1051 patients with PTC were performed. (*A, B*) The analysis results of patients with PTC of all types and only patients with conventional-variant PTC, respectively. In each panel, the patients were divided into 4 genotype groups: no mutation (*black line*), *BRAF* V600E only (*green line*), *TERT* promoter mutation only (*blue line*), and genetic duet of the 2 coexisting mutations (*red line*). (*Adapted from* Liu R, Bishop J, Zhu G, et al. Mortality risk stratification by combining *BRAF* V600E and *TERT* promoter mutations in papillary thyroid cancer: genetic duet of *BRAF* and *TERT* promoter mutations in thyroid cancer mortality. JAMA Oncol 2017;3(2):206; with permission.)

PDTC and ATC, and rarely in CPTC, and virtually none in TCPTC.[1] A significant association between *RAS* and *TERT* promoter mutations in thyroid cancer was reported in several studies, particularly in FTC and FVPTC.[15,42,48] This genetic duet of *RAS* and *TERT* promoter mutations was also shown to be associated with poor clinical outcomes of thyroid cancer, including robustly increased disease recurrence and patient mortality.[15,42,48] Some previous studies showed an association between *RAS* mutation and poor clinicopathologic outcomes in FTC[50] and PDTC.[51,52] It is possible that this effect of *RAS* mutation was actually the effect of the genetic duet of *RAS* and *TERT* promoter mutations because *RAS* mutation alone often occurs in benign follicular adenoma and low-risk DTC. *TERT* promoter mutations are fairly common in FTC and very common in PDTC and ATC.[8,11,15] The genetic duet of *RAS* and *TERT* promoter mutations is thus probably common and constitutes an important genetic background for the aggressiveness of these cancers. In fact, the duet of *RAS* and *TERT* promoter mutations was shown to be highly concordant between primary and matched metastatic FTC and associated with ominous clinical outcomes.[15] The molecular mechanism for this synergism between *RAS* and *TERT* promoter mutations in driving thyroid cancer aggressiveness remains to be elucidated, but it likely involves also the MAP kinase/ROS/GABP/TERT pathway used by the duet of *BRAF* V600E and *TERT* promoter mutations because RAS can also activate the MAP kinase pathway albeit less robustly. Because *RAS* and *BRAF* mutations are mutually exclusive,[1,13] their synergism with *TERT* promoter mutations represents a complementary mechanism of the 2 mutations to each other in driving the aggressiveness of thyroid cancer.

Other Oncogenic Genetic Alterations in Thyroid Cancer

There are some other oncogenic genetic alterations that play a role in thyroid cancer aggressiveness and may potentially have prognostic values. Among them are *TP53*, *EIF1A*, and β-*catenin* mutations, which occur commonly in PDTC and ATC, but very rarely in DTC.[53–60] This distribution pattern suggests that these genetic alterations are involved in the development of aggressiveness of thyroid cancer and their occurrence, if ever, in DTC likely has a strong prognostic power for poor prognosis. However, the rareness of these mutations in DTC suggests that their clinical utility in the risk stratification of DTC is practically limited.

Genomic and large-scale genetic studies in recent years have unveiled overwhelming new findings in thyroid cancer.[54,59,60] Large-scale epigenetic studies have similarly uncovered tremendous molecular information in thyroid cancer, such as aberrant microRNA and methylation.[23,54,61] These are now bringing in a potentially exciting opportunity for discovering new prognostic molecular markers in thyroid cancer. Nevertheless, the biological functions of the new gonomic/genetic/epigenetic molecular changes in thyroid cancer are largely undefined. Unlike *BRAF* V600E and *TERT* promoter mutations, most of these new molecular markers have limited clinical prognostic potential in thyroid cancer. Some of the common genetic rearrangements, such as *RET/PTC* and *PAX8/PPAR*γ, have no apparent impact on the development of aggressiveness of thyroid cancer and thus have a limited prognostic value.[1,13]

CLINICAL APPLICATION OF PROGNOSTIC GENETIC MARKERS IN THYROID CANCER

Given the strong association of some of the oncogenic genetic markers, particularly *BRAF* V600E and *TERT* promoter mutations, with poor clinical outcomes and their relatively common occurrence, their prognostic application in thyroid cancer has robust clinical utility. However, depending on the genetic type and clinical setting, these mutations do not necessarily always herald ominous outcomes of thyroid cancer. Therefore, their prognostic use should not be indiscriminative but should be tailored to meet individualized need in specific clinical settings. A good utility of prognostic genetic markers is that they can be a "tiebreaker" when a physician is faced with ambiguity from conventional clinicopathologic risk assessment in treatment decision making for thyroid cancer. In this context, it is also important to emphasize that the high negative predictive values (NPVs) of these genetic markers for poor prognosis of thyroid cancer make a negative genetic test equally valuable. The following specific clinical settings exemplify the clinical application of prognostic genetic markers, particularly *BRAF* V600E and *TERT* promoter mutations, in thyroid cancer.

General Consideration of Clinical Application of High-Risk Prognostic Genetic Markers

From the above discussion on the robust oncogenic role of the high-risk genetic alterations in the aggressiveness of thyroid cancer, including high patient mortality, it is reasonable to recommend that their existence in DTC should generally favor more aggressive treatment. These include the genetic duet of *BRAF* V600E and *TERT* promoter mutations, the genetic duet of *RAS* and *TERT* promoter mutations, and the rare *TP53*, *EIF1A*, and β-*catenin* mutations. Specifically, it is reasonable to recommend total thyroidectomy for all patients with DTC harboring such genetic markers, even in cases of PTMC. Therapeutic and prophylactic neck dissections and RAI ablation will be usually reasonable in such patients. Because only 7.7% of PTC on average harbor the genetic duet of *BRAF* V600E and *TERT* promoter mutations,[11] if guided by this genetic duet, less than 10% of patients with PTC overall will be treated relatively aggressively. Because high-risk genetic alterations are very rare in PTMC, only a small number of patients with PTMC will be treated aggressively based on them. In PTC greater than 1.0 to 2.0 cm, particularly tumors greater than 2.0 cm, prophylactic central neck dissection may be reasonable given the fact that large tumors are particularly associated with increased disease recurrence in the presence of BRAF V600E mutation,[62] and the high-risk genetic alterations are often associated with RAI refractoriness of recurrent disease,[1,24,63] thus making initial elimination of metastatic lymph nodes particularly important. Patients with FTC harboring high-risk genetic alterations, such as *TP53*, *EIF1A*, and β-*catenin* mutations as well as the genetic duet of *RAS* and *TERT* promoter mutations, similarly favor aggressive treatments.

Clinical Application of BRAF V600E in Solitary Intrathyroidal Papillary Thyroid Cancer

It is generally acceptable to treat clinically apparent invasive/metastatic thyroid cancer with relatively aggressive approaches, such as total thyroidectomy and, in appropriate settings, therapeutic/prophylactic neck dissections and radioiodine ablation. However, how to treat intrathyroidal PTC, that is, PTC without extrathyroidal invasion, lymph node metastasis, and distant metastasis, is not completely agreed upon among physicians. The current American Thyroid Association guidelines recommend lobectomy as an alternative option to total thyroidectomy for solitary intrathyroidal PTC (SI-PTC) of 1 to 4 cm in size.[5] This recommendation is somehow controversial as it may not be a straightforward effort to decide lobectomy versus total thyroidectomy in an individual patient because such apparently clinically low-risk thyroid cancer may not uniformly turn out to be free of poor clinical outcomes. A recent multicenter study shed light on tackling this dilemma using *BRAF* V600E as a prognostic genetic marker to guide better risk stratification in such patients.[62] In this study, the recurrence rates of SI-PTC greater than 1.0 cm, particularly tumors greater than 2.0 cm, were 20% to 30% versus recurrence rates of only 2% to 3% in matched wild-type *BRAF* SI-PTC, with NPVs of *BRAF* V600E for recurrence being 97% to 98% or 100% if only structural recurrence was considered. Remarkably, this was true even in SI-PTC greater than 4.0 cm. For intrathyroidal PTMC, structural recurrence rates were both low in *BRAF* V600E patients and wild-type *BRAF* patients, being only 1% to 2%. Given these findings, decision making on SI-PTC can now be more accurate if BRAF status is included in prognostic consideration: it is reasonable to treat wild-type *BRAF* SI-PTC of any tumor size, even tumors greater than 4.0 cm, with thyroid lobectomy; *BRAF* V600E-positive SI-PTC greater than 1.0 cm, particularly tumors greater than 2.0 cm, should be treated aggressively, with total thyroidectomy and prophylactic neck dissection, followed by RAI ablation if indicated. *BRAF* mutation-positive SI-PTC greater than 1.0 cm and ≤4.0 cm account for 23.1% and mutation-positive SI-PTC greater than 2.0 cm and ≤4.0 cm account for 8.3% of all cases of SI-PTC. Thus, only a small minority of SI-PTC needs to be treated aggressively. Given the low recurrence rates, SI-PTC less than 2.0 cm, particularly tumors less than 1.0 cm (ie, low-risk PTMC), may be treated with lobectomy regardless of the *BRAF* status. With this *BRAF* status-guided strategy, the vast majority of SI-PTC patients can be treated with thyroid lobectomy only, which is associated with fewer surgical complications and a good chance of the patient staying euthyroid, obviating life-long thyroid hormone replacement. Conservative active surveillance of BRAF mutation-negative SI-PTC <1.0 cm may be a reasonable alternative management option (see below for further discussion).

Clinical Application of BRAF V600E in Clinically Low-Risk Papillary Thyroid Microcarcinoma

It is widely agreed upon that clinically aggressive PTMC should be generally treated as for large PTC. Controversy exists, however, on how to treat clinically low-risk PTMC, that is, PTMC without extrathyroidal extension, lymph node metastasis, distant metastasis, and other aggressive features. Most physicians currently favor surgery as a preferred treatment option for such PTMC, usually lobectomy.[5] In recent years, nonsurgical active surveillance has become an alternative option acceptable to some physicians for clinically low-risk PTMC.[5] This is primarily based on several prospective Japanese studies showing that clinically low-risk PTMC in the vast majority of patients remained indolent without serious clinical consequence after active surveillance for an average of 5 to 6 years.[64–66] However, it has been well known that a small percentage of cases of PTMC present with significant tumor aggressiveness and even patient mortality, and all large PTC have grown from PTMC. A major challenge is that no clinical features can reliably differentiate the relatively small number of patients with PTMC with disease destined to progress from the larger population of patients harboring inherently indolent PTMCs. Thus, there is concern about whether indiscriminate active surveillance of all clinically low-risk PTMC, particularly for long term (eg, decades), is a reasonable strategy because serious disease progression, such as metastasis, may occur even if tumor size may remain relatively stable.

Knowledge of the *BRAF* status may now help facilitate decision making on such PTMC. As discussed above, mortality risk is extremely low in wild-type *BRAF* PTC in general regardless of tumor size and even lower in clinically low-risk PTMC. Even recurrence rate is extremely low in clinically low-risk wild-type *BRAF* PTC, including PTMC.[62] Thus, active surveillance for clinically low-risk wild-type *BRAF* PTMC seems to be reasonable and has the advantage of avoiding surgical complications and preserving normal thyroid functions. Given the lack of specific long-term prospective data, it is less clear, however, whether long-term active surveillance is reasonable for clinically low-risk but *BRAF* V600E-positive PTMC. The recent study on SI-PTC showed no significant impact of *BRAF* V600E on structural recurrence of clinically low-risk PTMC treated with thyroidectomy.[62] It is possible, however, that because surgical removal of PTMC at an early stage before *BRAF* V600E had sufficient time to exert adverse effects, there were no serious clinical consequences, even recurrence. The outcomes of increase in tumor size may potentially be problematic in the presence of *BRAF* V600E. As discussed above, in clinically low-risk SI-PTC, *BRAF* V600E was associated with robustly increased recurrence in tumors greater than 1.0 cm, particularly tumors greater than 2.0 cm, even after total thyroidectomy.[62] Theoretically, if given sufficient time, *BRAF* V600E may cause consequences, such as metastasis. Currently, there is no consensus on what is the appropriate size PTMC can be allowed to grow to before triggering thyroidectomy during active surveillance. If allowing *BRAF* V600E-positive but clinically apparent low-risk PTMC to grow to greater than 1.0 cm, particularly 2.0 cm, there may be a substantially increased risk of serious consequence, such as incurable RAI-refractory metastatic disease and even perhaps mortality. In contrast, some increase in tumor size (eg, >3 mm), which could trigger a decision to operate PTMC in patients under currently suggested active surveillance,[64–66] may not be as worrisome as currently thought if *BRAF* mutation is absent.

There is a well-known synergism between *BRAF* V600E and invasive tumor behaviors (eg, extrathyroidal invasion, lymph node metastasis, and distant metastasis) in adversely affecting PTC-related mortality.[27] Thus, surgical treatment rather than active surveillance of *BRAF* V600E-positive and clinically low-risk PTMC before the mutation has sufficient time to exert adverse actions seems to be reasonable. In such case, however, thyroid lobectomy may be just sufficient at this early stage of the disease when *BRAF* V600E does not exert adverse actions yet.[62] This seems to be practical because only a small minority of thyroid cancers is clinically low-risk PTMC harboring *BRAF* V600E mutation.[62] As discussed in the early section above, clinically low-risk PTMC, if ever found to harbor high-risk genetic alterations (eg, duets of *BRAF* V600E/*RAS* and *TERT* promoter mutations, *TP53*, *EIF1A*, and β-*catenin* mutations), should be most reasonably treated relatively aggressively (eg, total thyroidectomy).

Clinical Application of Prognostic Genetic Markers in Follicular Thyroid Cancer

Unlike PTC in which the prognostic value of *BRAF* V600E has been well characterized, molecular prognostication has been less well defined in FTC. Nevertheless, a few genetic markers are prognostically promising for FTC. *RAS* mutation was previously reported to be associated with aggressive behaviors of FTC.[50] *RAS* and *TERT* promoter mutations are both common in FTC, and there is a significant association between them.[11,15,42,48] In analogy with the robust prognostic value of the genetic duet of *BRAF* V600E and *TERT* promoter mutations in PTC, it is possible that the genetic duet of *RAS* and *TERT* promoter mutations may have an important prognostic value in FTC. In fact, this has been well demonstrated in DTC, including FTC, in several studies.[15,42,48] Therefore, the duet of *RAS* and *TERT* promoter mutations is an important genetic background and prognostic genetic pattern for poor clinical outcomes of FTC. It is thus reasonable to aggressively treat FTC harboring the genetic duet of *RAS* and *TERT* promoter mutations, including, for example, total thyroidectomy and RAI ablation. Other high-risk genetic alterations, such as *TP53*, *EIF1A*, and β-*catenin* mutations, if ever found, should be treated as important genetic predictors for poor clinical outcomes of FTC and favor aggressive treatment.

Application of Prognostic Genetic Markers in Predicting Radioiodine Refractoriness of Thyroid Cancer

Since it was first reported in 2005 that *BRAF* V600E was associated with recurrence of PTC and RAI refractoriness and hence incurability of recurrent PTC,[24] numerous studies have confirmed this finding and demonstrated impaired or even absent expression of the thyroid iodide-metabolizing genes, that is, genes for thyroid-stimulating hormone receptor, sodium/iodide symporter, thyroperoxidase, thyroglobulin (Tg), thyroid transcription factor 1, and PAX8 transcription factor, in PTC harboring *BRAF* V600E.[1,7,13,14] A direct functional link between BRAF V600E and the impairment of thyroid iodide-metabolizing gene expression was the demonstration that introduced expression of BRAF V600E in normal thyroid cells caused silencing of thyroid iodide-metabolizing genes; cessation of the expression of BRAF V600E or inhibition of the BRAF/MAP kinase pathway could restore the expression of thyroid genes.[67] This was later recapitulated in animal models[68] and even human patients: treatment of patients carrying RAI-refractory PTC with an inhibitor of the MAP kinase pathway could restore RAI avidity of the tumor.[69] Recent studies demonstrated that *TERT* promoter mutations may also be associated with impairment or loss of RAI avidity and, in fact, the genetic duet of *BRAF* V600E and *TERT* promoter mutations was most robustly associated with RAI refractoriness of metastatic PTC.[63] Pediatric PTC is generally highly curable with RAI treatment, consistent with its low prevalence of *BRAF* V600E[13] and very rare occurrence of *TERT* promoter mutations.[70] Because *BRAF* V600E is associated with increased risk of RAI refractoriness of recurrent disease of PTC, mostly recurrent metastatic lymph nodes, a positive test for *BRAF* V600E, particularly the genetic duet of *BRAF* V600E and *TERT* promoter mutations, favors thorough therapeutic neck dissection and, in appropriate cases, prophylactic neck dissection, to minimize the risk of the development of RAI-refractory recurrent disease. Prophylactic neck dissection is particularly applicable to *BRAF* mutation-positive PTC greater than 2.0 cm as discussed in the above sections. However, even with impairment of RAI avidity, *BRAF* V600E-positive PTC still should be treated with RAI ablation when clinically indicated because RAI avidity loss is often partial. Also, as the mutation-positive cancer has an increased risk for disease recurrence and even mortality, patients need to be effectively monitored in the follow-up surveillance following total thyroidectomy. Thus, a reliable specific Tg test is particularly important, which is made possible with RAI ablation of normal thyroid tissues. It is not clear at this time whether a higher dose of RAI may be beneficial to *BRAF* V600E-positive PTC given the impairment of RAI avidity in such cancer.

Application of Prognostic Genetic Markers in Differentiated Thyroid Cancer Already with Clinically Apparent Aggressiveness

Genetic markers may even be prognostically useful in DTC that already shows clinically apparent aggressiveness, such as extrathyroidal invasion, lymph nodes metastasis, and distant metastasis. Even though aggressive initial treatment is generally needed in such patients, the outcomes from the current standard treatments may be different depending on the genotype of *BRAF* and *TERT* in the tumor. In the absence of *BRAF* V600E and *TERT* promoter mutations, the mortality of PTC, particularly CPTC and FVPTC, is extremely low, whereas, in contrast, the genetic duet of *BRAF* V600E and *TERT* promoter mutations was associated with robustly high mortality in a manner independent of conventional clinicopathologic risk factors.[39] The genetic duet of *RAS* and *TERT* promoter mutations has similar prognostic value.[15,42,48] Also, as discussed above, these mutations are strongly associated with loss of RAI avidity and hence often treatment failure of recurrent disease. Thus, even the initial clinical presentation of the tumor aggressiveness is similar in patients, the disease prognosis can be different in such patients depending on whether there are these mutations. Therefore, these genetic markers still have values in assisting prognostic evaluation of clinically apparent aggressive DTC. Existence of these genetic markers implies increased risk of therapeutic failure of the current treatment and emphasizes the importance of complete eradication of the disease in the initial treatment and the need for subsequent vigilant active surveillance for disease recurrence.

Potential Prognostic Value of Genetic Markers in Anaplastic Thyroid Cancer and Poorly Differentiated Thyroid Cancer

Although ATC is generally an extremely aggressive cancer, its aggressiveness seems to be differentiable by certain genetic patterns. For example, *TERT* promoter mutation-positive ATC was found to be more commonly associated with distant metastasis,[43] which is likely to be translated into accelerated mortality. The genetic duet of *BRAF* V600E and *TERT* promoter mutations is likely to represent a genetic background for more aggressiveness of ATC. *RAS* mutation was reported to be associated with increased aggressiveness of PDTC.[51,52] It is likely that this effect of *RAS* mutation originates from the genetic duet of *RAS* and *TERT* promoter mutations as discussed above. Therapeutically, *BRAF* V600E-positive ATC has recently been demonstrated to have a remarkable response to the combination treatment with BRAF V600E and MEK inhibitors,[71] promoting an expedited approval by the Food and Drug Administration of the combination use of the BRAF V600E inhibitor dabrafenib and the MEK inhibitor trametinib for the treatment of BRAF V600E-positive ATC. Thus, testing of certain genetic markers in ATC may have both prognostic and predictive values. This may likely become true also for PTC.

Special Consideration of RAS Mutation in Several Clinical Settings

Because *RAS* mutations can occur in both benign and malignant thyroid neoplasms, its value as a diagnostic and prognostic marker by itself had been uncertain until recently.[72] It has been recently demonstrated that long-term follow-up of cytologically benign but *RAS* mutation-positive thyroid nodules had no clinical consequence, and *RAS* mutation alone in DTC was usually associated with low-risk disease with excellent clinical outcomes.[73] As discussed above, it is the genetic duet of *RAS* and *TERT* promoter mutations that is robustly associated with poor clinical outcomes of DTC.[15,42,48] Given these and other studies, the following recommendations for RAS mutation alone as recently proposed[72] may be reasonable to consider for thyroid neoplasms that are negative for other high-risk genetic alterations (eg, *TERT* promoter mutation) unless clinically suggested otherwise: (1) cytologically benign but *RAS* mutation-positive thyroid nodules can be nonsurgically managed with long-term surveillance; (2) *RAS* mutation-positive thyroid nodules with cytologic atypia of

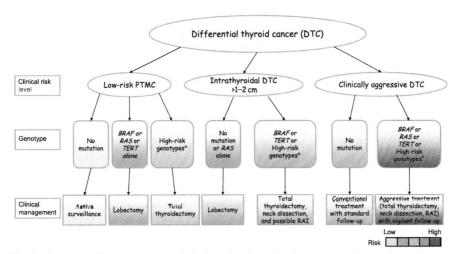

Fig. 3. Summary of the suggested clinical application of major prognostic genetic markers in thyroid cancer. The diagram shows how thyroid cancer at different clinical risk levels in various clinical settings can be appropriately treated with the guidance of specific individual genotypes. [a]High-risk genotypes include the duet of *BRAF* V600E/*RAS* and *TERT* promoter mutations, *TP53*, *EIF1A*, β-*catenin* mutations, and so forth.

undetermined significance or follicular neoplasm may be treated surgically with limited extent (eg, lobectomy); (3) clinically low-risk but *RAS* mutation-positive DTC can be generally treated with limited extent (eg, lobectomy).

SUMMARY

The value of prognostic genetic marker-based risk stratification and precision management of thyroid cancer is widely appreciated. Well-characterized and clinically applicable prognostic genetic markers are best exemplified by *BRAF* V600E and *TERT* promoter mutations. The genetic duet of *BRAF* V600E/*RAS* and *TERT* promoter mutations has particularly robust prognostic power for poor clinical outcomes of DTC. The NPVs of these prognostic genetic markers are equally important clinically. Appropriate application of these prognostic markers can particularly improve the precision of management decision making for thyroid cancer in currently controversial areas, such as thyroid lobectomy versus total thyroidectomy, prophylactic neck discussion versus no neck dissection, RAI ablation versus no RAI ablation, and nonsurgical active surveillance versus surgical treatment. A suggested approach for the clinical application of prognostic genetic markers in DTC is illustrated in **Fig. 3**. In this approach, the best prognostic utility of the genetic markers in guiding the treatment of thyroid cancer can be achieved in a clinical risk level-based and genotype-individualized manner.

REFERENCES

1. Xing M. Molecular pathogenesis and mechanisms of thyroid cancer. Nat Rev Cancer 2013;13(3):184–99.
2. Mao Y, Xing M. Recent incidences and differential trends of thyroid cancer in the USA. Endocr Relat Cancer 2016;23(4):313–22.
3. Shi X, Liu R, Basolo F, et al. Differential clinicopathological risk and prognosis of major papillary thyroid cancer variants. J Clin Endocrinol Metab 2016;101(1): 264–74.
4. Lloyd RV, Osamura RY, Klöppel G, et al, editors. WHO classification of tumours of endocrine organs. 4th edition. Lyon (France): International Agency for Research on Cancer (IARC); 2017.
5. Haugen BR, Alexander EK, Bible KC, et al. 2015 American Thyroid Association Management Guidelines for adult patients with thyroid nodules and differentiated thyroid cancer: The American Thyroid Association Guidelines Task Force on thyroid nodules and differentiated thyroid cancer. Thyroid 2016;26(1):1–133.
6. Noone AM, Howlader N, Krapcho M, et al. SEER cancer statistics review, 1975-2015. Bethesda (MD): National Cancer Institute; 2018. Available at: https://seer.cancer.gov/csr/1975_2015/. based on November 2017 SEER data submission, posted to the SEER web site.
7. Xing M, Haugen BR, Schlumberger M. Progress in molecular-based management of differentiated thyroid cancer. Lancet 2013;381(9871):1058–69.
8. Alzahrani AS, Alsaadi R, Murugan AK, et al. TERT promoter mutations in thyroid cancer. Horm Cancer 2016;7(3):165–77.
9. D'Cruz AK, Vaish R, Vaidya A, et al. Molecular markers in well-differentiated thyroid cancer. Eur Arch Otorhinolaryngol 2018;275(6):1375–84.
10. Li F, Chen G, Sheng C, et al. BRAFV600E mutation in papillary thyroid microcarcinoma: a meta-analysis. Endocr Relat Cancer 2015;22(2):159–68.
11. Liu R, Xing M. TERT promoter mutations in thyroid cancer. Endocr Relat Cancer 2016;23(3):R143–55.

12. Tufano RP, Teixeira GV, Bishop J, et al. BRAF mutation in papillary thyroid cancer and its value in tailoring initial treatment: a systematic review and meta-analysis. Medicine (Baltimore) 2012;91(5):274–86.

13. Xing M. BRAF mutation in thyroid cancer. Endocr Relat Cancer 2005;12(2): 245–62.

14. Xing M. BRAF mutation in papillary thyroid cancer: pathogenic role, molecular bases, and clinical implications. Endocr Rev 2007;28(7):742–62.

15. Sohn SY, Park WY, Shin HT, et al. Highly concordant key genetic alterations in primary tumors and matched distant metastases in differentiated thyroid cancer. Thyroid 2016;26(5):672–82.

16. Cohen Y, Xing M, Mambo E, et al. BRAF mutation in papillary thyroid carcinoma. J Natl Cancer Inst 2003;95(8):625–7.

17. Fukushima T, Suzuki S, Mashiko M, et al. BRAF mutations in papillary carcinomas of the thyroid. Oncogene 2003;22(41):6455–7.

18. Kimura ET, Nikiforova MN, Zhu Z, et al. High prevalence of BRAF mutations in thyroid cancer: genetic evidence for constitutive activation of the RET/PTC-RAS-BRAF signaling pathway in papillary thyroid carcinoma. Cancer Res 2003; 63(7):1454–7.

19. Namba H, Nakashima M, Hayashi T, et al. Clinical implication of hot spot BRAF mutation, V599E, in papillary thyroid cancers. J Clin Endocrinol Metab 2003; 88(9):4393–7.

20. Soares P, Trovisco V, Rocha AS, et al. BRAF mutations and RET/PTC rearrangements are alternative events in the etiopathogenesis of PTC. Oncogene 2003; 22(29):4578–80.

21. Xu X, Quiros RM, Gattuso P, et al. High prevalence of BRAF gene mutation in papillary thyroid carcinomas and thyroid tumor cell lines. Cancer Res 2003; 63(15):4561–7.

22. Davies H, Bignell GR, Cox C, et al. Mutations of the BRAF gene in human cancer. Nature 2002;417(6892):949–54.

23. de la Chapelle A, Jazdzewski K. MicroRNAs in thyroid cancer. J Clin Endocrinol Metab 2011;96(11):3326–36.

24. Xing M, Westra WH, Tufano RP, et al. BRAF mutation predicts a poorer clinical prognosis for papillary thyroid cancer. J Clin Endocrinol Metab 2005;90(12): 6373–9.

25. Kim TY, Kim WB, Rhee YS, et al. The BRAF mutation is useful for prediction of clinical recurrence in low-risk patients with conventional papillary thyroid carcinoma. Clin Endocrinol (Oxf) 2006;65(3):364–8.

26. Xing M, Alzahrani AS, Carson KA, et al. Association between BRAF V600E mutation and recurrence of papillary thyroid cancer. J Clin Oncol 2015;33(1):42–50.

27. Xing M, Alzahrani AS, Carson KA, et al. Association between BRAF V600E mutation and mortality in patients with papillary thyroid cancer. JAMA 2013;309(14): 1493–501.

28. Greider CW, Blackburn EH, Identification of a specific telomere terminal transferase activity in Tetrahymena extracts. Cell 1985;43(2 Pt 1):405–13.

29. Szostak JW, Blackburn EH. Cloning yeast telomeres on linear plasmid vectors. Cell 1982;29(1):245–55.

30. Low KC, Tergaonkar V. Telomerase: central regulator of all of the hallmarks of cancer. Trends Biochem Sci 2013;38(9):426–34.

31. Horn S, Figl A, Rachakonda PS, et al. TERT promoter mutations in familial and sporadic melanoma. Science 2013;339(6122):959–61.

32. Huang FW, Hodis E, Xu MJ, et al. Highly recurrent TERT promoter mutations in human melanoma. Science 2013;339(6122):957–9.
33. Liu X, Bishop J, Shan Y, et al. Highly prevalent TERT promoter mutations in aggressive thyroid cancers. Endocr Relat Cancer 2013;20(4):603–10.
34. Bell RJ, Rube HT, Kreig A, et al. The transcription factor GABP selectively binds and activates the mutant TERT promoter in cancer. Science 2015;348(6238): 1036–9.
35. Borah S, Xi L, Zaug AJ, et al. TERT promoter mutations and telomerase reactivation in urothelial cancer. Science 2015;347(6225):1006–10.
36. Bu R, Siraj AK, Divya SP, et al. Telomerase reverse transcriptase mutations are independent predictor of disease-free survival in Middle Eastern papillary thyroid cancer. Int J Cancer 2018;142(10):2028–39.
37. Jin L, Chen E, Dong S, et al. BRAF and TERT promoter mutations in the aggressiveness of papillary thyroid carcinoma: a study of 653 patients. Oncotarget 2016;7(14):18346–55.
38. Landa I, Ganly I, Chan TA, et al. Frequent somatic TERT promoter mutations in thyroid cancer: higher prevalence in advanced forms of the disease. J Clin Endocrinol Metab 2013;98(9):E1562–6.
39. Liu R, Bishop J, Zhu G, et al. Mortality risk stratification by combining BRAF V600E and TERT promoter mutations in papillary thyroid cancer: genetic duet of BRAF and TERT promoter mutations in thyroid cancer mortality. JAMA Oncol 2017;3(2):202–8.
40. Liu X, Qu S, Liu R, et al. TERT promoter mutations and their association with BRAF V600E mutation and aggressive clinicopathological characteristics of thyroid cancer. J Clin Endocrinol Metab 2014;99(6):E1130–6.
41. Melo M, da Rocha AG, Vinagre J, et al. TERT promoter mutations are a major indicator of poor outcome in differentiated thyroid carcinomas. J Clin Endocrinol Metab 2014;99(5):E754–65.
42. Shen X, Liu R, Xing M. A six-genotype genetic prognostic model for papillary thyroid cancer. Endocr Relat Cancer 2017;24(1):41–52.
43. Shi X, Liu R, Qu S, et al. Association of TERT promoter mutation 1,295,228 C>T with BRAF V600E mutation, older patient age, and distant metastasis in anaplastic thyroid cancer. J Clin Endocrinol Metab 2015;100(4):E632–7.
44. Xing M, Liu R, Bishop J. TERT promoter and BRAF mutations cooperatively promote papillary thyroid cancer-related mortality. Thyroid 2014;24(S1):A–131.
45. Xing M, Liu R, Liu X, et al. BRAF V600E and TERT promoter mutations cooperatively identify the most aggressive papillary thyroid cancer with highest recurrence. J Clin Oncol 2014;32(25):2718–26.
46. Griewank KG, Murali R, Puig-Butille JA, et al. TERT promoter mutation status as an independent prognostic factor in cutaneous melanoma. J Natl Cancer Inst 2014;106(9) [pii:dju246].
47. Rusinek D, Pfeifer A, Krajewska J, et al. Coexistence of TERT promoter mutations and the BRAF V600E alteration and its impact on histopathological features of papillary thyroid carcinoma in a selected series of Polish patients. Int J Mol Sci 2018;19(9):2647.
48. Song YS, Lim JA, Choi H, et al. Prognostic effects of TERT promoter mutations are enhanced by coexistence with BRAF or RAS mutations and strengthen the risk prediction by the ATA or TNM staging system in differentiated thyroid cancer patients. Cancer 2016;122(9):1370–9.
49. Liu R, Zhang T, Zhu G, et al. Regulation of mutant TERT by BRAF V600E/MAP kinase pathway through FOS/GABP in human cancer. Nat Commun 2018;9(1):579.

50. Fukahori M, Yoshida A, Hayashi H, et al. The associations between RAS mutations and clinical characteristics in follicular thyroid tumors: new insights from a single center and a large patient cohort. Thyroid 2012;22(7):683–9.
51. Garcia-Rostan G, Zhao H, Camp RL, et al. ras mutations are associated with aggressive tumor phenotypes and poor prognosis in thyroid cancer. J Clin Oncol 2003;21(17):3226–35.
52. Volante M, Rapa I, Gandhi M, et al. RAS mutations are the predominant molecular alteration in poorly differentiated thyroid carcinomas and bear prognostic impact. J Clin Endocrinol Metab 2009;94(12):4735–41.
53. Alzahrani AS, Murugan AK, Qasem E, et al. Absence of EIF1AX, PPM1D, and CHEK2 mutations reported in Thyroid Cancer Genome Atlas (TCGA) in a large series of thyroid cancer. Endocrine 2019;63(1):94–100.
54. Cancer Genome Atlas Research Network. Integrated genomic characterization of papillary thyroid carcinoma. Cell 2014;159(3):676–90.
55. Donghi R, Longoni A, Pilotti S, et al. Gene p53 mutations are restricted to poorly differentiated and undifferentiated carcinomas of the thyroid gland. J Clin Invest 1993;91(4):1753–60.
56. Fagin JA, Matsuo K, Karmakar A, et al. High prevalence of mutations of the p53 gene in poorly differentiated human thyroid carcinomas. J Clin Invest 1993;91(1):179–84.
57. Garcia-Rostan G, Camp RL, Herrero A, et al. Beta-catenin dysregulation in thyroid neoplasms: down-regulation, aberrant nuclear expression, and CTNNB1 exon 3 mutations are markers for aggressive tumor phenotypes and poor prognosis. Am J Pathol 2001;158(3):987–96.
58. Garcia-Rostan G, Tallini G, Herrero A, et al. Frequent mutation and nuclear localization of beta-catenin in anaplastic thyroid carcinoma. Cancer Res 1999;59(8):1811–5.
59. Landa I, Ibrahimpasic T, Boucai L, et al. Genomic and transcriptomic hallmarks of poorly differentiated and anaplastic thyroid cancers. J Clin Invest 2016;126(3):1052–66.
60. Pozdeyev N, Gay LM, Sokol ES, et al. Genetic analysis of 779 advanced differentiated and anaplastic thyroid cancers. Clin Cancer Res 2018;24(13):3059–68.
61. Faam B, Ghaffari MA, Ghadiri A, et al. Epigenetic modifications in human thyroid cancer. Biomed Rep 2015;3(1):3–8.
62. Huang Y, Qu S, Zhu G, et al. BRAF V600E mutation-assisted risk stratification of solitary intrathyroidal papillary thyroid cancer for precision treatment. J Natl Cancer Inst 2018;110(4):362–70.
63. Yang X, Li J, Li X, et al. TERT promoter mutation predicts radioiodine-refractory character in distant metastatic differentiated thyroid cancer. J Nucl Med 2017;58(2):258–65.
64. Ito Y, Miyauchi A, Inoue H, et al. An observational trial for papillary thyroid microcarcinoma in Japanese patients. World J Surg 2010;34(1):28–35.
65. Ito Y, Miyauchi A, Kihara M, et al. Patient age is significantly related to the progression of papillary microcarcinoma of the thyroid under observation. Thyroid 2014;24(1):27–34.
66. Sugitani I, Toda K, Yamada K, et al. Three distinctly different kinds of papillary thyroid microcarcinoma should be recognized: our treatment strategies and outcomes. World J Surg 2010;34(6):1222–31.
67. Liu D, Hu S, Hou P, et al. Suppression of BRAF/MEK/MAP kinase pathway restores expression of iodide-metabolizing genes in thyroid cells expressing the V600E BRAF mutant. Clin Cancer Res 2007;13(4):1341–9.

68. Chakravarty D, Santos E, Ryder M, et al. Small-molecule MAPK inhibitors restore radioiodine incorporation in mouse thyroid cancers with conditional BRAF activation. J Clin Invest 2011;121(12):4700–11.
69. Ho AL, Grewal RK, Leboeuf R, et al. Selumetinib-enhanced radioiodine uptake in advanced thyroid cancer. N Engl J Med 2013;368(7):623–32.
70. Alzahrani AS, Qasem E, Murugan AK, et al. Uncommon TERT promoter mutations in pediatric thyroid cancer. Thyroid 2016;26(2):235–41.
71. Subbiah V, Kreitman RJ, Wainberg ZA, et al. Dabrafenib and trametinib treatment in patients with locally advanced or metastatic BRAF V600-mutant anaplastic thyroid cancer. J Clin Oncol 2018;36(1):7–13.
72. Xing M. Clinical utility of RAS mutations in thyroid cancer: a blurred picture now emerging clearer. BMC Med 2016;14:12.
73. Medici M, Kwong N, Angell TE, et al. The variable phenotype and low-risk nature of RAS-positive thyroid nodules. BMC Med 2015;13:184.

Conventional Thyroidectomy in the Treatment of Primary Thyroid Cancer

Benjamin R. Roman, MD, MSHP[a], Gregory W. Randolph, MD[b],*,
Dipti Kamani, MD[b]

KEYWORDS

- Thyroidectomy • Thyroid surgery • Thyroid anatomy • Recurrent laryngeal nerve
- Thyroid cancer • Intraoperative neuro monitoring

KEY POINTS

- Conventional thyroidectomy is the most common, time-tested, and preferred management approach for thyroid carcinoma.
- Three recent developments—the new American Thyroid Association 2015 guidelines, 2017 Bethesda classification and the introduction of NIFTP—have further refined indications for surgery related to thyroid cancer and nodules.
- Detailed preoperative evaluation is important for judging the indication and extent of surgery and to prepare for shared decision-making and preoperative counseling with the patient.
- Although surgeons may have personal preferences, the basic steps of conventional thyroidectomies remain the same.
- Strong knowledge of head and neck anatomy, meticulous surgery, and planning an optimal surgery based on preoperatively identified disease extent are important for achieving good outcomes.

INTRODUCTION

In 2018, 53,990 new cases of thyroid cancer are expected to be diagnosed in the United States,[1] making it the fifth most common cancer in women and twelfth most common cancer overall. The increasing incidence of thyroid cancer has been well-documented in recent decades, with population-level estimates of new cases cresting

---

Disclosure Statement: The authors have nothing to disclose.
[a] Department of Surgery, Division of Head and Neck, Memorial Sloan Kettering Cancer Center, 1275 York Avenue, Room C-1075, New York, NY 10065, USA; [b] Department of Otolaryngology, Division of Thyroid and Parathyroid Endocrine Surgery, Massachusetts Eye and Ear Infirmary, 243 Charles Street, Boston, MA 02114, USA
* Corresponding author.
E-mail address: Gregory_Randolph@meei.harvard.edu

at 64,300 in 2016.[2] Recent evidence suggests a plateau in the incidence of thyroid cancer,[3,4] which is further supported by decreasing population estimates provided by the American Cancer Society since 2016. The large majority of new cases of thyroid cancer in the United States are due to papillary thyroid cancer (PTC). More than one-half of new cases of thyroid cancer detected today are PTC that are 1.5 cm or less in size.[5] Follicular thyroid carcinoma, medullary thyroid carcinoma, poorly differentiated cancers, and anaplastic thyroid cancers complete the list of other primary thyroid malignancies and seem to be relatively not involved in the increased incidence, which is centered on PTC.

Surgical removal has long been the traditional approach for management of thyroid cancer. In the nineteenth and twentieth centuries, the safety and reliability of surgical extirpation of the thyroid gland was refined and standardized by William Kocher, and popularized in the United States by William S. Halsted. Although active surveillance is a new and reasonable choice for select cases of PTC,[6,7] surgery as the primary treatment modality has stood the test of time. The conventional thyroidectomy procedure remains the most common and preferred management strategy for thyroid carcinoma today with an excellent complication profile, cervical scar acceptance, and surgical outcomes including survival and recurrence.

This article focuses on conventional surgical management of thyroid cancer, reviewing long-standing principles and practices. It also covers newer controversies and techniques, including changes in the indications for thyroidectomy, intraoperative management of the recurrent and superior laryngeal nerves (SLNs) and parathyroid glands, extent of thyroidectomy, and the importance of outcomes measurement and quality improvement. Elsewhere in this issue of *Endocrinology & Metabolism Clinics,* other articles specifically address management of lymph nodes and neck dissection in thyroid cancer, and nonconventional approaches to thyroidectomy, including robotic and other endoscopic approaches.

INDICATIONS

Conventional thyroidectomy related to cancer is usually performed for one of several reasons. These include (a) diagnostic removal of a thyroid lobe for a nodule suspicious for cancer, (b) treatment of a biopsy-proven thyroid cancer, (c) "completion thyroidectomy" after hemithyroidectomy for thyroid cancer, to facilitate the administration of radioactive iodine and otherwise streamline cancer follow-up, (d) treatment of recurrent thyroid cancer, and (e) prophylactic removal of a thyroid gland in a patient with a known genetic mutation predisposing them to the development of thyroid cancer.

Three recent developments have further refined indications for surgery related to thyroid cancer and nodules. These include the updated American Thyroid Association 2015 guidelines for the management of thyroid nodules and cancers, updated Bethesda classification criteria for thyroid fine needle aspiration (FNA) biopsy, and the renaming of some lesions previously called cancer to noninvasive follicular thyroid neoplasm with papillary-like nuclear features (NIFTP).

The new American Thyroid Association 2015 guidelines contained 2 notable changes to recommendations regarding management of thyroid nodules and guidelines[7] (**Table 1**). First, highly suspicious nodules are recommended to have FNA biopsy only if they are greater than 1 cm in size; in other words, any thyroid nodule less than 1 cm in size is not required to undergo biopsy, even if highly suspicious in appearance, as long it is it is centered within the thyroid rather than at the periphery. Second, an active surveillance management approach was endorsed for the first time for select patients.

Table 1 **Notable changes in ATA 2015 guidelines regarding management of thyroid nodules and cancer**	
New ATA 2015 Recommendations	**Text of the Recommendation**
No biopsy of nodules <1 cm	Thyroid nodule diagnostic FNA is recommended for: A. Nodules >1 cm in greatest dimension with high suspicion sonographic pattern B. Nodules >1 cm in greatest dimension with intermediate suspicion sonographic C. Nodules >1.5 cm in greatest dimension with low suspicion sonographic pattern Thyroid nodule diagnostic FNA may be considered for: D. Nodules >2 cm in greatest dimension with very low suspicion sonographic pattern (eg, spongiform). Observation without FNA is also a reasonable option Thyroid nodule diagnostic FNA is not required for: E. Nodules that do not meet the above criteria. F. Nodules that are purely cystic.
Active surveillance endorsed	A cytology diagnostic for a primary thyroid malignancy will almost always lead to thyroid surgery. However, an active surveillance management approach can be considered as an alternative to immediate surgery in: A. Patients with very low risk tumors (eg, papillary microcarcinomas) B. Patients at high surgical risk because of comorbid conditions C. Patients expected to have a relatively short remaining life span D. Patients with concurrent medical or surgical issues that need to be addressed before thyroid surgery.

Abbreviations: ATA, american thyroid association; FNA, fine needle aspiration.

In 2017, the Bethesda classification system for FNA biopsy of thyroid nodules was updated from its original 2009 version, reflecting newer data about the risk of cancer (**Table 2**).[8,9] In addition, the 2017 edition made modifications in the evidence-based usual management recommendations associated with each category. Specifically, the recommendation for Bethesda III nodules (atypia of undetermined significance or follicular lesion of undetermined significance) in 2009 was repeat FNA, whereas in 2017 it is repeat FNA, molecular testing, or lobectomy. The recommendation for Bethesda IV nodules (follicular neoplasm or suspicious for follicular neoplasm) in 2009 was surgical lobectomy, whereas in 2017 it is molecular testing or lobectomy. The recommendation for Bethesda V and VI nodules (suspicious for malignancy; malignant) has always been surgery. In 2017, a lobectomy rather than total thyroidectomy is presented as an option for either category.

In 2016, a new name—NIFTP—for an old clinical thyroid entity was coined by an international group of thyroid pathologists, endocrinologists, and surgeons.[10] Before this, the entity had carcinoma in the name—encapsulated follicular variant of papillary thyroid carcinoma. This group reviewed cases of this entity and found that, compared with cases where the tumor was not encapsulated, there were no deaths, recurrences, or metastases, and that a change in nomenclature was therefore indicated. Notably, the diagnosis of NIFTP cannot be made with certainty without diagnostic surgical lobectomy, and so the renaming of the entity does not significantly change the

Table 2
Bethesda system for reporting thyroid cytopathology, comparing 2009 and 2017 versions

Diagnostic Category	2009 Risk of Malignancy (%)	2017 Risk of Malignancy, if NIFTP ≠ CA (%)	2017 Risk of Malignancy, if NIFTP = CA (%)	2009 Usual Management	2017 Usual Management
I. Nondiagnostic or unsatisfactory	1–4	5–10	5–10	Repeat FNA with ultrasound guidance	Repeat FNA with ultrasound guidance
II. Benign	0–3	0–3	0–3	Clinical follow-up	Clinical and sonographic follow-up
III. Atypia of undetermined significance or follicular lesion of undetermined significance	~5–15	6–18	~10–30	Repeat FNA	Repeat FNA, molecular testing, or lobectomy
IV. Follicular neoplasm or suspicious for a follicular neoplasm	15–30	10–40	25–40	Surgical lobectomy	Molecular testing, lobectomy
V. Suspicious for malignancy	60–75	45–60	50–75	Near-total thyroidectomy or surgical lobectomy	Near-total thyroidectomy or lobectomy
VI. Malignant	97–99	94–96	97–99	Near-total thyroidectomy	Near-total thyroidectomy or lobectomy

Abbreviation: FNA, fine needle aspiration.

indications for surgery. Nonetheless, as noted in **Table 2**, it does change the preoperative risk of cancer based on whether NIFTP is considered cancer, and this may therefore change decision making regarding indications for surgery. The presence of NIFTP, owing to its designation as a noncancer entity, will mainly affect the clinical management with a reduction in the offering of additional management such as completion surgery, T4 suppression, and Radioactive Iodine (RAI) treatment.[11]

PREOPERATIVE EVALUATION

Before undertaking thyroid surgery, it is important to review the indications for surgery, as well as to envision the extent of surgery needed. Careful preoperative evaluation of the patient's history and symptoms, physical examination findings, ultrasound examination or other imaging results, and cytology including molecular diagnostics if performed, are critical to decision making. These factors contribute to decisions about the extent of surgery. A related point of importance is appropriate laryngeal examination to determine preoperative function of the vocal cords, which can influence the extent of surgery, preoperative counseling, and intraoperative considerations.

EXTENT OF SURGERY: HISTORY, PHYSICAL EXAMINATION, IMAGING, AND CYTOLOGY

The extent of surgery is based on a review of all available data contributing to the diagnosis/suspicion of carcinoma, as well as to the extent of the disease. The history should include patient's age and gender (higher risk of malignancy for patients <20 years or >60 years; men have a higher risk), family history of thyroid cancer or familial syndromes predisposing to cancer (familial papillary carcinoma, Cowden syndrome, multiple endocrine neoplasia type 2A or 2B), and a history of ionizing radiation exposure, especially in childhood. The review of symptoms should include a history of rapidly growing thyroid mass, new-onset breathy hoarseness, and the presence of neck masses.

On physical examination, palpation of the thyroid must be performed with attention to the presence of the nodule, including its size, firmness, and fixation to the larynx or overlying skin. Examination of the lateral neck for lymph node metastasis should focus on levels 2 to 4 medial to the sternocleidomastoid muscle. Especially important is laryngoscopy for the presence of vocal cord paralysis (VCP), as discussed elsewhere in this article.

Laboratory findings should be reviewed. Although thyroid-stimulating hormone is typically assessed, thyroglobulin and thyroglobulin antibodies, calcitonin, and carcinoembryonic antigen are typically not offered for the routine thyroid nodule workup. Elevated thyroid-stimulating hormone values are associated with an increased risk of malignancy.

Imaging typically includes ultrasound examination; ultrasound findings such as solid nodule, irregular margins, microcalcifications, central blood flow, and a taller than wider shape also increase the risk of malignancy. Ultrasound features of extrathyroidal extension of a tumor should be noted, as well as findings of lymph nodes suspicious for metastasis, both in the central compartment and trachea–esophageal groove, and in the lateral necks. A computed tomography scan is also recommended, preoperative ultrasound examination, and a computed tomography scan are found to be complimentary especially in the presence of nodal metastasis.[12] The bulk of the nodal disease in PTC is in the central neck, which is not viewed very well by ultrasound examination, specifically in cases where the thyroid gland is still in situ.[12]

FNA cytology results and molecular diagnostics also influence the likelihood of malignancy and extent of planned surgery. Anything less than a Bethesda VI diagnosis of thyroid carcinoma, as long as there are no other concerning findings (VCP, lymph node metastases), usually prompts a diagnostic thyroid lobectomy as the planned extent of surgery. When a preoperative diagnosis of thyroid carcinoma is certain or if there are other concerning findings that may warrant future radioactive iodine administration, the extent of surgery may include total thyroidectomy and appropriate lymph node dissection. Cytopathology and molecular diagnostic considerations are reviewed in more detail elsewhere in this issue.

PREOPERATIVE LARYNGEAL EXAMINATION

Special attention should be paid to examining laryngeal function before undertaking thyroid surgery.[13] This is important for several reasons. (1) VCP may be present without voice changes, and may be an indication of more aggressive malignancy.[14] (2) The presence of VCP influences preoperative counseling about surgical risks. (3) Intraoperative considerations for monitoring and extent of surgery may be influenced by preoperative vocal cord function. (4) Postoperative examination of laryngeal function, both for quality assessment and documenting complications of surgery, requires a preoperative baseline. (5) Also, from a medicolegal standpoint, preoperative vocal cord function documentation can help to avoid false accusation in the setting of iatrogenic VCP.

Several large medical and surgical societies have recently published guidelines and statements on this subject, for both preoperative and postoperative laryngeal examination. The American Head and Neck Society Consensus Statement suggests that preoperative laryngeal examination should be performed on all patients undergoing thyroid surgery who are at high risk for nerve injury (preoperative voice abnormalities, history of cervical or upper chest surgery, thyroid cancer with known posterior extension, or extensive cervical node metastases).[15] The American Academy of Otolaryngology-Head and Neck Surgery recommends preoperative laryngoscopy when the voice is abnormal, if there is preoperative suspicion of malignancy with extrathyroidal extension, or if there is a history of surgery in which the vagus or recurrent laryngeal nerve (RLN) was at risk.[16]

SURGERY FOR THYROID CANCER

Successful completion of thyroid surgery requires careful attention to detail and planned steps based on surgical principles. The surgeon should consider how to manage and monitor the RLN intraoperatively, and should pay particular attention to parathyroid preservation, SLN preservation, and complete surgical extirpation of the carcinoma. Other intraoperative considerations include appropriate use of frozen section to guide decision making as well as the decision to proceed with planned contralateral surgery. At the end of the procedure, a careful documentation of intraoperative surgical findings should be performed. Neck dissection indications and techniques are important for complete management of thyroid cancer and are detailed elsewhere in this issue.

STEPS AND SURGICAL PRINCIPLES

The patient is placed in supine position, with the neck extended and arms tucked and padded at the patient's side. Reverse Trendelenburg (head higher than feet) positioning can decrease venous pressure (**Fig. 1**). Careful communication with the anesthesiologist regarding the type of endotracheal tube and the avoidance of long-lasting paralytic agents when intraoperative nerve monitoring (IONM) is used before induction is important.[17] The neck is prepped and draped widely to include the chin, lateral necks, shoulders, and upper chest. Even in the setting of a small, minimally invasive thyroid surgery, this wide area prepping allows optimal and symmetric positioning of this incision parallel to the normal skin creases in the most optimal position approximately 1 finger breadth below the cricoid cartilage.

The incision for thyroidectomy is best placed in or parallel to a horizontal skin crease for optimal cosmetic result, ideally 1 cm inferior to the cricoid cartilage, overlying the thyroid isthmus (**Fig. 2**). However, modification of the location of the incision may be appropriate to ensure it is in a deep skin crease. Regardless of which thyroid lobe is to be removed, the incision is placed in the midline. Surgeons may differ on the length of the incision, with 4 cm being the usual shortest incision. Longer incisions are certainly appropriate depending on surgeon preference for exposure, because of large tumors, inclusion of the lateral neck dissection, or patient anatomy.

Subplatysmal flaps are raised superiorly and inferiorly, leaving the anterior jugular veins down. The midline raphe between the strap muscles is incised, revealing the thyroid isthmus, cricoid cartilage, and the tissue inferior to the thyroid in the central compartment. Next, the sternohyoid muscle on the initial operative side is lifted away from the thyroid gland to reveal the deeper and slightly more lateral sternothyroid

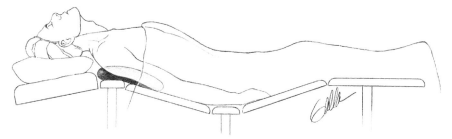

Fig. 1. Reverse Trendelenburg with extended neck position for thyroidectomy. (*From* Randolph GW, editor. Surgery of the thyroid and parathyroid glands. Philadelphia: Saunders; 2013; with permission.)

muscle, which lies directly over the thyroid gland. The sternothyroid muscle inserts on the thyroid cartilage lamina and covers the superior pole of the thyroid gland. Careful dissection of the muscle superiorly off the thyroid gland, or division of the upper head of this muscle, allows exposure for addressing the superior pole vessels and external branch of the spear laryngeal nerve. If the sternothyroid muscle seems to be adherent to the thyroid gland, there may be extrathyroidal extension of the malignancy. In this case, the muscle should be left on the gland and cut at its upper and lower ends to allow the invaded section of muscle to remain en bloc adherent to the thyroid. There should be no hesitation in removing the strap muscles, either to aid in exposure or because of possible malignant infiltration, because this maneuver has no significant impact on function or cosmetic appearance.[18] As dissection proceeds laterally, the thyroid lobe can be pulled and rotated medially, revealing the middle thyroid vein on the anterior lateral surface of the gland, which can be ligated safely at this point (**Fig. 3**).

The next step varies based on the surgeon's preference. Some address the inferior pole and lower parathyroid, whereas some address the superior pole, SLN, and upper parathyroid gland. Others partially mobilize the gland at both the inferior and superior poles before retracting the gland medially to identify the RLN. Regardless of the approach, these next steps should identify and preserve both the superior and inferior parathyroid glands, the SLN, and the RLN.

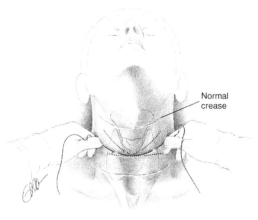

Normal
crease

Fig. 2. The thyroidectomy incision is marked and fashioned symmetrically in the natural skin crease in the neck. (*From* Randolph GW, editor. Surgery of the thyroid and parathyroid glands. Philadelphia: Saunders; 2013; with permission.)

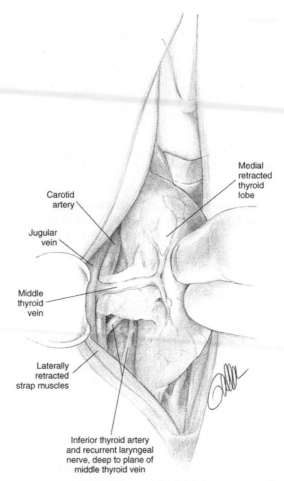

Medial retracted thyroid lobe

Carotid artery

Jugular vein

Middle thyroid vein

Laterally retracted strap muscles

Inferior thyroid artery and recurrent laryngeal nerve, deep to plane of middle thyroid vein

Fig. 3. The thyroid gland is retracted anteriorly and medially, exposing the posterior surface of thyroid gland. This helps in the identification of the middle thyroid vein(s), which is (are) then ligated and divided. (*From* Randolph GW, editor. Surgery of the thyroid and parathyroid glands. Philadelphia: Saunders; 2013; with permission.)

Identification of the parathyroid glands is aided by knowing their likely anatomic locations, and noting their brown-red mottled color, distinct organoid shape, and sharp edge compared with the surrounding fat (**Table 3**) In general, preservation of the parathyroid glands is accomplished by dissecting on the capsule of the thyroid gland.

The parathyroid glands location relate to their embryologic pathway of migration. The superior parathyroids arise from the fourth branchial pouch and lie more posteriorly/deeply in the neck, behind the upper pole of the thyroid gland. They are located within 1 cm of the articulation of the cricoid and thyroid cartilages or 1 cm cranial to the intersection of the inferior thyroid artery and RLN. The inferior parathyroids arise from the third branchial pouch and are located more superficially/anteriorly in the neck (often tracking with the thymus) compared with the superior parathyroids, although their exact position is more variable. Usually, they are located within 1 cm lateral and inferior to the inferior thyroid pole. Occasionally, they will remain

Table 3
Distinguishing characteristics of parathyroid glands

Structure	Color	Firmness	Shape	Discrete Sliding Movement	Vascular Hilum
Parathyroid gland	Tan, brown, salmon	Soft	Elliptical, flat	Yes	Yes
Thyroid	Red	Yes	Varies	No	No
Fat	Bright yellow	No	Amorphous	No	No
Lymph node	White-gray to red	Yes	Spherical to elliptical	+/−	No
Thymus	White-yellow	No	Amorphous	No	No

undescended, or stop in their descent along the pathway between the carotid bifurcation and the lower neck. Pyrtek and Painter[19] have described specific locations of the parathyroid glands relative to the plane in which RLN tracks in the neck. If the course of RLN in the neck is visualized to represent the coronal plane, then the inferior parathyroid glands are found ventral or anterior to the plane and the superior parathyroid glands are found dorsal or posterior to the RLN plane (**Fig. 4**). The SLN can be preserved by meticulous dissection of the upper pole. It is important to retract the upper end of the sternothyroid muscle laterally or to divide the upper end of this muscle for greater visualization, while putting medial traction on the thyroid–larynx complex

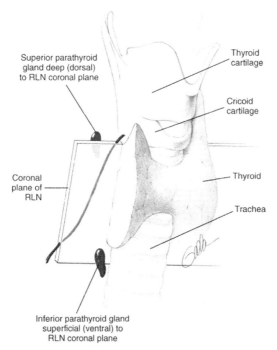

Fig. 4. Respective positions of the superior (dorsal) and inferior (ventral) parathyroid glands relative to the coronal plane represented by the recurrent laryngeal nerve (RLN) course in the neck. (*From* Randolph GW, editor. Surgery of the thyroid and parathyroid glands. Philadelphia: Saunders; 2013; with permission.)

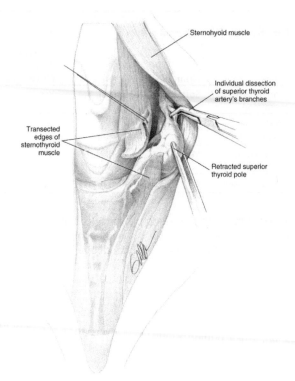

Fig. 5. Sternothyroid muscle transection provides better exposure of the superior pole region, superior thyroid artery's branches are ligated individually. (*From* Randolph GW, editor. Surgery of the thyroid and parathyroid glands. Philadelphia: Saunders; 2013; with permission.)

(**Fig. 5**). The SLN branches from the vagus nerve and runs inferomedially to the larynx, where it divides into an internal branch that penetrates the larynx and an external branch (external branch of the SLN [EBSLN]) that runs superficial to the inferior constrictor muscle and innervates the cricothyroid muscle (**Fig. 6**). In approximately 20% of cases, the EBSLN is vulnerable to surgical injury crossing the superior thyroid artery vessels at or below the level of the superior pole of the thyroid (type 2b).[20] The EBSLN can often be identified visually overlying the cricothyroid muscle or can be identified with electrical stimulation. It should be noted that 20% of EBSLN are subfascial and hence cannot be identified visually, and neuromonitoring can identify 100% of EBSLN resulting in twitching of the cricothyroid muscle.[21] In this way, division of the superior thyroid artery vessels can be safely accomplished.

The RLN can be identified and preserved by knowledge of its anatomy, use of high-yield dissection techniques and by using IONM. IONM is described in a separate section elsewhere in this article. Anatomically, the right RLN branches from the vagus nerve behind the subclavian artery and enters the base of the neck at the thoracic inlet in a more lateral location compared with the left RLN, which branches from the vagus anterior to the aortic arch and wraps posteriorly under the arch. Thus, the right RLN tracks obliquely from the neck base to the laryngeal entry point, assuming a paratracheal position only in the last 1 cm of its course, and the left RLN tracks more vertically from neck base to laryngeal entry point, lying, medially within the tracheoesophageal groove for most of its course in the neck (**Fig. 7**). Posterior to the thyroid gland, at the

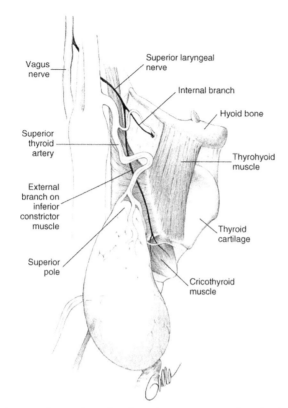

Fig. 6. Superior laryngeal nerve branches from the vagus nerve, then divides into an internal branch that enters the larynx and an external branch that courses superficial to the inferior constrictor muscle to innervate the cricothyroid muscle. (*From* Randolph GW, editor. Surgery of the thyroid and parathyroid glands. Philadelphia: Saunders; 2013; with permission.)

lower edge of the cricoid cartilage, the RLN courses under the lower fibers of the inferior constrictor muscle and behind the cricothyroid articulation, where it enters the larynx. Displacement of RLN by a large goiter, the presence of extralaryngeal RLN branching, and a nonrecurrent RLN can make RLN identification difficult.[22]

Surgeons have different techniques for identifying and preserving this nerve (**Fig. 8**). A lateral approach involves finding the nerve through medial traction of the lobe after mobilization of the inferior and superior poles. In this approach, the nerve can be found near the inferior thyroid artery, crossing either anterior or posterior to it. An inferior approach is best used for revision cases or large goiters, which involves "triangulating" the nerve as described by Loré and colleagues[23]. The advantage of this approach is finding the nerve before it has branched, and usually outside the previously dissected field in cases of previous surgery. The superior approach involves identifying the nerve at its laryngeal entry. The advantage of this approach is that there is less variation in its location, near the inferior cornu of the thyroid cartilage, which can be easily palpated. This method is a reliable way to identify the nerve in difficult cases, revision surgery, or large goiters. A disadvantage of this approach is that the nerve may have branched when identified, putting nonidentified branches at risk, and this area may be vascular around Berry's ligament.

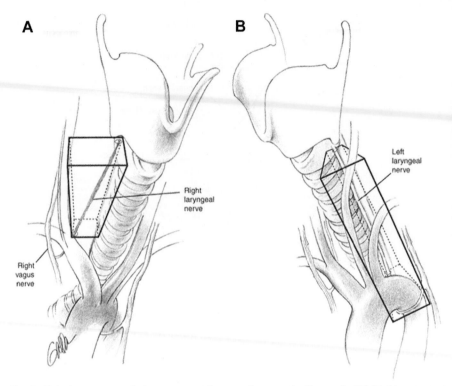

Fig. 7. Relative courses of the recurrent laryngeal nerves in the neck: (A) Right recurrent laryngeal nerve; (B) Left recurrent laryngeal nerve. (*From* Randolph GW, editor. Surgery of the thyroid and parathyroid glands. Philadelphia: Saunders; 2013; with permission.)

After removal of the first thyroid lobe, frozen section may be used, and contralateral lobe dissection may be performed. These issues are addressed in separate sections elsewhere in this article. At the conclusion of surgery, the thyroid specimen should be examined for parathyroid glands on its surface, and they should be autotransplanted if identified and confirmed to be parathyroid gland by frozen section. The parathyroid gland is minced and then placed into the sternocleidomastoid muscle, marking the location with a permanent stitch, and documenting it in the operative report. Hemostasis is confirmed via a Valsalva maneuver, the wound is copiously irrigated, and then closed. Drains are usually not used. During closure, the strap muscles are approximated in the midline to prevent scarring of the skin to the trachea.

INTRAOPERATIVE MONITORING OF THE RECURRENT LARYNGEAL NERVE

The reported incidence of RLN injury and postoperative vocal cord dysfunction varies, the underlying reasons include the variability in identifying temporary and permanent paralysis; the methods, timing and thoroughness of laryngeal evaluation; and differences in reporting between high- and low-volume surgeons and hospitals. Permanent paralysis occurs in approximately 1% to 2% of cases performed by high-volume surgeons.[24]

Although the studies have reported overall lower rates of VCP with IONM, the difference is not statistically significant in these studies.[25] This finding is largely due to

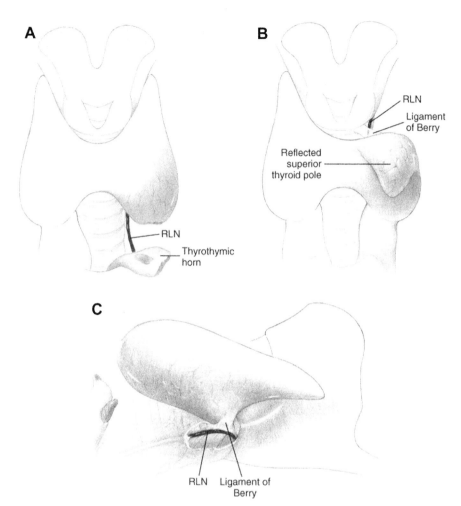

Fig. 8. (*A*) Inferior, (*B*) superior, and (*C*) lateral surgical approaches to the recurrent laryngeal nerve. (*From* Randolph GW, editor. Surgery of the thyroid and parathyroid glands. Philadelphia: Saunders; 2013; with permission.)

inadequate power. Dralle and colleagues[26] have shown that an adequately powered study would need 9 million patients per arm for benign goiter and 40,000 patients per arm for thyroid cancer. Notably, studies have shown that IONM improves rate of postoperative VCP in certain high-risk surgeries such as revision surgeries, surgeries for malignancy, and for large goiters.[27,28] The potential benefits of IONM include neural identification/neural mapping, aid in dissection, and prognostication of postoperative neural function and injury lesion site identification.[22]

The dominant technique for IONM is intermittent monitoring through endotracheal-tube based electrodes. Standardization in IONM application is important, and the systematic application and interpretation of IONM has been detailed in IONM guidelines published by the International Neural Monitoring Study Group.[29] Recent advancements in IONM include continuous neural vagal monitoring (continuous IONM), which decreases the risk of injury to the RLN in between intermittent stimulations and monitoring of the EBSLN, allowing for the identification of all EBSLNs including visually unidentifiable subfascial EBSLN.[30,31]

THE USE OF INTRAOPERATIVE FROZEN SECTION AND CONTRALATERAL SURGERY CONSIDERATIONS

Frozen section analysis of tissue during thyroid surgery may have some benefit, but careful thought and decision making should be used. The usefulness of frozen section is well-established for confirmation of parathyroid tissue (eg, when a devascularized parathyroid gland is being autotransplanted into a muscle). Similarly, frozen section has undoubted usefulness in confirming lymph node metastasis, especially when suspicious lymph nodes are encountered intraoperatively; this technique facilitates decision making regarding the extent of needed lymph node dissection.

The usefulness of frozen section performed on a thyroid lobe for decision making about contralateral lobectomy is debatable. In general, after a thyroid lobe with the index nodule or cancer has been removed, the contralateral lobe may be considered for removal for several reasons: (a) when postoperative radioactive iodine is needed, (b) to facilitate malignancy surveillance with thyroglobulin levels, and (c) when the patient and surgeon have decided to remove contralateral nodularity.

The guideline recommendations for the use of radioactive iodine have changed, leading to fewer indications for contralateral thyroidectomy; in addition, hemithyroidectomy for malignancy is now accepted for low-risk tumors. Because of this change, the need for frozen section analysis and intraoperative decision making about contralateral lobectomy is often negated. Even when intraoperative findings suggest the need for postoperative radioactive iodine treatment, the decision to proceed with contralateral lobectomy is usually made without frozen section of the first removed lobe.

Frozen section for thyroid nodules, rather than cancer, may be of some usefulness, but only in rare scenarios; usually, only a diagnostic hemithyroidectomy is planned in such cases. If there are intraoperative findings of extrathyroidal extension possibly requiring radioactive iodine, confirming malignancy intraoperatively is important before proceeding with contralateral lobectomy. An important caveat is that nodules diagnosed as follicular and Hurthle cell neoplasms on FNA cannot easily be diagnosed as malignant on frozen section, because a careful analysis of capsular and vascular invasion is usually necessary, which requires permanent pathologic analysis. This situation is in contrast with PTC, which can more easily be diagnosed on frozen section.

Safety and the need for contralateral lobectomy must also be considered before proceeding. Specifically, it is important to confirm that contralateral lobectomy is necessary, with indications described elsewhere in this article. Regarding safety, it is important to confirm the intact status of the RLN on the dissected side, because bilateral RLN injury, although rare, may require tracheotomy. Ipsilateral weak RLN may be a reason to defer contralateral lobectomy until the nerve has recovered. In addition, it is important to confirm that the parathyroid glands on the ipsilateral side are intact. If both parathyroid glands were removed or damaged and contralateral lobectomy is not crucial to facilitate radioactive iodine, contralateral thyroidectomy should be deferred.

DOCUMENTING SURGICAL FINDINGS

Careful documentation of surgical findings in the operative report is necessary for many reasons, including communicating the factors related to the risk of recurrence with the endocrinologist, to help make the decisions about radioactive iodine. This documentation also provides relevant findings for future surgical planning if ever needed. Synoptic reporting in electronic records may help to ensure that all appropriate information is collected. This documentation should include nodule/tumor size, location, invasion of structures and extrathyroidal extension, completeness of resection, and location/extent of lymphadenopathy. In addition, the status of the RLN, EBSLN, and parathyroid glands should be documented.

POSTOPERATIVE MANAGEMENT
Calcium Management

If hemithyroidectomy has been performed, the contralateral parathyroids remain undisturbed and there is no risk of hypocalcemia. Total thyroidectomy, however, can cause temporary or permanent hypocalcemia. Surgeons and institutions differ an exact management of this potential complication. On 1 end of the spectrum, some programs perform a preoperative assessment and correction of vitamin D and calcium levels, or provide postoperative prophylactic oral supplementation. On the other end of the spectrum, postoperative serum calcium levels are checked and supplementation with calcium and calcitriol is given only if levels are low or there are symptoms of hypocalcemia. For severe postoperative hypocalcemia, intravenous calcium gluconate may be given in addition to oral supplementation. Most commonly, patients requiring only routine oral supplementation can be weaned within 4 weeks. Permanent hypocalcemia is defined as requiring medications 1 year after surgery, and is a rare complication.

Postoperative Laryngeal Examination

After thyroid surgery, voice changes are not uncommon, and may be related to endotracheal intubation, injury or scar of strap muscles or laryngeal musculature including the cricothyroid muscle, or to RLN or EBSLN injury. It is important to distinguish these causes through laryngeal examination, because their treatment will vary. Specifically, if there is RLN injury, there are additional potential diagnostic and treatment modalities that may be used, which are beyond the scope of this article.

Another important reason to consider routine postoperative laryngeal examination in all patients undergoing thyroid surgery relates to the importance of outcomes assessment and continuous quality improvement. Many patients will not have any symptoms of voice changes postoperatively, but careful examination may reveal some dysfunction in vocal cord mobility. It behooves the surgeon to learn this information to consider adjustments to surgical technique in future cases.

OUTCOMES MEASUREMENT AND IMPROVEMENT

As surgeons progress through their careers, they should undertake continuous learning and improvement in technique to drive better outcomes for their patients. This learning is not possible without objective and ongoing scrutiny of their outcomes. Perioperative quality assessment is now in place at many institutions, guided by regulatory requirements and an evolving culture of quality measurement and improvement. In addition to institutional or practice-specific data collection, there are ongoing efforts to establish national or regional registries of quality data, to have benchmarks for performance comparison. Today, some registries in Europe are widely accepted, including those maintained by the British Association of Endocrine and Thyroid Surgeons and the Scandinavian Quality Register for Thyroid and Parathyroid Surgery. In the United States, quality registries specifically addressing quality issues in thyroid surgery are not widely used, but are likely to be more commonly used in the future.

REFERENCES

1. American Cancer Society. Cancer facts & figures 2018. Atlanta (GA): American Cancer Society; 2018.
2. American Cancer Society. Cancer facts & figures 2016. Atlanta (GA): American Cancer Society; 2016.
3. Shi LL, DeSantis C, Jemal A, et al. Changes in thyroid cancer incidence, post-2009 American Thyroid Association guidelines. Laryngoscope 2017;127(10):2437–41.
4. Roman BR, Morris LG, Davies L. The thyroid cancer epidemic, 2017 perspective. Curr Opin Endocrinol Diabetes Obes 2017;24(5):332–6.
5. Davies L, Welch HG. Current thyroid cancer trends in the United States. JAMA Otolaryngol Head Neck Surg 2014;140(4):317–22.
6. Tuttle RM, Fagin JA, Minkowitz G, et al. Natural history and tumor volume kinetics of papillary thyroid cancers during active surveillance. JAMA Otolaryngol Head Neck Surg 2017;143(10):1015–20.
7. Haugen BR, Alexander EK, Bible KC, et al. 2015 American Thyroid Association management guidelines for adult patients with thyroid nodules and differentiated thyroid cancer: the American Thyroid Association guidelines task force on thyroid nodules and differentiated thyroid cancer. Thyroid 2016;26(1):1–133.
8. Cibas ES, Ali SZ. The Bethesda system for reporting thyroid cytopathology. Thyroid 2009;19(11):1159–65.
9. Cibas ES, Ali SZ. The 2017 Bethesda system for reporting thyroid cytopathology. Thyroid 2017;27(11):1341–6.
10. Nikiforov YE, Seethala RR, Tallini G, et al. Nomenclature revision for encapsulated follicular variant of papillary thyroid carcinoma: a paradigm shift to reduce over-treatment of indolent tumors. JAMA Oncol 2016;2(8):1023–9.
11. Ferris RL, Nikiforov Y. AHNS series: do you know your guidelines? AHNS endocrine section consensus statement: state-of-the-art thyroid surgical recommendations in the era of noninvasive follicular thyroid neoplasm with papillary-like nuclear features. Head Neck 2018;40(9):1881–8.
12. Lesnik D, Cunnane ME, Zurakowski D, et al. Papillary thyroid carcinoma nodal surgery directed by a preoperative radiographic map utilizing CT scan and ultrasound in all primary and reoperative patients. Head Neck 2014;36(2):191–202.
13. Randolph GW. The importance of pre- and postoperative laryngeal examination for thyroid surgery. Thyroid 2010;20(5):453–8.
14. Randolph GW, Kamani D. The importance of preoperative laryngoscopy in patients undergoing thyroidectomy: voice, vocal cord function, and the preoperative detection of invasive thyroid malignancy. Surgery 2006;139(3):357–62.
15. Sinclair CF, Bumpous JM, Haugen BR, et al. Laryngeal examination in thyroid and parathyroid surgery: an American Head and Neck Society consensus statement: AHNS consensus statement. Head Neck 2016;38(6):811–9.
16. Chandrasekhar SS, Randolph GW, Seidman MD, et al. Clinical practice guideline: improving voice outcomes after thyroid surgery. Otolaryngol Head Neck Surg 2013;148(6 Suppl):S1–37.
17. Macias AA, Eappen S, Malikin I, et al. Successful intraoperative electrophysiologic monitoring of the recurrent laryngeal nerve, a multidisciplinary approach: the Massachusetts Eye and Ear Infirmary monitoring collaborative protocol with experience in over 3000 cases. Head Neck 2016;38(10):1487–94.
18. Phillips DE, Charters P. Strap muscles in thyroid surgery: to cut or not to cut? Ann R Coll Surg Engl 1993;75(5):378.

19. Pyrtek L, Painter RL. An anatomic study of the relationship of the parathyroid glands to the recurrent laryngeal nerve. Surg Gynecol Obstet 1964;119:509–12.
20. Cernea CR, Ferraz AR, Nishio S, et al. Surgical anatomy of the external branch of the superior laryngeal nerve. Head Neck 1992;14(5):380–3.
21. Darr EA, Tufano RP, Ozdemir S, et al. Superior laryngeal nerve quantitative intraoperative monitoring is possible in all thyroid surgeries. Laryngoscope 2014;124(4):1035–41.
22. Randolph GW, editor. Surgery of the thyroid and parathyroid glands. 1st edition. Philadelphia: Saunders-Elsevier Science; 2003.
23. Loré JM Jr, Kim DJ, Elias S. Preservation of the laryngeal nerves during total thyroid lobectomy. Ann Otol Rhinol Laryngol 1977;86(6 Pt 1):777–88.
24. Eisele D. Complication of thyroid surgery. In: Eisele D, editor. Complications in head and neck surgery. St Louis (MO): Mosby; 1993. p. 493–516.
25. Higgins TS, Gupta R, Ketcham AS, et al. Recurrent laryngeal nerve monitoring versus identification alone on post-thyroidectomy true vocal fold palsy: a meta-analysis. Laryngoscope 2011;121(5):1009–17.
26. Dralle H, Sekulla C, Haerting J, et al. Risk factors of paralysis and functional outcome after recurrent laryngeal nerve monitoring in thyroid surgery. Surgery 2004;136(6):1310–22.
27. Randolph GW, Shin JJ, Grillo HC, et al. The surgical management of goiter: part II. Surgical treatment and results. Laryngoscope 2011;121(1):68–76.
28. Chan WF, Lang BH, Lo CY. The role of intraoperative neuromonitoring of recurrent laryngeal nerve during thyroidectomy: a comparative study on 1000 nerves at risk. Surgery 2006;140(6):866–72 [discussion: 872–3].
29. Randolph GW, Dralle H, Abdullah H, et al. Electrophysiologic recurrent laryngeal nerve monitoring during thyroid and parathyroid surgery: international standards guideline statement. Laryngoscope 2011;121(Suppl 1):S1–16.
30. Phelan E, Schneider R, Lorenz K, et al. Continuous vagal IONM prevents recurrent laryngeal nerve paralysis by revealing initial EMG changes of impending neuropraxic injury: a prospective, multicenter study. Laryngoscope 2014;124(6):1498–505.
31. Barczynski M, Randolph GW, Cernea CR, et al. External branch of the superior laryngeal nerve monitoring during thyroid and parathyroid surgery: International Neural Monitoring Study Group standards guideline statement. Laryngoscope 2013;123(Suppl 4):S1–14.

Neck Dissection in the Surgical Treatment of Thyroid Cancer

Ahmad M. Eltelety, MBBCh, MSc, MD-PhD, MRCS(ENT)[a,b],
David J. Terris, MD[c,*]

KEYWORDS

- Thyroidectomy • Neck dissection • Lymph node • Metastasis • Thyroid cancer

KEY POINTS

- The incidence of thyroid cancer is increasing owing to the prevalence of imaging, especially high-resolution ultrasound examination of the neck.
- Papillary thyroid cancer is the most common thyroid malignancy.
- Thyroid cancer is commonly found to have regional cervical neck metastasis.
- The management of the neck has long been a topic of considerable debate.
- Adherence to the most up-to-date and evidence-based practices leads to optimal patient outcomes.

INTRODUCTION

The continued growth of radiographic diagnostic modalities has led to a tremendous increase in the number of patients diagnosed with thyroid nodules.[1] Most of these are smaller than 1 cm and they are usually asymptomatic. This overdetection coupled with widely available ultrasound-guided fine needle aspiration has resulted in a surge in the diagnosis of what is now known as papillary thyroid microcarcinoma. Approximately 64,300 patients were diagnosed with thyroid cancer in the United States in 2016.[2] Papillary thyroid cancer (PTC) is by far the commonest thyroid malignant neoplasm, representing at least 75% of this population.[3] It has a very high tendency to metastasize to the regional cervical lymph nodes. There is significant variability in the reported incidence of regional neck disease associated with PTC, ranging between 30% and

[a] Endocrine Head and Neck Surgery, Otolaryngology Department, Medical College of Georgia, Augusta University, 1120 Fifteenth Street, DP-4109, Augusta, GA 30912-4060, USA; [b] Otolaryngology Department, Cairo University, ElManial, Cairo 11562, Arab Republic of Egypt; [c] Otolaryngology Department, Augusta University, Thyroid and Parathyroid Center, 1120 Fifteenth Street, BP-4109, Augusta, GA 30912-4060, USA
* Corresponding author.
E-mail address: dterris@augusta.edu

Endocrinol Metab Clin N Am 48 (2019) 143–151
https://doi.org/10.1016/j.ecl.2018.11.004
0889-8529/19/© 2018 Elsevier Inc. All rights reserved.

80%. Despite this fact, the prognosis of well-differentiated thyroid cancer is usually excellent, with long-term survival rates exceeding 90%.[4]

DECISION MAKING
Central Neck Dissection

Prophylactic

Prophylactic central neck dissection (CND) implies the removal of the lymph nodes of the central neck compartment in the absence of preoperative clinical or radiologic or intraoperative evidence of pathologic lymphadenopathy.[5] Despite earlier recommendations favoring this approach, the most recent American Thyroid Association guidelines (2015) advocate against the routine practice of prophylactic CND in small PTC tumors (T1 and T2). Although prophylactic CND may be acceptable in patients with large tumors (T3 and T4), the reality is that occult nodal disease is unlikely to be a driver of the clinical outcome of patients with advanced primary disease.[6] Importantly, none of these recommendations are based on a grade A level of evidence.

It is notable that even microcarcinomas (<1 cm) have a high incidence of regional microscopic lymph nodes metastasis, yet this rarely affect the long-term patient outcome and prognosis.[7–9] Furthermore, there is no evidence from United States-based institutions that prophylactic CND confers an impact on survival. Historically, the Japanese have approached the central neck compartment more aggressively and have been in favor of prophylactic CND based on limited evidence of better outcomes.[10 11] However, the most recent trend—even in that country—has been for less aggressive surgery, and even no surgery at all (active surveillance).[15]

The movement 15 years ago toward aggressive initial primary and nodal surgical management in a quest to minimize the likelihood of recurrence has given way to multiple reports confirming the safety of reoperative central neck nodal surgery in experienced hands.[16–18] Therefore, we need not subject a large majority of patients (who would otherwise never manifest with neck disease) to an operation that increases the risks of recurrent nerve injury and especially parathyroid (PTH) gland injury.[19–26]

Medullary thyroid carcinoma (MTC) is more likely to present at a later stage and, therefore, a clinically negative neck (cN0) is less common. The surgical management is considerably more aggressive and includes elective removal of the central compartment nodes even if they are cN0.[27,28]

Therapeutic

Therapeutic CND implies the removal of lymph nodes that are deemed to be pathologic either by preoperative clinical examination, radiologic evaluation, or intraoperative inspection and palpation.[5] There is consensus that any pathologic lymph nodes in the central compartment should be addressed by surgical removal. The practice of only removing the grossly visible lymph node (so-called berry picking) is no longer endorsed. Compartment-oriented surgery leads to better survival outcomes and reduced recurrence rates.[5,29,30] The principal consideration while performing a therapeutic CND is whether to do a unilateral or bilateral surgery. A proposed classification system for the extent of CND was adopted by Carty and colleagues,[5] which clarifies the nodal basins that constitute a dissection and allows for either a unilateral or bilateral paratracheal lymph node dissection. The surgeon should describe in detail the type of neck dissection, the laterality, and the excised nodal basins.

Therapeutic CND is generally performed in the same setting as the total thyroidectomy (TT). Unilateral CND is preferred to bilateral CND if the disease is limited to one paratracheal nodal basin. This helps reduce the incidence of postoperative hypocalcemia (transient or permanent) and reduces the risk for bilateral recurrent laryngeal nerve (RLN) injury with potential respiratory compromise. Bilateral CND is oncologically appropriate when there is gross involvement of both paratracheal areas, because in this case the benefit of operating on both sides outweighs the risks of surgical complications. The benefit of therapeutic CND is based mainly on reducing the incidence of disease recurrence, thereby avoiding the morbidity that may accompany revision surgical procedures. There is evidence to suggest prolonged patient survival.[30–32]

Lateral Neck Dissection

Prophylactic

It is generally accepted that there is no role for prophylactic lateral neck dissection (LND) in the management of PTC. Although 25% of patients who have clinically negative neck nodes (cN0) have microscopic disease in the lateral nodal chains, these metastases rarely present clinically if all grossly visible disease is addressed properly. Consequently, there is no evidence that elective neck dissection of the lateral nodes confers any improvement in prognosis and outcome, and the morbidity of prophylactic LND surpasses the benefits even in experienced hands.

There is some degree of controversy when dealing with medullary thyroid cancer. There are 3 principal strategies for managing the clinically negative lateral nodal basins in patients with MTC. For patients who do not have lateral neck metastasis, 1 report confirms that there is no statistical difference between patients who were managed by observation of their lateral nodes and those who underwent elective LND.[33] Others have adopted a more proactive approach when dealing with the same group of patients; for example, de Groot and colleagues[34] advocate managing the neck with central, bilateral lateral, and upper mediastinal dissections to decrease the risk of locoregional recurrence. A cautious approach is recommended by the American Thyroid Association. Patients with MTC and no evidence of regional or systemic metastasis should undergo TT and CND without the need for LND. The presence of clinically evident nodal disease in the central compartment—but not the lateral compartment—does not warrant prophylactic LND, even though a minority of the Task Force favored prophylactic LND at this stage. To resolve this conflict, it was agreed that patients with familial MTC and high levels of calcitonin or with a palpable thyroid nodule should be managed by TT, CND, and bilateral prophylactic LND. Patients with sporadic MTC greater than 2 cm and central neck disease may be managed with TT, CND, and ipsilateral prophylactic LND.[27]

Therapeutic

Therapeutic LND is the recommended approach for patients known to have PTC and grossly identifiable lateral neck disease. In this case, surgery generally includes removal of levels IIa, III, IV, and Vb, based on the usual pattern of lymphatic spread for PTC. Superior pole lesions tend to spread to level II nodes, whereas cancers in the remaining parts of the gland tend to metastasize to levels III and IV. Involvement of levels IIb and Va are as low as 6% and 11%, respectively. Elective dissection of level Vb is indicated because there is a high risk of level Vb involvement with large and advanced primary tumors (T4 and tumors >4 cm) and in the presence of positive level IV nodes.[35,36]

It is notable that the presence of nodal disease independently affects survival for patients who are older than 45 years. Patients younger than 45 years may also have higher mortality risk when compared with those who do not have nodal disease; these patients are considered to be in the intermediate and high-risk groups.[6,13,31,37] Because patients with lateral neck disease are at higher risk for mortality, most of them are offered radioactive iodine (RAI) postoperatively and therefore TT is coupled with the LND.[38]

Morbidity resulting from LND is low and the procedure can be performed safely when done for appropriately indicated lateral neck disease.[39] Nodal invasion of the sternocleidomastoid (SCM) or the neurovascular structures adjacent to the lateral distribution of lymph nodes is rare. More conservative procedures like berry picking are associated with a high rate of recurrence.[40] Although the pattern of lymphatic spread for PTC is from medial to lateral, skip metastasis to the lateral compartment does occur in a significant portion of patients. Therefore, an elective CND need not be performed in patients with lateral neck disease in the absence of clinical or radiologic evidence of involvement.[41] If LND is to be performed for regional recurrence after TT and RAI, multiple nodal involvement is expected and so comprehensive neck dissection is warranted to minimize the risk of residual or recurrent disease.[42]

Patients with MTC who have palpable cervical lymphadenopathy have a 47% incidence of contralateral lymphadenopathy. For this reason, these patients may elect to undergo bilateral LND in an effort to decrease the risk of locoregional recurrence.[27]

KEY TECHNICAL ASPECTS

A comprehensive description of the performance of neck dissections is beyond the scope of this monograph, and the reader is referred to other excellent materials for this purpose.[43–45] Rather, the pertinent considerations and key steps are shared here based on evidence and experience.

Central Compartment Surgery

CND is generally performed after TT. The dissection starts with removal of the prelaryngeal lymph nodes superiorly and extends inferiorly to the pretracheal lymph nodes to the level of the innominate artery. Paratracheal lymph node dissection usually starts superiorly at the level of the cricoid cartilage and continues inferiorly to the innominate artery on the right and the intersection between the innominate artery and the trachea on the left. Importantly, paratracheal lymph nodes on the right side are located posterior to the RLN, related to its more oblique course in the central neck, and may be present posterior to the carotid artery on both sides. The RLNs should be dissected fully with the least amount of traction possible. Although efforts to maintain the PTH glands in situ should be exercised, the reality is that it is difficult to accomplish a thorough CND while also preserving the blood supply to the inferior PTH glands. Because nodal metastasis predicts nodal recurrence, there should be a low threshold for autografting at least 1 inferior PTH gland into a muscle away from the oncologic field in anticipation of the need for future surgeries. The superior PTH gland (especially on the side contralateral to the cancer) can usually be preserved in situ.[22,46] Hypoparathyroidism and consequent hypocalcemia is a recognized complication of TT (between 6.4% and 21.6% during primary surgery and even higher in revision cases when scarring and fibrosis make it more difficult to identify and preserve the PTH glands); however, the concurrent performance of CND with TT leads to an increase in this incidence. The specimen should be thoroughly examined before being removed from the sterile field for any PTH tissue that will then be amenable to autotransplantation. Postoperative management is focused on the prophylactic treatment of hypocalcemia for 3 weeks without the need for laboratory assessment.[47]

Lateral Compartment Surgery

The LND begins with subplatysmal flap elevation, which is no longer needed for a simple thyroidectomy. The deep investing fascia is incised over the SCM and represents the lateral border of the dissection. The superior border is the submandibular gland

and digastric tendon. The inferior limit of dissection is the clavicle. Lymph node-bearing fat is removed from the area lateral to the lateral border of the sternohyoid and medial to the posterior border of the SCM, with special attention to skeletonizing the internal jugular vein. The spinal accessory nerve should be identified and protected. The specimen is delivered from the posterior level Vb to the anterior neck triangle deep to the SCM and may be removed in 1 or sometimes 2 specimens.[40]

The levels of the neck are marked on the specimen with a corresponding number of skin staples to facilitate assessment by pathology.

REVISION SURGERY

Rising thyroglobulin levels (in the absence of thyroglobulin antibodies) coupled with structurally identifiable disease (usually seen on ultrasound examination) warrants fine needle aspiration. If malignancy is confirmed, then revision surgery may be considered. Needle washout for thyroglobulin may be useful to confirm metastatic PTC, especially in the lateral neck.[17] Review of the previous operative notes and pathology reports may be of benefit in planning the reoperative surgery. Particular points of interest are the functional status of the RLNs, the integrity of the PTH glands, completeness of resection of disease, and the occurrence of any complications.[16]

For central compartment reoperation, the lateral back door approach may be helpful in avoiding scarring from the prior surgery. Dissection may be done in the potential space medial to the SCM and lateral to the strap muscles or between the sternohyoid and sternothyroid strap muscles. Efforts should be made to identify the RLN in the tracheoesophageal groove or just before its entrance into the larynx. The strap muscles may be excised if needed for expediency or if they are adherent to the tumor.

The use of a laryngeal nerve monitor is advisable in the reoperative setting; however, it should not replace the anatomic identification of the nerve. There are 2 locations where the RLN is commonly identified in revision surgery. Superiorly at the lower border of the inferior constrictor muscle is the most distal point at which the nerve can be seen. Identification of the nerve at this area is preferable if there is extensive recurrence or fibrosis in the lower surgical field or the superior mediastinum. By contrast, if identification of the nerve superiorly proves to be difficult for the same reasons, the nerve can be identified low in the surgical field at the thoracic inlet, and below the region of the prior dissection. Importantly, scar tissue may cause the nerve to assume an abnormal location at the anterior wall of the trachea. In this case, the nerve can be easily injured at this position so in revision surgery care should be taken before proceeding to dissection at the anterior tracheal wall.[48]

If the recurrence is found in the lateral nodal basin, a selective compartmental dissection is usually performed. Well-differentiated thyroid cancer rarely metastasizes to level I nodes and there is no need to perform any dissection in this area in most of the cases. As with primary surgery, the dissection should therefore include removal of levels IIa, III, IV, and Vb if possible. Compartment-oriented surgery is recommended to decrease the incidence of additional recurrences with their associated morbidity.[29] In very rare circumstances, sternal split (either partial or complete) in conjunction with a thoracic surgeon may be needed if there is meaningful involvement of the superior mediastinum.

COMPLICATIONS: PREVENTION AND MANAGEMENT
Chyle Fistula

Chyle fistula (also called chyle leak) is a risk with neck dissection and is particularly common in the setting of left-sided PTC level IV metastasis (which is often matted directly in the region where the thoracic duct empties into the internal jugular vein). Initial treatment is usually conservative with a low-fat diet, total parenteral nutrition, and a compression bandage. This method is sufficient in most of the low-volume output cases. Failure of conservative management (and especially when the daily output exceeds 500 mL, causing a risk of electrolyte depletion) may trigger the need for more aggressive intervention including reoperation with ligation of the thoracic duct, negative pressure wound therapy, and the use of somatostatin analog therapy, which has been associated with varying degrees of success.[49–51]

Spinal Accessory Nerve Syndrome

Shoulder dysfunction is a common complication after LND even when the accessary nerve is able to be preserved. The reported incidence ranges between 30% and 40% for patients undergoing LND with preservation of the XIth nerve, and it has various clinical presentations. The patient usually reports shoulder drop, a constant dull ache, a decreased range of motion in lateral abduction, and joint stiffness. The fact that this syndrome may occur despite the structural preservation of the nerve has led to the conclusion that other factors may be contributing to the condition. Proposed etiologies are cervical plexus injury and temporary dysfunction of the shoulder girdle muscles. Immobility may eventually result in joint stiffness and adhesive capsulitis. Early rehabilitation and physiotherapy with passive motion of the shoulder can decrease the postoperative shoulder symptoms. Low-dose botulinum toxin injection in the distribution of the nerve was proved to be effective in managing the condition in some patients with minimal side effects.[52,53]

Major Vascular Injury

Although uncommon, major vascular injuries are among the fatal complications that should be considered in every patient undergoing neck dissection. The first priority remains the airway, then breathing, and finally the circulation. Fluid resuscitation, preferably by activating the massive transfusion protocol, and O-negative blood transfusion may be needed. The immediate steps needed in the event of an injured vessel include proximal control, distal control, flow restoration as early as possible, and consideration of a temporary vascular shunt if necessary. Definitive treatment options include ligation, repair, and bypass. A vascular surgeon may be needed, depending on the circumstances. Interventional procedures are gaining popularity and stenting of partially injured or threatened vessels may be appropriate. A collaborative effort offers the patient the best chances for a successful outcome.[54]

SUMMARY

Neck dissection is sometimes necessary in the surgical treatment of thyroid cancer. CND is now rarely performed prophylactically, but is essential if the patient has clinical or radiologic evidence of central compartment disease. Its performance may increase the incidence of hypoparathyroidism and, therefore, hypocalcemia. LND should be performed by experienced surgeons and compartment-oriented dissection is advocated to achieve optimal oncologic results.

REFERENCES

1. Jemal A, Siegel R, Ward E, et al. Cancer statistics, 2010. CA Cancer J Clin 2010; 60(5):277–300.
2. Siegel RL, Miller KD, Jemal A. Cancer statistics. CA Cancer J Clin 2016;66(1): 7–30.

3. Sherman SI. Thyroid carcinoma. Lancet 2003;361(9356):501–11.
4. Ort S, Goldenberg D. Management of regional metastases in well-differentiated thyroid cancer. Otolaryngol Clin North Am 2008;41(6):1207–18.
5. Carty SE, Cooper DS, Doherty GM, et al. Consensus statement on the terminology and classification of central neck dissection for thyroid cancer. Thyroid 2009;19(11):1153–9.
6. Haugen BR, Alexander EK, Bible KC, et al. 2015 American Thyroid Association management guidelines for adult patients with thyroid nodules and differentiated thyroid cancer: the American Thyroid Association guidelines task force on thyroid nodules and differentiated thyroid cancer. Thyroid 2016;26(1):1–133.
7. Trivizki O, Amit M, Fliss DM, et al. Elective central compartment neck dissection in patients with papillary thyroid carcinoma recurrence. Laryngoscope 2013;123(6): 1564–8.
8. De Carvalho AY, Chulam TC, Kowalski LP. Long-term results of observation vs prophylactic selective level VI neck dissection for papillary thyroid carcinoma at a cancer center. JAMA Otolaryngol Head Neck Surg 2015;141(7):599–606.
9. Shah MD, Hall FT, Eski SJ, et al. Clinical course of thyroid carcinoma after neck dissection. Laryngoscope 2003;113(12):2102–7.
10. Dubernard X, Dabakuyo S, Ouedraogo S, et al. Prophylactic neck dissection for low-risk differentiated thyroid cancers: risk-benefit analysis. Head Neck 2016; 38(7):1091–6.
11. Pitoia F, Ward L, Wohllk N, et al. Recommendations of the Latin American Thyroid Society on diagnosis and management of differentiated thyroid cancer. Arq Bras Endocrinol Metabol 2009;53(7):884–7.
12. Perros P, Colley S, Boelaert K, et al. Guidelines for the management of thyroid cancer. Clin Endocrinol (Oxf) 2014;81(s1):1–122.
13. Pacini F, Schlumberger M, Dralle H, et al. European consensus for the management of patients with differentiated thyroid carcinoma of the follicular epithelium. Eur J Endocrinol 2006;154(6):787–803.
14. Takami H, Ito Y, Okamoto T, et al. Therapeutic strategy for differentiated thyroid carcinoma in japan based on a newly established guideline managed by Japanese society of thyroid surgeons and Japanese association of endocrine surgeons. World J Surg 2011;35(1):111–21.
15. Oda H, Miyauchi A, Ito Y, et al. Incidences of unfavorable events in the management of low-risk papillary microcarcinoma of the thyroid by active surveillance versus immediate surgery. Thyroid 2016;26(1):150–5.
16. Pai SI, Tufano RP. Reoperation for recurrent/persistent well-differentiated thyroid cancer. Otolaryngol Clin North Am 2010;43(2):353–63.
17. Scharpf J, Tuttle M, Wong R, et al. Comprehensive management of recurrent thyroid cancer: an American Head and Neck Society Consensus Statement. Head Neck 2016;38(12):1862–9.
18. Clayman GL, Agarwal G, Edeiken BS, et al. Long-term outcome of comprehensive central compartment dissection in patients with recurrent/persistent papillary thyroid carcinoma. Thyroid 2011;21(12):1309–16.
19. Grant CS, Stulak JM, Thompson GB, et al. Risks and adequacy of an optimized surgical approach to the primary surgical management of papillary thyroid carcinoma treated during 1999-2006. World J Surg 2010;34(6):1239–46.
20. Kutler DI, Crummey AD, Kuhel WI. Routine central compartment lymph node dissection for patients with papillary thyroid carcinoma. Head Neck 2012;34(2): 260–3.

21. Roh JL, Park JY, Park C II. Total thyroidectomy plus neck dissection in differentiated papillary thyroid carcinoma patients: pattern of nodal metastasis, morbidity, recurrence, and postoperative levels of serum parathyroid hormone. Ann Surg 2007;245(4):604–10.
22. Cavicchi O, Piccin O, Caliceti U, et al. Transient hypoparathyroidism following thyroidectomy: a prospective study and multivariate analysis of 604 consecutive patients. Otolaryngol Head Neck Surg 2007;137(4):654–8.
23. Lee YS, Kim SW, Kim SW, et al. Extent of routine central lymph node dissection with small papillary thyroid carcinoma. World J Surg 2007;31(10):1954–9.
24. Torlontano M, Crocetti U, Augello G, et al. Comparative evaluation of recombinant human thyrotropin-stimulated thyroglobulin levels, 131I whole-body scintigraphy, and neck ultrasonography in the follow-up of patients with papillary thyroid microcarcinoma who have not undergone radioiodine therapy. J Clin Endocrinol Metab 2006;91(1):60–3.
25. Pacini F, Molinaro E, Castagna MG, et al. Recombinant human thyrotropin-stimulated serum thyroglobulin combined with neck ultrasonography has the highest sensitivity in monitoring differentiated thyroid carcinoma. J Clin Endocrinol Metab 2003;88(8):3668–73.
26. Bonnet S, Hartl D, Leboulleux S, et al. Prophylactic lymph node dissection for papillary thyroid cancer less than 2 cm: implications for radioiodine treatment. J Clin Endocrinol Metab 2009;94(4):1162–7.
27. Dackiw APB. The surgical management of medullary thyroid cancer. Otolaryngol Clin North Am 2010;43(2):305–74.
28. Liao S, Shindo M. Management of well-differentiated thyroid cancer. Otolaryngol Clin North Am 2012;45(5):1163–79.
29. Shaha AR. Revision thyroid surgery - technical considerations. Otolaryngol Clin North Am 2008;41(6):1169–83.
30. Agrawal N, Evasovich MR, Kandil E, et al. Indications and extent of central neck dissection for papillary thyroid cancer: an American Head and Neck Society Consensus Statement. Head Neck 2017;39(7):1269–79.
31. Zaydfudim V, Feurer ID, Griffin MR, et al. The impact of lymph node involvement on survival in patients with papillary and follicular thyroid carcinoma. Surgery 2008;144(6):1070–8.
32. Yd P, Smith D, Ld W, et al. The implication of lymph node metastasis on survival in patients with well-differentiated thyroid cancer. Am Surg 2005;71(9):731–5.
33. Pena I, Clayman GL, Grubbs EG, et al. Management of the lateral neck compartment in patients with sporadic medullary thyroid cancer. Head Neck 2018;40(1):79–85.
34. de Groot JWB, Links TP, Sluiter WJ, et al. Locoregional control in patients with palpable medullary thyroid cancer: results of standardized compartment-oriented surgery. Head Neck 2007;29(9):857–63.
35. Lombardi D, Paderno A, Giordano D, et al. Therapeutic lateral neck dissection in well-differentiated thyroid cancer: analysis on factors predicting distribution of positive nodes and prognosis. Head Neck 2018;40(2):242–50.
36. Khafif A, Medina JE, Robbins KT, et al. Level V in therapeutic neck dissections for papillary thyroid carcinoma. Head Neck 2013;35(4):605–7.
37. Adam MA, Pura J, Goffredo P, et al. Presence and number of lymph node metastases are associated with compromised survival for patients younger than age 45 years with papillary thyroid cancer. J Clin Oncol 2015;33(21):2370–5.
38. Nixon IJ, Shaha AR, Patel SG. Surgical diagnosis. Frozen section and the extent of surgery. Otolaryngol Clin North Am 2014;47(4):519–28.

39. Kupferman ME, Patterson DM, Mandel SJ, et al. Safety of modified radical neck dissection for differentiated thyroid carcinoma. Laryngoscope 2004;114(3): 403–6.
40. Schoppy DW, Holsinger FC. Management of the neck in thyroid cancer. Otolaryngol Clin North Am 2014;47(4):545–56.
41. Fritze D, Doherty GM. Surgical management of cervical lymph nodes in differentiated thyroid cancer. Otolaryngol Clin North Am 2010;43(2):285–300.
42. Wu G, Fraser S, Pai S, et al. Determining the extent of lateral neck dissection necessary to establish regional disease control and avoid reoperation after previous total thyroidectomy and radioactive iodine for papillary thyroid cancer. Head Neck 2012;34(10):1418–21.
43. Walsh NJ, Talukder AM, Terris DJ. Central neck dissection: the five key steps. VideoEndocrinology 2018;5(3).
44. Hughes DT, Doherty GM. Central neck dissection for papillary thyroid cancer. Cancer Control 2011;18(2):83–8.
45. Uchino S, Noguchi S, Yamashita H, et al. Modified radical neck dissection for differentiated thyroid cancer: operative technique. World J Surg 2004;28(12): 1199–203.
46. Ondik MP, McGinn J, Ruggiero F, et al. Unintentional parathyroidectomy and hypoparathyroidism in secondary central compartment surgery for thyroid cancer. Head Neck 2010;32(4):462–6.
47. Singer MC, Bhakta D, Seybt MW, et al. Calcium management after thyroidectomy: a simple and cost-effective method. Otolaryngol Head Neck Surg 2012;146(3): 362–5.
48. Richer SL, Wenig RL. Changes in surgical anatomy following thyroidectomy. Otolaryngol Clin North Am 2008;41(6):1069–78.
49. Kadota H, Kakiuchi Y, Yoshida T. Management of chylous fistula after neck dissection using negative-pressure wound therapy: a preliminary report. Laryngoscope 2012;122(5):997–9.
50. Valentine CN, Barresi R, Prinz RA. Somatostatin analog treatment of a cervical thoracic duct fistula. Head Neck 2002;24(8):810–3.
51. Swanson MS, Hudson RL, Bhandari N, et al. Use of octreotide for the management of chyle fistula following neck dissection. JAMA Otolaryngol Head Neck Surg 2015;141(8):723–7.
52. Salerno G, Cavaliere M, Foglia A, et al. The 11th nerve syndrome in functional neck dissection. Laryngoscope 2002;112(7):1299–307.
53. Wittekindt C, Liu W-C, Preuss SF, et al. Botulinum Toxin A for neuropathic pain after neck dissection: a dose-finding study. Laryngoscope 2006;116(7):1168–71.
54. Tisherman SA. Management of major vascular injury: open. Otolaryngol Clin North Am 2016;49(3):809–17.

Conventional Robotic Endoscopic Thyroidectomy for Thyroid Cancer

Meghan E. Garstka, MD, MS, Ehab S. Alameer, MD,
Saad Al Awwad, MD, Emad Kandil, MD, MBA*

KEYWORDS

- Robotic endoscopic thyroidectomy • Thyroid cancer • Conventional

KEY POINTS

- The conventional robotic endoscopic remote access techniques detailed in this article have been discussed in a series of increasing volumes in the literature, including for the treatment of thyroid cancer.
- Lower-volume centers now perform most robotic thyroidectomies in the United States and are responsible for recent increases in utilization patterns despite higher complication rates.
- These trends highlight the importance of increasing surgeon exposure to and experience with these techniques in order to improve procedure safety.
- Additional large-volume, multicenter studies to define patients who will most benefit from these conventional robotic endoscopic procedures for thyroid cancer are needed.

INTRODUCTION

The application of surgical technology to conventional thyroidectomy has allowed for the development of multiple minimally invasive approaches to the thyroid gland. In the early 2000s, Miccoli and colleagues[1] developed and reported on their results with the minimally invasive endoscopic thyroidectomy, which gained significant interest in the United States.[2–4] Surgeons also applied endoscopic technology to initial attempts at remote access thyroidectomy with extracervical approaches to the thyroid gland through incisions in the anterior chest, breast, or axilla.[5] It was thought that such extracervical, "scarless in the neck" approaches would be desirable for many patients interested in cosmesis and desiring to avoid an anterior cervical neck incision, including young patients and patients with a history of keloid or hypertrophic scars.

The authors have nothing to disclose.
Department of Surgery, Tulane University School of Medicine, 1430 Tulane Avenue, SL-22, New Orleans, LA 70112, USA
* Corresponding author.
E-mail address: ekandil@tulane.edu

Endocrinol Metab Clin N Am 48 (2019) 153–163
https://doi.org/10.1016/j.ecl.2018.10.005
0889-8529/19/© 2018 Elsevier Inc. All rights reserved.

However, initial work with endoscopic thyroidectomy demonstrated that these approaches proved to be limited by 2-dimensional visualization and rigid instruments.[5] The introduction of robotic technology to thyroidectomy, in particular through the transaxillary approach, as pioneered by Chung and colleagues,[6,7] and the facelift or retroauricular approach, as described by Terris and colleagues,[8] provided 3-dimensional visualization and multiarticulated endoscopic arms, which proved ideal for the limited workspace of the neck.

Development of multiple robotic-assisted surgery techniques occurred quickly, prompting the American Thyroid Association (ATA) to issue a statement on this topic in 2016.[9] In this statement, the investigators acknowledged that remote-access thyroid surgery has a role when performed by experienced surgeons in select circumstances. The investigators also recommended adherence to strict selection criteria defined by ongoing quality outcomes research. At the time of publication of this ATA statement, the 4 most commonly used robotic-assisted approaches to thyroidectomy in the United States were the endoscopic breast approach, the endoscopic and robotic bilateral axillo-breast approach, the endoscopic and robotic transaxillary approach, and the endoscopic and robotic facelift (retroauricular) approach. With the introduction of transoral endoscopic thyroidectomy, these robotic-assisted approaches may be considered the "conventional" approaches. In this article, the authors discuss the use of conventional robotic endoscopic thyroidectomy for the treatment of thyroid cancer.

PATIENT SELECTION

In general, for the 2 most commonly performed conventional robotic endoscopic thyroidectomy techniques in the United States, the robotic-assisted gasless transaxillary and retroauricular approaches, "ideal" patients are typically young and women and have small or average body mass indices (BMIs) less than 30 kg/m^2. However, the authors showed that these can be done in North American patients with BMI greater than 40 kg/m^2.[10] These techniques may be considered especially in patients meeting such criteria with a history of keloid or hypertrophic scar formation. For the transaxillary approach, patients also must not have anatomic or pathologic contraindications to the required procedural positioning, such as rotator cuff pathology or cervical spine stenosis. Older or obese patients may undergo these procedures safely by experienced surgeons. Because of the learning curve associated with these procedures, conservative patient selection is recommended for surgeons new to these techniques.

Similarly, with regards to patient selection and thyroid pathology, although partial thyroidectomy is recommended as the procedure for surgeons new to the conventional robotic endoscopic techniques, recent studies have reported success in total thyroidectomy and neck dissection for those experienced with these techniques.[11,12] Performance of procedures of increasing complexity has allowed for the expansion of clinical pathology successfully treated by these procedures. Absolute clinical contraindications to robotic thyroidectomy remain, including large substernal or retropharyngeal goiters, T3 thyroid cancer or any suspicious gross invasion, and medullary thyroid cancer.[13] Relative clinical contraindications have previously included nodules greater than 5 cm, large goiters with volumes greater than 40 mL, known T2 well-differentiated thyroid cancer, Hashimoto thyroiditis, and Grave's disease, as well as obesity, a history of previous neck surgery, or radiation. However, the authors and others have demonstrated the safety and feasibility of these conventional robotic-assisted remote access approaches for patients with Hashimoto thyroiditis, Grave's disease, and advanced thyroid cancer.[11,12,14–17]

THYROID CANCER AND CONVENTIONAL ROBOTIC ENDOSCOPIC SURGERY

Initial experience with the techniques of conventional robotic endoscopic thyroidectomy was first reported from centers in Asia. In 2013, Lee and colleagues[11] noted similar oncologic outcomes and safety, similar recovery of neck and shoulder disability, and better quality-of-life outcomes, including better cosmetic results, reductions in neck sensory changes, and reduced swallowing discomfort in patients undergoing robotic thyroidectomy, including those with modified radical neck dissection. In 2016, the same group also reported 5-year surgical outcomes with similar long term-oncologic quality for patients undergoing robotic-assisted versus conventional open thyroidectomy with central compartment node dissection.[12] In 2017, Kim and colleagues[18] reported similar perioperative and 5-year oncologic outcomes for robotic-assisted and conventional open thyroidectomy with modified radical neck dissection. Most recently, Professor Chung's group from South Korea published data on a series of 5000 gasless transaxillary thyroidectomies, from which 4767 patients demonstrated malignancy on final pathology from surgery.[19] The investigators of this study noted that they have tried to improve remote access thyroidectomy using the gasless transaxillary technique and have achieved acceptable surgical outcomes, and that although large numbers of retrospective patient series have been published on this approach, reproducibility remains an issue, and proper training with sufficient experience will lead to the ideal applications of this technique.

In a recent study, the investigators of this article further evaluated the safety and feasibility of robotic-assisted thyroid surgery for the population undergoing procedures for well-differentiated thyroid cancer in the Western population at the authors' North American institution from 2015 to 2017.[20] They noted that for the 144 surgeries for thyroid cancer performed at the authors' institution over this time period, including 35 (24.3%) robotic-assisted gasless transaxillary procedures, there were no significant differences in estimated blood loss, operative times, complication rates, specimen sizes, positive microscopic margins, number of lymph nodes removed with associated lymph node dissections, patient follow-up duration, or clinical recurrence rates between the 2 groups. However, overall length of stay was shorter for robotic-assisted surgery. The authors concluded that in their North American population, the conventional robotic endoscopic approach of gasless transaxillary thyroidectomy for thyroid cancer was feasible and oncologically sound for a select group of well-differentiated patients with thyroid cancer, much as in the Asian experience. However, additional larger, multi-institutional studies are also needed in the Western population.

OVERVIEW OF RETROAURICULAR (FACELIFT) TECHNIQUE

Steps in a standard conventional robotic endoscopic retroauricular (facelift) thyroidectomy procedure are as follows:

- The patient undergoes general anesthesia and is intubated with an electromyographic (EMG) endotracheal tube for intraoperative recurrent laryngeal nerve monitoring.
- Positioning is supine with arms tucked bilaterally on the operating table. The head is rotated slightly 20° to 30° to the contralateral side of the planned incision. The hair at the base of the occipital hairline is shaved 1 cm posteriorly along the planned incision.
- The inferior end of the incision is marked at the inferior extent of the lobule in the postauricular crease and is carried superiorly and posteriorly into the shaved

region of the occipital hairline in a gentle curve (**Fig. 1**). The incision is infiltrated with local anesthetic, and the neck is prepared and draped in a sterile fashion.

- The skin is incised with a scalpel, and electrocautery is used to develop a subplatysmal flap, exposing the sternocleidomastoid (SCM) muscle; dissection continues anteriorly and inferiorly along the SCM muscle.
- The great auricular nerve is identified, and dissection superior to this reveals the external jugular vein and the anterior border of the SCM. If necessary for exposure, the external jugular vein can be divided.
- Dissection continues down to the anteromedial border of the SCM to the clavicle and reveals a muscular triangle bordered by the SCM, the omohyoid, and the sternohyoid muscles. The omohyoid, sternohyoid, and sternothyroid muscles are retracted ventrally, exposing the ipsilateral superior pole of the thyroid gland, and the superior pedicle is isolated.
- The self-retaining modified thyroidectomy or Chung retractor (Marina Medical, Sunrise, FL, USA) is secured on the contralateral side of the operating table and positioned to retract the strap muscles ventrally. A Singer hook (Medtronic, Jacksonville, FL, USA) or Army-Navy retractor is attached to a Greenberg retractor (Codman & Shurtleff, Inc, Raynham, MA, USA) and secured to the ipsilateral side of the operating table and serves to retract the SCM laterally and dorsally. Alternatively, a modified approach creates the plane between the 2 heads of the SCM.
- The Da Vinci robot system (Intuitive, Sunnyvale, CA, USA) is positioned in the operative field contralateral to the incision. The endoscopic camera in the "30° down" configuration is introduced first into the incision. A vessel sealer device and a Maryland grasper are placed in arms 2 and 3 and brought into the operative field under direct visualization. The vessel sealer is usually placed in the surgeon's dominant hand.
- The upper thyroid pole is retracted ventrally and inferiorly, exposing the superior thyroid vessels, which are dissected and divided near the capsule. The gland is then retracted medially, allowing for identification of the recurrent laryngeal nerve in the tracheoesophageal groove. The nerve monitor is used to confirm integrity of the nerve, which is dissected along its path until the insertion into the cricothyroid muscle. The superior and inferior parathyroid glands are identified and preserved.
- The inferior thyroid pedicle is then dissected and divided, and the thyroid is dissected from the trachea. The isthmus is divided, and the thyroid is removed. Integrity of the recurrent laryngeal nerve and hemostasis is verified.

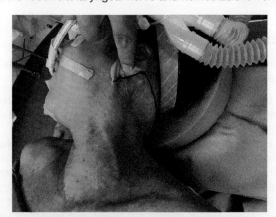

Fig. 1. Preoperative view of retroauricular or "facelift" incision.

- If used, a drain is placed posterior to the retroauricular incision. The incision is closed in 2 layers. Interrupted absorbable subdermal sutures are placed, and the skin is closed with interrupted or running absorbable sutures, or nonabsorbable interrupted sutures, which must be removed in clinic (**Fig. 2**).
- When appropriate, excision of redundant skin can be performed before closure, allowing for a simultaneous "facelift" procedure.

Overview of Transaxillary Technique

Steps in a standard conventional robotic endoscopic transaxillary thyroidectomy procedure are as follows:

- The patient is positioned supine and undergoes general anesthesia and intubation with an EMG endotracheal tube for intraoperative nerve monitoring. The neck is slightly extended with a shoulder roll, and the arm ipsilateral to the lesion or the larger lobe of the thyroid is placed cephalad and flexed above the head into the modified Ikeda's arm position (**Fig. 3**). The contralateral arm is padded and tucked. The investigators routinely use somatosensory evoked potentials (SSEP; Biotronic, Ann Arbor, MI, USA) to monitor the median and ulnar nerve signals (**Fig. 4**). Intraoperative ultrasound is performed after positioning.
- To mark the inferior point of the incision, a transverse line is drawn from the sternal notch, laterally to the axilla. The superior point of the incision is marked with a 60° oblique line from the thyrohyoid membrane to the axilla (**Fig. 5**).
- These points are connected with a longitudinal mark approximately 2 inches in length running along the border of the pectoralis major muscle. The neck and anterior chest are prepared and draped, and the incision site is infiltrated with local anesthetic and then incised.
- Monopolar electrocautery is used to dissect through the subcutaneous tissues of the incision in order to expose the lateral border of the pectoralis major muscle and continues cephalad toward the clavicle in order to create a flap in the subplatysmal plane, superficial to the pectoralis fascia. This may require the extender tip of the electrocautery.
- Lighted breast retractors are used to facilitate flap creation. The clavicle is identified and followed medially to the sternal notch, leading to identification of the ipsilateral SCM muscle. The sternal (medial) and clavicular (lateral) heads of the SCM are identified.
- The avascular plane, which exists between the sternal and clavicular heads of the SCM, can be developed with electrocautery or a vessel sealer and anterior retraction of the sternal head of the SCM, exposing the omohyoid muscle.

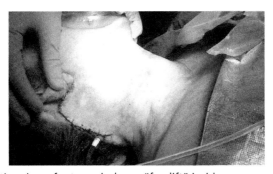

Fig. 2. Postoperative view of retroauricular or "facelift" incision.

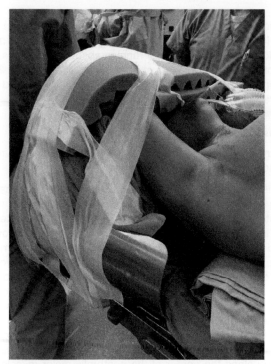

Fig. 3. Modified Ikeda arm position for transaxillary thyroidectomy.

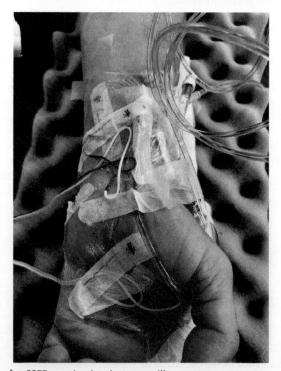

Fig. 4. Electrodes for SSEP monitoring in transaxillary surgery.

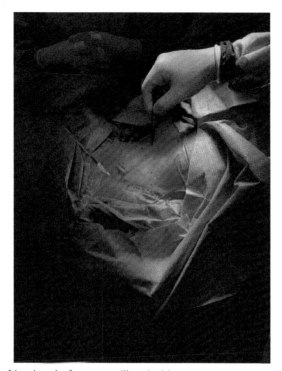

Fig. 5. Marking of landmarks for transaxillary incision.

- Dissection of the uppermost fibers of the omohyoid muscle with electrocautery or a vessel sealer will reveal the superior pole of the thyroid gland. The surgeon must avoid damage to the internal jugular vein. Once the superior pole is exposed, a self-retaining Chung retractor or modified thyroidectomy retractor (Marina Medical, Sunrise, FL, USA) is mounted to the contralateral side of the operating table and used to lift the strap muscles anteriorly (**Fig. 6**).
- The Da Vinci surgical robot is brought into the operative field from the contralateral side (**Fig. 7**). The dual-channel camera configured in the "30° down" mode is

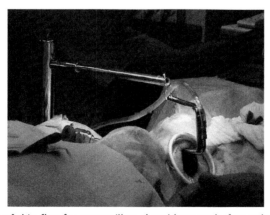

Fig. 6. Retraction of skin flap for transaxillary thyroidectomy before robot docking.

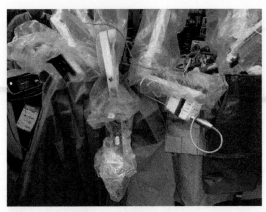

Fig. 7. Robot docked for transaxillary procedure.

docked first in the central position. A second and third arm are placed with instruments to the right or the left of the central camera arm under direct visualization. The investigators place a sealing device on the surgeon's dominant side and a Maryland dissector in the contralateral arm. With a fourth arm, the Prograsper can be placed on the upper edge of the incision, to the same side of the lesion in relation to the blade of the self-retaining retractor.

- The assisting surgeon inserts a laparoscopic suction/irrigation device through the axillary incision. This serves also to retract the clavicular SCM head or trachea downward during the dissection. The assistant is also responsible for placement of the nerve monitoring device and can troubleshoot robotic arm positioning and maintenance.
- The vagus nerve is stimulated in the carotid sheath. If a bilateral dissection or neck dissection is planned, an electrode may be placed on the vagus nerve for continuous nerve monitoring. The upper pole of the thyroid (**Fig. 8**) is retracted medially and inferiorly, and the superior thyroid vessels are dissected and divided close to the thyroid to avoid injury to the external branch of the superior laryngeal nerve. The superior pole is freed from the cricothyroid muscle, and the superior parathyroid gland is identified and preserved.

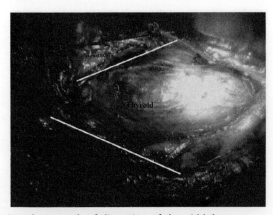

Fig. 8. Intraoperative photograph of dissection of thyroid lobe.

- The thyroid is retracted medially, and the middle thyroid vein is dissected and divided. The recurrent laryngeal nerve is identified at the tracheoesophageal groove and is carefully followed until insertion into the cricothyroid muscle. The functional integrity of the recurrent laryngeal nerve once identified is confirmed.
- The inferior pedicle is dissected and divided. The inferior parathyroid is identified and preserved. The inferior thyroid is dissected medially to the recurrent laryngeal nerve and is shaved from the trachea until reaching the contralateral side. The thyroid lobe and isthmus are divided, and the specimen is extracted.
- If a central lymph node dissection is incorporated into the procedure, the central lymph nodes are dissected en bloc circumferentially from the nerve and removed en bloc with the thymus and the thyroid.
- For total thyroidectomy, once the ipsilateral lobe has been removed, subcapsular dissection of the contralateral lobe from the trachea is performed. When the contralateral tracheoesophageal groove is reached, the recurrent laryngeal nerve is identified and stimulated. The superior and inferior pedicles are dissected and ligated; the recurrent laryngeal nerve is traced to the cricothyroid membrane, and the remaining thyroid is dissected and extracted through the axillary incision.
- Final stimulation of the recurrent laryngeal and vagus nerves is performed, and hemostasis is ensured. A drain is placed, and the axillary incision is closed in 2 layers with interrupted subcutaneous and continuous subcuticular closure (**Fig. 9**).

COMPLICATIONS

Complications for the conventional robotic endoscopic procedures discussed here include not only those observed with conventional cervical procedures, such as

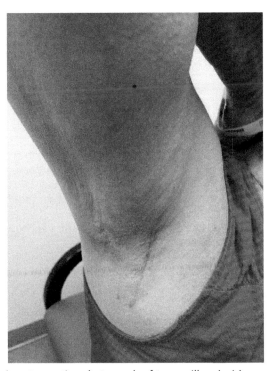

Fig. 9. Well-healed postoperative photograph of transaxillary incision.

recurrent laryngeal nerve injury, postoperative pain, neck hematoma, wound infection, and hypocalcemia, but also those unique to the type of access technique, such as brachial plexus neuropraxia for the transaxillary technique.[8] Reported rates of transient recurrent laryngeal nerve palsies range from 1% to 3%, with around 0.3% permanent injuries. Rates of hematoma have been reported to be approximately 1%, and brachial plexus neuropraxia is about 2.2%, which can be eliminated with the use of SSEP to monitor for radial, ulnar, and median nerves. A recent study at the authors' institution evaluated a series of 137 robotic transaxillary surgeries using SSEP monitoring performed on 123 patients. Seven patients (5.1%) developed significant changes, and immediate arm repositioning resulted in recovery of signals and complete return to baseline parameters with no postoperative positional brachial plexus injuries.[21]

SUMMARY

The conventional robotic endoscopic remote access techniques detailed in this article have been discussed in a series of increasing volumes in the literature, including for the treatment of thyroid cancer. It should be noted that there was a change in procedure volume performed in the United States after Intuitive Surgical Inc, the manufacturer of the Da Vinci surgical system, changed support and training policies for these procedures in October 2011.[22] Lower-volume centers now perform most robotic thyroidectomies in the United States and are responsible for recent increases In utilization patterns despite higher complication rates. These trends highlight the importance of increasing surgeon exposure to and experience with these techniques in order to improve procedure safety. Additional large-volume, multicenter studies to define patients who will most benefit from these conventional robotic endoscopic procedures for thyroid cancer are needed.

REFERENCES

1. Miccoli P, Bellantone R, Mourad M, et al. Minimally invasive video-assisted thyroidectomy: multiinstitutional experience. World J Surg 2002;26(8):972–5.
2. Terris DJ, Gourin CG, Chin E. Minimally invasive thyroidectomy: basic and advanced techniques. Laryngoscope 2006;116(3):350–6.
3. Duke WS, White JR, Waller JL, et al. Endoscopic thyroidectomy is safe in patients with a high body mass index. Thyroid 2014;24(7):1146–50.
4. Duke WS, White JR, Waller JL, et al. Six-year experience with endoscopic thyroidectomy: outcomes and safety profile. Ann Otol Rhinol Laryngol 2015;124(11): 915–20.
5. Bomeli SR, Duke WS, Terris DJ. Robotic facelift thyroid surgery. Gland Surg 2015; 4(5):403–9.
6. Mohamed HE, Kandil E. Robotic trans-axillary and retro-auricular thyroid surgery. J Surg Oncol 2015;112(3):243–9.
7. Yoon JH, Park CH, Chung WY. Gasless endoscopic thyroidectomy via an axillary approach: experience of 30 cases. Surg Laparosc Endosc Percutan Tech 2006; 16(4):226–31.
8. Terris DJ, Singer MC, Seybt MW. Robotic facelift thyroidectomy: patient selection and technical considerations. Surg Laparosc Endosc Percutan Tech 2011;21(4): 237–42.
9. Berber E, Bernet V, Fahey TJ 3rd, et al, American Thyroid Association Surgical Affairs Committee. American Thyroid Association Statement on Remote-Access Thyroid Surgery. Thyroid 2016;26(3):331–7.

10. Kandil EH, Noureldine SI, Yao L, et al. Robotic transaxillary thyroidectomy: an examination of the first one hundred cases. J Am Coll Surg 2012;214(4):558–64 [discussion: 564–6].
11. Lee J, Kwon IS, Bae EH, et al. Comparative analysis of oncological outcomes and quality of life after robotic versus conventional open thyroidectomy with modified radical neck dissection in patients with papillary thyroid carcinoma and lateral neck node metastases. J Clin Endocrinol Metab 2013;98(7):2701–8.
12. Lee SG, Lee J, Kim MJ, et al. Long-term oncologic outcome of robotic versus open total thyroidectomy in PTC: a case-matched retrospective study. Surg Endosc 2016;30(8):3474–9.
13. Bhatia P, Mohamed HE, Kadi A, et al. Remote access thyroid surgery. Gland Surg 2015;4(5):376–87.
14. Kandil E, Noureldine S, Abdel Khalek M, et al. Initial experience using robot-assisted transaxillary thyroidectomy for Graves' disease. J Visc Surg 2011;148(6):e447–51.
15. Noureldine SI, Yao L, Wavekar RR, et al. Thyroidectomy for Graves' disease: a feasibility study of the robotic transaxillary approach. ORL J Otorhinolaryngol Relat Spec 2013;75(6):350–6.
16. Kang SW, Chung WY. Transaxillary single-incision robotic neck dissection for metastatic thyroid cancer. Gland Surg 2015;4(5):388–96.
17. Noureldine SI, Jackson NR, Tufano RP, et al. A comparative North American experience of robotic thyroidectomy in a thyroid cancer population. Langenbecks Arch Surg 2013;398(8):1069–74.
18. Kim MJ, Lee J, Lee SG, et al. Transaxillary robotic modified radical neck dissection: a 5-year assessment of operative and oncologic outcomes. Surg Endosc 2017;31(4):1599–606.
19. Kim MJ, Nam KH, Lee SG, et al. Yonsei experience of 5000 gasless transaxillary robotic thyroidectomies. World J Surg 2018;42(2):393–401.
20. Garstka M, Mohsin K, Ali DB, et al. Well-differentiated thyroid cancer and robotic transaxillary surgery at a North American institution. J Surg Res 2018;228:170–8.
21. Huang S, Garstka M, Murcy M, et al. Somatosensory evoked potential: preventing brachial plexus injury in transaxillary robotic surgery. Laryngoscope, in press.
22. Hinson AM, Kandil E, O'Brien S, et al. Trends in robotic thyroid surgery in the United States from 2009 through 2013. Thyroid 2015;25(8):919–26.

Transoral Endoscopic Thyroidectomy for Thyroid Cancer

Isariya Jongekkasit, MD, FRCST, Pornpeera Jitpratoom, MD, FRCST,
Thanyawat Sasanakietkul, MD, FRCST,
Angkoon Anuwong, MD, FRCST*

KEYWORDS

- Transoral endoscopic thyroidectomy, vestibular approach • TOETVA
- Thyroid cancer • Safety • Feasibility • Central node dissection • Outcomes
- Surgical technique

KEY POINTS

- There is no significant difference between outcome and postoperative complication in transoral endoscopic thyroidectomy, vestibular approach (TOETVA), with better cosmetic outcomes, compared with an open technique.
- TOETVA can be done in low-risk differentiated thyroid cancer (DTC) where size does not exceed 2 cm.
- There is no limitation for performing central cervical lymph node dissection in TOETVA.
- Long-term study of safety and feasibility of TOETVA in low-risk DTC is to be further studied.

INTRODUCTION

Differentiated thyroid cancer (DTC) is the most common form of thyroid cancer. A conventional open thyroidectomy is the standard surgical procedure since 1906, developed by Emil Theodor Kocher.[1] However, an open thyroidectomy leaves a noticeable scar on the anterior neck, which is a concerning issue for women, who represent most patients with DTC. Thanks to the development of endoscopic surgery, surgeons can perform thyroidectomy from remote site without leaving any visible scar on the neck. There are numerous remote-access approaches that have been developed for thyroid surgery over the past 2 decades, although, nearly all of them still leave a visible scar somewhere on the body just not in the anterior neck region. Only transoral endoscopic thyroidectomy (TOET) can truly called scarless surgery. There are

Disclosure Statement: The authors have nothing to disclose.
Minimally Invasive and Endocrine Surgery Division, Department of Surgery, Police General Hospital, 492/1, Rama 1 Road, Pathumwan, Bangkok 10330, Thailand
* Corresponding author.
E-mail address: noii167@hotmail.com

Endocrinol Metab Clin N Am 48 (2019) 165–180
https://doi.org/10.1016/j.ecl.2018.11.009
0889-8529/19/© 2019 Elsevier Inc. All rights reserved.

endo.theclinics.com

number of different techniques for TOET, but the TOET, vestibular approach (TOETVA) is the most cited technique because of its the low complication rate and excellent surgical outcomes.[2–7]

DEVELOPMENT OF TRANSORAL ENDOSCOPIC THYROIDECTOMY, VESTIBULAR APPROACH

The concept of thyroid surgery via natural orifice transluminal endoscopic surgery was developed by Witzel and colleagues.[8] In their report, the TOET was performed in 2 cadavers and 10 living pigs via the sublingual route. Many attempts had been tried to propose different techniques of TOET via the sublingual route in Germany and China; however, all were associated with a high complication rate.[9] As a result, it is no longer performed in clinical practice.

The oral vestibular approach was first described by Richmon and colleagues.[10] They first performed transoral robotic-assisted thyroidectomy with a sublingual approach and found out later that moving the camera to the oral vestibule was a superior approach. Nakajo and colleagues[11] performed transoral video-assisted neck surgery, a gasless technique, in 8 cases. Wang and colleagues[6] reported another vestibular approach with CO_2 insufflation in 12 patients. Both Nakajo and colleagues[11] and Wang and colleagues[6] reported complication of mental nerve injuries, which was a major concern for patients and surgeons.

The first TOETVA article that claimed to have no mental nerve injury and low postoperative complication was published by Anuwong.[12] From 60 patients who underwent TOETVA, none of patients had mental nerve injury and only 2 patients experienced transient recurrent laryngeal nerve (RLN) injury, which completely resolved afterward. To date, more than 800 cases of TOETVA have been performed at the Police General Hospital, Thailand. The technique is described step by step in the technique section.

Although there are many articles that report on the safety and feasibility of TOETVA in both thyroid and parathyroid diseases, there is scarce literature on the long-term outcomes of this technique. But now it can be assumed that TOETVA is an alternative treatment for both benign and malignant thyroid disease in addition to parathyroid disease, that has excellent outcome from surgical and aesthetics aspects (Fig. 1).

ROLE OF TRANSORAL ENDOSCOPIC THYROIDECTOMY, VESTIBULAR APPROACH IN DIFFERENTIATED THYROID CANCER

There are many articles that tried describe patient selection criteria for TOETVA and other endoscopic thyroidectomy techniques for benign thyroid disease, and concluded that it is safe to perform TOETVA for a benign thyroid lesion that is smaller than 8 to 10 cm. However, the size of the thyroid gland that can be removed via 2.0 to 2.5-cm wound without the risk of rupturing of the thyroid capsule should not exceed 3 to 4 cm.[13] With the increasing utility of advanced imaging technologies and development of an early screening test, the incidence of small-sized thyroid cancer has increased significantly in many parts of the world, especially in Asia.[14–19] With all of the known facts about the limitations and outcomes of TOETVA and the natural history of thyroid disease, TOETVA can be performed for small-sized, low-risk patients with DTC. It suggests that patients with a 2 cm or smaller lesion and have low-risk DTC can be managed by lobectomy via the TOETVA technique with adequate pathologic and oncological outcomes without any risk of capsular violation of the tumor.[20] After that article there were many attempts to prove the safety and

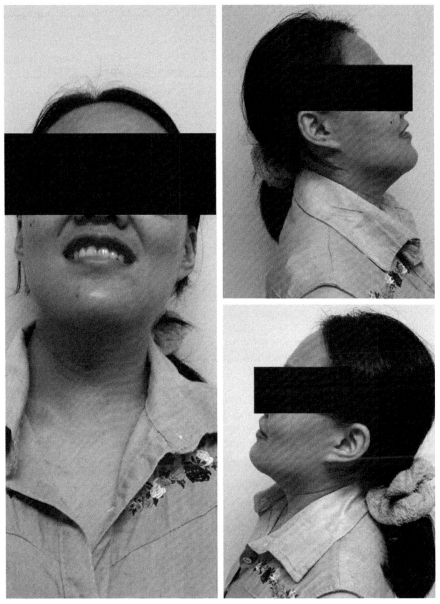

Fig. 1. The neck of a patient with PTC who underwent TOETVA with bilateral central neck dissection on her postoperative day 7. There was no complication after the surgery, such as RLN injury, or hypoparathyroidism. Postoperative serum Tq is less than 0 1 ng/mL. The patient was satisfied with the cosmetic outcome. There was no scar, no hematoma, or no bruise left on her anterior neck region.

feasibility of TOETVA in small-sized DTC as shown in **Table 1**. However, most of the studies were case series, most likely because of the novelty of the technique, concern of inadequate oncological resection, and lack of long-term follow-up. There are several scientific studies showing that other approaches of endoscopic remote-

Table 1
TOETVA experiences in thyroid cancer

Author, Year	Approach	Number of Patients	Diagnosis	Type of Surgery	Lymph Node Station
Yang et al,[38] 2015	ETOVA	4	PTC	Total	CND
Wang et al,[6] 2016	TOETVA	10	PTC	Lobectomy	CND
Anuwong,[12] 2016	TOETVA	2	MicroPTC	Lobectomy	CND
Dionigi et al,[3] 2017	TOETVA	2	MicroPTC	Lobectomy	CND
Wu et al,[39] 2017	Breast combine oral	6	PTC	Total	CND
Chai et al,[28] 2017	TOETVA	10	MicroPTC	Lobectomy	CND
Anuwong et al,[13] 2018	TOETVA	26	MicroPTC	Lobectomy	CND

Abbreviations: CND, central lymph node dissection; ETOVA, endoscopic thyroidectomy via oral vestibular approach; PTC, papillary thyroid cancer; TOETVA, transoral endoscopic thyroidectomy, vestibular approach.

access thyroidectomy have revealed no significant difference in outcome in terms of safety and adequacy of oncological outcomes when comparing them with conventional open thyroidectomy. When comparing the value of postoperative thyroglobulin and results of postoperative scans from TOETVA case series with other endoscopic remote-access thyroidectomy studies,[21] it can be implied that TOETVA has no significant difference between safety and oncological adequacy outcomes compared with other routes of thyroidectomy.

Older studies claim that routine central lymph node dissection (RCLD) in treatment of DTC has higher morbidity and did not demonstrate any benefits in terms of long-term survival, but it cannot be denied that up to 80% of patients with papillary thyroid cancer (PTC) have been reported to have at least cervical lymph node micrometastases, even in a clinically node-negative low-risk small PTC case that was smaller than 2 cm. As most PTCs have low aggressive behavior, a low locoregional recurrence rate, with need of long-term follow-up (more than 20 years) altogether, and with the presence of new emerging TOETVA technique that has been described for less than a decade, the author recommends doing RCLD in every thyroid cancer case for the best long-term result for the patients. Another reason that make us feel very comfortable to ensure all surgeons perform RCLD is no report claimed to have permanent RLN injury in performing one side TOETVA, which is the main reason for not doing the RCLD.[22–27] In terms of technical aspect, there is no technical significant difference in central neck dissection between open thyroidectomy and TOETVA. Recently, Chai and colleagues[28] reported that the mean number of retrieved lymph nodes from central neck dissection from TOETVA in papillary thyroid microcarcinoma was 2.7 ± 1.7, without any permanent injury to RLN, only 2 of 7 patients had transient vocal cord palsy, which all recovered in 3 months.

TOETVA is now performed only for low-risk DTC that is smaller than 2 cm. We recommend for patients to undergo TOETVA lobectomy of the affected side, including isthmectomy, to limit postoperative complications. In cases in which there are other lesions in the other side that is still suitable for TOETVA or it is a patient's preference, against our advice, such cases can undergo simultaneous total TOETVA and RCLD.

SURGICAL ASPECT OF TRANSORAL ENDOSCOPIC THYROIDECTOMY, VESTIBULAR APPROACH

Patient Selection for Transoral Endoscopic Thyroidectomy, Vestibular Approach in Patients with Differentiated Thyroid Cancer

Indication for transoral endoscopic thyroidectomy, vestibular approach

- Patients with low-risk, DTC with tumor size that is smaller than 2 cm and no evidence of extracapsular involvement from the imaging study.
- No history of prior neck surgery or radiation (except for completion thyroidectomy from prior TOETVA within 2 weeks or more than 2 months)

Contraindication for transoral endoscopic thyroidectomy, vestibular approach

- Those with severe medical comorbidities who cannot tolerate general anesthesia
- Medullary or anaplastic thyroid cancer
- Evidence of lateral cervical lymph node involvement
- Oral cavity infection, such as abscess
- Active perioral and labial infection, such as herpes simplex infection
- Evidence of preoperative RLN palsy
- History of chin augmentation by silicone implantation of fillers (relative contraindication)

Preoperative Preparation

Preoperative ultrasound with lymph node mapping is routinely performed. Computed tomography scan should be used in every case to evaluate extracapsular extension, adjacent organ involvement, and distance metastasis. Preoperative indirect laryngoscopy or fiberoptic laryngoscopic examination is performed to assess vocal cord function. Dental consultation is obtained if the patient has not seen a dentist in the past few months. The patient is admitted to the hospital a day before surgery. Prophylactic perioperative antibiotics are administered before surgery (amoxicillin/clavulanic acid 1.2 g).

Surgical Technique

The patient is paced in the supine position, slight neck extension position. A neuromonitoring endotracheal tube is used for intubation either via oral route or nasal route. We prefer left-sided nasotracheal intubation, as most surgeons are right handed, and this will prevent any limitation of movement of instruments. The sterile sticker is draped

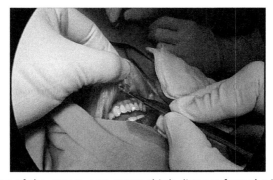

Fig. 2. The incision of the camera port at two-thirds distance from the inner lower lip to frenulum.

over the upper face. The area encompassing the nipple to the forehead is prepped with hibiscrub solution and hibitane solution in water. The lower lip is everted to expose the lower vestibule. The first incision is made transversely and centrally at two-thirds of the distance between the inferior labial frenulum and the edge of the lower lip. The length of the first incision can vary between 1.5 and 2.5 cm depending on the size of the thyroid gland (**Fig. 2**). An energy device may be used to create the chin flap by cutting through the mentalis muscle until the lower border of the angle of the chin. The Veress needle No.18 is inserted through the first incision for injection of a solution of 0.1% adrenaline 1 mL with 500 mL of normal saline solution into the subplatysmal plane as called as a hydrodissection. To complete hydrodissection, we usually use the solution approximately 30 to 50 mL per case and infiltrate the solution in a fan shape along the anterior border of the sternocleidomastoid muscle from one side to the other and downward to the sternal notch. The Kelly clamp is inserted for dilating the central incision. The fulcrum of the Kelly clamp should be placed at the tip of the chin to make the optimum dilatation for the tract (**Fig. 3**). The blunt tip dilator (Angkoon dilator) is inserted into the subplatysmal plane for space creation along the infiltrated field (**Fig. 4**). A 10-mm trocar is inserted through the first incision as a camera port. The hanging stitch is made at 1 cm below the tip of the trocar for preventing acute angle of the skin flap in front of the port. Two of 5-mm working trocars were inserted at both lateral side of oral vestibule, in the area of the imaginary line from the incisor in the right angle up just below the inner lip (**Fig. 5**). Again, hydrodissection is performed in the same fashion as in the midline incision but only downward to a level of an angle of the mandible. Both of the 5-mm ports and the camera port are parallel to each other, with very few degrees of medial deviation. We use a 10-mm, 30° camera system. A Maryland dissector is inserted into both lateral trocars and brought into view by puncturing through the fibrous tissue at the main surgical field. The fibrous tissue is also cleared by an electrocautery device or any other type of vascular sealing system. The subplatysmal space creation extends to the anterior border of both sides of the sternocleidomastoid muscles and a sternal notch. Strap muscles are divided in the midline from the sternal notch up to the level of cricoid cartilage (**Fig. 6**). The lateral mobilization of the affected side of the thyroid gland from the strap muscles was done until the carotid sheath is met (**Fig. 7**). The vagus nerve is tested via a neuromonitoring probe at the lateral side of the carotid sheath. Isthmectomy is always performed, by using a vascular sealing system, as a first step of the true dissection of the gland even in a case that requires total thyroidectomy (**Fig. 8**). We recommend performing isthmectomy and cut some anterior part of the Berry ligament not farther than

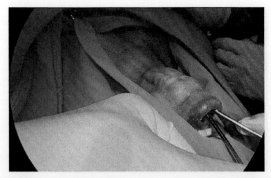

Fig. 3. Dilatation of the tract at a camera port by using a Kelly clamp. A fulcrum of Kelly clamp should be at the tip of the chin and dilate the tract at a subplatysmal plane.

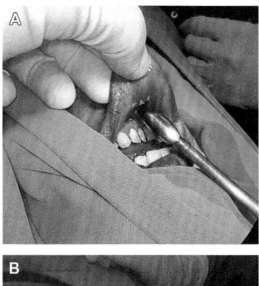

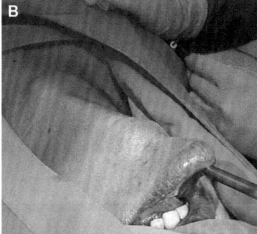

Fig. 4. How to apply a blunt tip dilator to create subplatysmal plane. A good dilator should be in the shape of nearly a point at the tip but not sharp, as shown in (A). (B) How to apply dilator in 3 directions like a fan shape between the border of both sternocleidomastoid muscles.

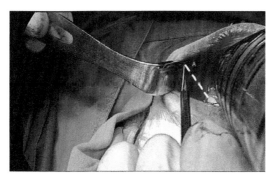

Fig. 5. An imaginary line from the incisor in the right angle up to inner lip, line A. We put 5 mm of working port at the end of this line at both sides to prevent mental nerve injury.

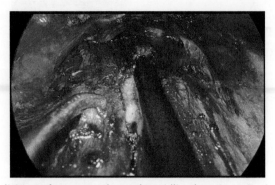

Fig. 6. A step of division of strap muscles at the midline by using a Bovie.

one-third of the anterior surface of the trachea to facilitate mobilization of the affected thyroid lobe in the next step to prevent unintentional rupture of the thyroid capsule. An additional lateral hanging stitch is placed from the outside to include the strap muscles to obtain better exposure of the superior pole (**Fig. 9**). After a good exposure of the superior pole is achieved, the superior thyroid artery and vein are gently dissected. The superior parathyroid gland is retracted down and preserved. Sometimes we might be able to see the external branch of the superior laryngeal nerve from this step (**Fig. 10**) or it can be tested by nerve stimulation at the cricothyroid muscle. After the superior parathyroid gland is preserved, the superior thyroid artery and vein are individually ligated and secured by either vascular sealing system or clip and then transected. This step is made easier by grasping the superior pole up by accessing into the Joll space (**Fig. 11**).

After transecting the superior thyroid vessels, the next step is to find the RLN and inferior parathyroid gland. The key to finding the RLN is to grasp the affected thyroid lobe to the opposite side. The RLN must be found at its insertion and traced down along it course until it runs down below the inferior pole (**Fig. 12**). From our experience, the incidence of nonrecurrent laryngeal nerve in TOETVA is comparable to the incidence during conventional open thyroidectomy at 0% to 4.76%. The RLN should be stimulated both at its proximal end, around insertion, and more distal to the dissection plane and collect the amount of the amplitude. The inferior parathyroid gland is usually located ventral to the RLN. After the RLN and inferior parathyroid gland are identified and preserved, the affected thyroid lobe is dissected from the Berry ligament

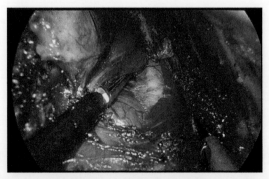

Fig. 7. Carotid artery that is the border of the lateral mobilization of the thyroid gland. We test a vagus nerve at the lateral boarder of the carotid artery.

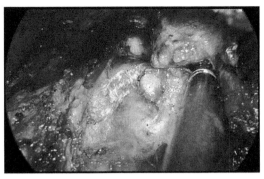

Fig. 8. How isthmectomy is done. We grasp the thyroid up and use vascular sealing equipment to cut the thyroid gland. The correct plane should show a white plane of pretracheal fascia.

by using the vascular sealing system. In this step, we suggest being very careful to gently push the nerve and parathyroid gland away from the affected thyroid lobe because these 2 structures may attach densely or may have anatomic distortion compared with the patient with a normal thyroid, because we have to preserve their function and also remove all of the affected thyroid gland out as much as possible. Care is taken not to injure the underlying trachea or the nerve. A safety distance, for preventing lateral heat spreading, from the vascular sealing system to the preserved tissue is at least 4 mm. After all of the specimens are dissected, the EndoCatch bag is inserted through the camera port. The specimen is gently removed altogether with the EndoCatch bag to prevent rupture of the thyroid capsule while extracting the specimen.

Most of the steps that were described previously, except flap dissection, are exactly the same steps compared with the open technique. The principle of the central lymph node dissection (CND) technique is also the same as in the open technique. There is no limitation in performing simultaneous prophylactic central neck dissection in the TOETVA procedure. All the fatty tissue and lymph nodes between the carotid sheath and esophagus can be removed from the RLN along the trachea and from the tracheoesophageal groove. The central neck dissection is continued into the superior mediastinum while dissecting along the RLN. The superior mediastinum nodes can be dissected by removing the upper thymus with the

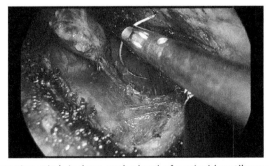

Fig. 9. A lateral hanging stitch is done at the level of a cricoid cartilage or superior pole as shown.

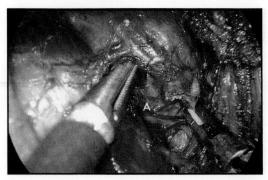

Fig. 10. The relation of the superior thyroid vessels and an external branch of superior laryngeal nerve (A).

adjacent fatty tissue after determining the position of the inferior parathyroid gland. Sometimes it is difficult to preserve the lower parathyroid gland, as it is indistinguishable from the surrounding fatty tissue and lymph nodes, in some cases. Although we perform only one side of the thyroid gland and injury to both the parathyroid gland on the affected side will not lead to postoperative hypoparathyroidism, we can also send a suspected parathyroid specimen for frozen section confirmation, and autotransplanted if necessary. The central neck node specimens are retrieved in a separate EndoCatch bag.

We ensure adequate hemostasis at the end of the procedure. The drain is rarely needed in this operation, although it can be placed in case bleeding is a concern, by placing another 5-mm trocar above the clavicle. A Redivac drain no. 10 is inserted into the trocar and placed in the surgical bed. The amplitude of nerve stimulation at RLN and vagus nerve is compared between preoperative and postoperative, respectively, to confirm function of the nerve. Strap muscles are reapproximated by using 3-0 continuous barbing suture or interrupted absorbable multifilament suture (**Fig. 13**). The central incision wound is closed by using 4-0 interrupted absorbable multifilament suture for the mentalis muscle layer. All other incisions at a level of mucosal and submucosal layers are closed by using 4-0 continuous locking absorbable multifilament suture (**Fig. 14**). The oral vestibule is irrigated by the hibitane in water solution. The

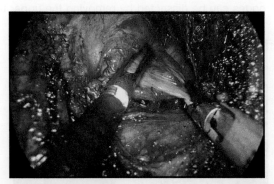

Fig. 11. A grasper in the left hand of the surgeon approaching superior lobe via the Joll space. The right hand of the surgeon with a vascular sealing device was trying to dissect the superior thyroid vessels and control it.

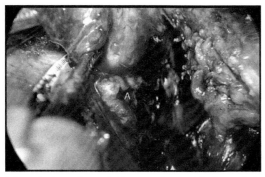

Fig. 12. The RLN (A) from its insertion, which runs along with thyroid gland downward into the chest.

chin, not the anterior neck, is compressed by a few pieces of 4 × 4 gauze for 24 hours postoperatively.

Postoperative Care

For general everyday life in the first week after the operation, we advise patients to use mouthwash in the morning, after every meal, and before bedtime. Brushing the teeth can be done gently or use a small toothbrush for children instead. Also, patients must avoid extremely hot and cold food or drinks, coughing, and massaging on the anterior neck area.

We allow patients sips of water immediately after the surgery (postoperative day 0). Acetaminophen is usually adequate for pain control. On postoperative day 1, the patient is ready to have a liquid diet in the morning and soft diet in the evening. The patient can be discharged home safely if there is no fever and pain is adequately controlled with oral pain medications.[29]

POSTOPERATIVE COMPLICATIONS AND QUALITY OF LIFE

The most concerning postoperative complication in TOETVA is an infection, because the operation might introduce infection from the contaminated area in the mouth into the sterile area in the neck. In the literature review, there was no infection in the oral vestibular approach.

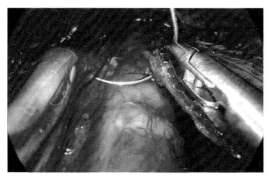

Fig. 13. After all the specimens were removed and hemostasis was secured, the strap muscles were reapproximate by 4-0 barbed suture continuous fashion, as shown.

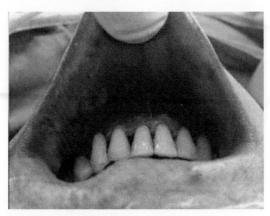

Fig. 14. The wounds inside the mouth after the operation was completed.

With other postoperative complications, such as RLN injury, hypoparathyroidism, and bleeding, there are no differences in prevalence of those complications when comparing TOETVA with open thyroidectomy. There is no limitation to using intraoperative neuromonitoring equipment to detect RLN or Indocyanine green (ICG) injection to help identify the parathyroid gland.[6,30–33] Chai and colleagues[28] reported a result of TOETVA in a case series of patients with DTC. There was zero postoperative bleeding, mental nerve injury, and permanent vocal cord palsy. Only 2 of 10 patients developed transient vocal cord palsy from laryngoscopy study and all resolved within 3 months.

There is some study showing that other route of endoscopic thyroidectomy seems to have more postoperative pain than open thyroidectomy on a basis of longer and larger flap dissection. Ha and colleagues[34] performed a cohort study on postoperative neck pain among open thyroidectomy, endoscopic gasless transaxillary, and robotic transaxillary approaches. They found that postoperative neck pain was significantly higher in endoscopic and robotic thyroidectomy groups than in the open thyroidectomy group, in term of absence or presence of neck pain ($P = .026$). However, there was no significant difference in pain scale score among the 3 groups ($P = .2$). The fact that the TOETVA technique has the shortest and smallest flap dissection compared with other endoscopic route, only around the chin is there more dissection compared with the open technique. Anuwong and colleagues[4] reported that mean postoperative pain score was as low as 2.41 ± 2.04,[2–7] 1.17 ± 1.4 (0–5), and 0.47 ± 0.83 (0–3) on the first, second, and third days, respectively.

It is no doubt that endoscopic thyroidectomy is equal to open thyroidectomy in terms of surgical outcome. Because of that, the aim of all endoscopic thyroid surgery should be focused on the satisfaction of the patient after the surgery. Quality of life after the surgery is one factor that should be mentioned. Patients with PTC who underwent endoscopic thyroidectomy showed significantly greater improvement in emotional function at 1 month ($P = .039$) and physical function at 3 months ($P = .042$) compared with patients who underwent open thyroidectomy.[35,36]

FOLLOW-UP AND SURVEILLANCE

According to the American Thyroid Association 2015 guidelines, follow-up and surveillance of patients depends on whether patients have undergone total TOETVA or less than that and which category of initial risk stratification system that patients

High Risk
Gross extrathyroidal extension,
incomplete tumor resection, distant metastases,
or lymph node >3 cm

Intermediate Risk
Aggressive histology, minor extrathyroidal
extension, vascular invasion,
or > 5 involved lymph nodes (0.2–3 cm)

Low Risk
Intrathyroidal DTC
≤ 5 LN micrometastases (< 0.2 cm)

FTC, extensive vascular invasion ($\approx$ 30–55%)
pT4a gross ETE ($\approx$ 30–40%)
pN1 with extranodal extension, >3 LN involved ($\approx$ 40%)
PTC, > 1 cm, TERT mutated ± BRAF mutated* (>40%)
pN1, any LN > 3 cm ($\approx$ 30%)
PTC, extrathyroidal, BRAF mutated* ($\approx$ 10–40%)
PTC, vascular invasion ($\approx$ 15–30%)
Clinical N1 ($\approx$20%)
pN1, > 5 LN involved ($\approx$20%)
Intrathyroidal PTC, < 4 cm, BRAF mutated* ($\approx$10%)
pT3 minor ETE ($\approx$ 3–8%)
pN1, all LN < 0.2 cm ($\approx$5%)
pN1, ≤ 5 LN involved ($\approx$5%)
Intrathyroidal PTC, 2–4 cm ($\approx$ 5%)
Multifocal PTMC ($\approx$ 4–6%)
pN1 without extranodal extension, ≤ 3 LN involved (2%)
Minimally invasive FTC ($\approx$ 2–3%)
Intrathyroidal, < 4 cm, BRAF wild type* ($\approx$ 1–2%)
Intrathyroidal unifocal PTMC, BRAF mutated*, ($\approx$ 1–2%)
Intrathyroidal, encapsulated, FV-PTC ($\approx$ 1–2%)
Unifocal PTMC ($\approx$ 1–2%)

Fig. 15. The risk of structural disease recurrence scale. *While analysis of BRAF and/or TERT status is not routinely recommended for initial risk stratification, 2015 ATA guideline have included these findings to assist clinicians in proper risk stratification in cases where this information is available. ETE, extrathyroidal extension; FTC, follicular thyroid carcinoma; FVPTC, follicular variant of papillary thyroid carcinoma; LN, lymph node; PTC, papillary thyroid carcinoma; PTMC, papillary thyroid microcarcinoma. (*Data from* Haugen BR, Alexander EK, Bible KC, et al. 2015 American Thyroid Association management guidelines for adult patients with thyroid nodules and differentiated thyroid cancer. Thyroid 2016;26(1):1–133.)

are in (**Fig. 15**). All the patient must be assigned for neck ultrasonography at 6 to 12 months and then periodically, depending on the patient's risk for recurrent disease and thyroglobulin (Tg) status (**Table 2**). For the low-risk patients who underwent less than total TOETVA, thyroid-stimulating hormone (TSH) may be maintained in the mid to lower reference range (0.5–2 mU/L) while surveillance is continued. Thyroid hormone therapy may not be needed if patients can maintain their serum TSH in this target range.

Every low-risk patient who has undergone total TOETVA must have postoperative serum Tg level checked and be assigned for postoperative diagnostic radioactive iodine whole-body scan (RAI WBS). Patients who have higher administered activities of RAI WBS without large remnant is suspected may receive a low-dose (30 mCi) RAI ablation. Routine RAI ablation is not recommended for low-risk patients with DTC. Serum level of Tg and TSH are used as bio-chemical markers for follow-up and surveillance of patients. For low-risk patients who have undetectable serum Tg levels (<0.2 ng/mL), TSH may be maintained at the lower end of the reference range (0.5–2 mU/L) while continuing surveillance. But for the low-risk patients who have low-level serum Tg levels, TSH may be maintained at or slightly below the lower limit of normal range (0.1–0.5 mU/L).[37] Further detail of surveillance evaluation of response to therapies is discussed in the following articles.

Table 2
Postoperative surveillance strategy based on American Thyroid Association risk category

Investigation	6 mo	12 mo	18 mo	24 mo
Thyroglobulin	All[a]	All[a]	All[a]	All[a]
Ultrasound neck	—	All[a]	—	All[a]
Diagnostic RAI scan	—	—	Intermediate/high risk	—
CT/MRI	—	High risk	—	High risk
PET scan	—	High risk	—	High risk

Abbreviations: CT, computed tomography; RAI, radioactive iodine.
[a] All: all low, intermediate, and high-risk patients.
Data from Momesso DP, Tuttle RM. Update on differentiated thyroid cancer staging. Endocrinol Metab Clin North Am 2014;43(2):401–21.

COMPLETION THYROIDECTOMY VIA TRANSORAL ENDOSCOPIC THYROIDECTOMY, VESTIBULAR APPROACH

Reoperative surgery sometimes can be a difficult situation and has a higher rate of postoperative complications because of the nature of the tissue-healing process. The golden period of reoperative surgery should be later than 6 weeks or within 2 weeks in every organ including the thyroid. Completion thyroidectomy via the TOETVA approach is a safe procedure. For the first 2 weeks, there is no increased difficulty, no significant adhesion when performing dissection. Good operative outcome was archived without other complications such RLN injury or hypoparathyroidism [21] Because DTC is a slow-growing cancer, sometimes a completion thyroidectomy after the lobectomy can be deferred for 6 weeks, if necessary, after the first operation without any change in course of the disease.

DISCUSSION

TOETVA is a new novel operation that offers the best cosmetic result. Many studies have shown the safety and feasibility of this technique in both benign and malignant lesions of the thyroid, although there is still a scarcity of long-term results in cancer series, as the procedure was described only recently. However, as the results from the literature show promising trends of safety and feasibility in oncologic validity, a larger series is required and long-term follow-up is necessary to understand the oncologic validity of this approach.

REFERENCES

1. Hannan SA. The magnificent seven. Int J Surg 2006;4:187–91.
2. Jitpratoom P, Ketwong K, Sasanakietkul T, et al. Transoral endoscopic thyroidectomy vestibular approach (TOETVA) for Graves' disease: a comparison of surgical results with open thyroidectomy. Gland Surg 2016;5(6):546–52.
3. Dionigi G, Lavazza M, Bacuzzi A, et al. Transoral endoscopic thyroidectomy vestibular approach (TOETVA): from A to Z. Surg Technol Int 2017;30:103–12.
4. Anuwong A, Sasanakietkul T, Jitpratoom P, et al. Transoral endoscopic thyroidectomy vestibular approach (TOETVA): indications, techniques and results. Surg Endosc 2018;32(1):456–65.
5. Le QV, Ngo DQ, Ngo QX. Transoral endoscopic thyroidectomy vestibular approach (TOETVA): a case report as new technique in thyroid surgery in Vietnam. Int J Surg Case Rep 2018;50:60–3.

6. Wang Y, Yu X, Wang P, et al. Implementation of intraoperative neuromonitoring for transoral endoscopic thyroid surgery: a preliminary report. J Laparoendosc Adv Surg Tech A 2016;26(12):965–71.

7. Yi JW, Yoon SG, Kim HS, et al. Transoral endoscopic surgery for papillary thyroid carcinoma: initial experiences of a single surgeon in South Korea. Ann Surg Treat Res 2018;95(2):73–9.

8. Witzel K, von Rahden BH, Kaminski C, et al. Transoral access for endoscopic thyroid resection. Surg Endosc 2008;22:1871–5.

9. Karakas E, Steinfeldt T, Gockel A, et al. Transoralparathyroid sugery, a new alternative or non sense? Langenbecks Arch Surg 2014;399:7415.

10. Richmon JD, Pattani KM, Benhidjeb T, et al. Transoral robotic assisted thyroidectomy a preclinical feasibility study in 2 cadavers. Head Neck 2011;33:330–3.

11. Nakajo A, Arima H, Hirata M, et al. Transoral video-assisted neck surgery (TO-VANS). A new transoral technique of endoscopic thyroidectomy with gasless premandible approach. Surg Endosc 2013;27:1105–10.

12. Anuwong A. Transoral endoscopic thyroidectomy vestibular approach: a series of the first 60 human cases. World J Surg 2016;40:491–7.

13. Anuwong A, Ketwong K, Jitpratoom P, et al. Safety and outcomes of the transoral endoscopic thyroidectomy vestibular approach. JAMA Surg 2018;153(1):21–7.

14. Park S, Oh CM, Cho H, et al. Association between screening and the thyroid cancer "epidemic" in South Korea: evidence from a nationwide study. BMJ 2016;355: i5745.

15. Davies L, Welch HG. Increasing incidence of thyroid cancer in the United states, 1973-2002. JAMA 2006;295:2164–7.

16. Kitahara CM, Sosa JA. The changing incidence of thyroid cancer. Nat Rev Endocrinol 2016;12(11):646–53.

17. Lim H, Devesa SS, Sosa JA, et al. Trends in thyroid cancer incidence and mortality in the United States, 1974-2013. JAMA 2017;317(13):1338–48.

18. La Vecchia C, Malvezzi M, Bosetti C, et al. Thyroid cancer mortality and incidence: a global overview. Int J Cancer 2015;136(9):2187–95.

10. Wiltshire JJ, Drake TM, Uttley L, et al. Systematic review of trends in the incidence rates of thyroid cancer. Thyroid 2016;26(11):1541–52.

20. Wu YJ, Chi SY, Elsarawy A, et al. What is the appropriate nodular diameter in thyroid cancer for extraction by transoral endoscopic thyroidectomy vestibular approach without breaking the specimens? A surgicopathologic study. Surg Laparosc Endosc Percutan Tech 2018. https://doi.org/10.1097/SLE.0000000000000563.

21. Razavi CR, Tufano RP, Russell JO. Completion thyroidectomy via the transoral endoscopic vestibular approach. Gland Surg 2018;7(Suppl 1):S77–9.

22. Agrawal N, Evasovich MR, Kandil E, et al. Indications and extent of central neck dissection for papillary thyroid cancer: an American Head and Neck Society Consensus Statement. Head Neck 2017;39(7):1269–79.

23. Gambardella C, Tartaglia E, Nunziata A, et al. Clinical significance of prophylactic central compartment neck dissection in the treatment of clinically node-negative papillary thyroid cancer patients. World J Surg Oncol 2016;14(1):247.

24. Deutschmann MW, Chin-Lenn L, Au J, et al. Extent of central neck dissection among thyroid cancer surgeons: cross-sectional analysis. Head Neck 2016; 38(Suppl 1):E328–32.

25. Chinn SB, Zafereo ME, Waguespack SG, et al. Long-term outcomes of lateral neck dissection in patients with recurrent or persistent well-differentiated thyroid cancer. Thyroid 2017;27(10):1291–9.

26. Lee YC, Na SY, Park GC, et al. Occult lymph node metastasis and risk of regional recurrence in papillary thyroid cancer after bilateral prophylactic central neck dissection: a multi-institutional study. Surgery 2017;161(2):465–71.

27. Zhao W, You L, Hou X, et al. The effect of prophylactic central neck dissection on locoregional recurrence in papillary thyroid cancer after total thyroidectomy: a systematic review and meta-analysis: pCND for the locoregional recurrence of papillary thyroid cancer. Ann Surg Oncol 2017;24(8):2189–98.

28. Chai YJ, Chung JK, Anuwong A, et al. Transoral endoscopic thyroidectomy for papillary thyroid microcarcinoma: initial experience of a single surgeon. Ann Surg Treat Res 2017;93(2):70–5.

29. Anuwong A, Kim HY, Dionigi G. Transoral endoscopic thyroidectomy using vestibular approach: updates and evidence. Gland Surg 2017;6(3):277–84.

30. Vidal Fortuny J, Belfontali V, Sadowski SM, et al. Parathyroid gland angiography with indocyanine green fluorescence to predict parathyroid function after thyroid surgery. Br J Surg 2016;103(5):537–43.

31. Zaidi N, Bucak E, Yazici P, et al. The feasibility of indocyanine green fluorescence imaging for identifying and assessing the perfusion of parathyroid glands during total thyroidectomy. J Surg Oncol 2016;113(7):775–8.

32. Yu HW, Chung JW, Yi JW, et al. Intraoperative localization of the parathyroid glands with indocyanine green and Firefly(R) technology during BABA robotic thyroidectomy. Surg Endosc 2017;31(7):3020–7.

33. Lavazza M, Liu X, Wu C, et al. Indocyanine green-enhanced fluorescence for assessing parathyroid perfusion during thyroidectomy. Gland Surg 2016;5(5): 512–21.

34. Ha TK, Kim DQ, Park HK, et al. Comparison of postoperative neck pain and discomfort, swallowing difficulty, and voice change after conventional open, endoscopic, and robotic thyroidectomy: a single-center cohort study. Front Endocrinol (Lausanne) 2018;9(418):1–6.

35. Lee MC, Park H, Lee BC, et al. Comparison of quality of life between open and endoscopic thyroidectomy for papillary thyroid cancer. Head Neck 2016;3: E827–31.

36. Wang LY, Ganly I. Nodal metastases in thyroid cancer: prognostic implication and management. Future Oncol 2016;12(7):981–94.

37. Haugen BR, Alexander EK, Bible KC, et al. 2015 American Thyroid Association Management guidelines for adult patients with thyroid nodules and differentiated thyroid cancer. Thyroid 2016;26(1):1–133.

38. Yang J, Wang C, Li J, et al. Complete endoscopic thyroidectomy via oral vestibular approach versus areola approach for treatment of thyroid diseases. J Laparoendosc Adv Surg Tech A 2015;25(6):470–6.

39. Wu GY, Fu JB, Lin FS, et al. Endoscopic central lymph node dissection via breast combined with oral approach for papillary thyroid carcinoma: a preliminary study. World J Surg 2017;41(9):2280–2.

Conventional Radioiodine Therapy for Differentiated Thyroid Cancer

Dorina Ylli, MD, PhD[a], Douglas Van Nostrand, MD[b],
Leonard Wartofsky, MD, MACP[a],*

KEYWORDS

- Radioiodine • Thyroid cancer • Therapy • Definitions • Indications • Dosages
- Dosimetry • Recombinant human TSH

KEY POINTS

- Radioiodine ablation, adjuvant therapy, and treatment remain indispensable components in the armamentarium for the management of patients with well-differentiated thyroid cancer, whether the dosages of radioiodine-131 (131-I) are selected by either empiric or dosimetric approaches.
- The development of recombinant human thyroid stimulating hormone offers patients a safe and effective alternative to thyroid hormone withdrawal in the detection of recurrent/residual thyroid cancer and facilitation of radioiodine ablation.
- With a thorough understanding of the various approaches along with consideration of the many factors that may alter the dosage of radioiodine, the health care team should optimally develop an appropriate personalized treatment plan.

INTRODUCTION

The first report of patients with thyroid cancer who were treated with radioiodine-131 (131-I) was in 1946.[1] Since then, radioiodine (RAI) has been an important and well-accepted component in the armamentarium for the treatment of patients who have well-differentiated thyroid cancer (WDTC). The objective of this article is to present an overview of the use of radioiodine in the treatment of WDTC. This article reviews (1) definitions; (2) staging; (3) the 2 principal approaches for the selection of

---

Disclosure Statement: Dr D. Van Nostrand is a speaker and consultant for Jubliant Draximage. Drs D. Ylli and L. Wartofsky has nothing to disclose.
[a] Thyroid Cancer Research Center, MedStar Health Research Institute, 110 Irving Street, Washington, DC 20010, USA; [b] Department of Nuclear Medicine, Nuclear Medicine Research, MedStar Health Research Institute and MedStar Washington Hospital Center, 110 Irving Street, Washington, DC 20010, USA
* Corresponding author.
E-mail address: Leonard.wartofsky@medstar.net

Endocrinol Metab Clin N Am 48 (2019) 181–197
https://doi.org/10.1016/j.ecl.2018.11.005
0889-8529/19/© 2018 Elsevier Inc. All rights reserved.

radioiodine dosage; (4) the objectives of ablation, adjuvant therapy, and treatment; (5) the indications for ablation, adjuvant therapy, and treatment; (6) the recommendations for the use of radioiodine therapy contained in the guidelines of the American Thyroid Association (ATA) and the Society of Nuclear Medicine and Molecular Imaging; (7) the use of recombinant human thyroid-stimulation hormone (rhTSH) in radioiodine therapy; and (8) the MedStar Washington Hospital Center approach to 131-I therapy.

DEFINITIONS

Given differences in terminology throughout the world, usage of several terms is defined as follows: *remnant ablation* is the use of 131-I to destroy normal residual functioning thyroid tissue with the objectives of (1) facilitating the interpretation of subsequent serum thyroglobulin (Tg) levels, (2) increasing the sensitivity of detection of locoregional and/or metastatic disease on subsequent follow-up RAI whole-body scans, (3) maximizing the therapeutic effect of any subsequent 131-I treatments and (4) facilitating a postablation scan that may identify additional sites of disease that were not identified on the preablation scan or suspected if a preablation scan was not performed.[2,3]

Adjuvant treatment is the use of 131-I to destroy unknown microscopic thyroid cancer and/or suspected but unproved residual thyroid cancer to potentially decrease recurrence and mortality from thyroid cancer.[2,3]

Treatment is the use of 131-I to destroy known locoregional and/or distant metastasis with the objectives of potential cure, reduced recurrence and mortality from thyroid cancer, and/or palliation.[2,3]

Confusion may arise from the use of the term, *131-I therapy*, generically for remnant ablation, adjuvant treatment, or treatment of known locoregional or distant metastases. Although many physicians may argue that this distinction in the definitions is not necessary, the authors believe that differential use of the terms helps communicate time and the primary objective of the therapeutic intervention as well as help with the development and application of guidelines. *Dosage* is referred to in this publication as the amount of radioiodine administered in millicuries (mCi) or becquerels (Bq), and the term may be used interchangeably with the term, *activity*. The term, *dose*, should be reserved to express the absorbed dose of radiation to an organ or tumor and is expressed in rads or grays (Gy).

STAGING

A large number of staging systems currently exist, including the age, metastases, extent of tumor, and size of tumor (AMES); tumor, node, metastases (TNM); Ohio State scoring system; age, grade of histology, extent, and size of tumor (AGES) system; metastases, age, completeness of resection, invasion, and size of tumor (MACIS) system; and National Thyroid Cancer Treatment Cooperative Study (NTCTCS) system. The TNM system was developed by the American Joint Commission on Cancer (AJCC) and is by the American Thyroid Association (ATA) for the management guidelines for WDTC. Note that the TNM system has undergone changes in the recent 8th edition of the *AJCC Cancer Staging Manual*.[4,5] The main changes consist of (1) raising the age cutoff from 45 years of age at diagnosis to 55 years of age and (2) removing regional lymph node metastases and microscopic extrathyroidal extension from the definition of T3 disease. These changes are expected to downstage a significant number of patients and will likely be incorporated in the next iteration of the ATA guidelines.[4,5]

APPROACHES FOR THE SELECTION OF RADIOIODINE DOSAGE (ACTIVITY) FOR ABLATION, ADJUVANT THERAPY, OR TREATMENT

A dosage of radioiodine may be selected by 1 of 2 methods: empiric or dosimetric (**Fig. 1**). The *empiric approach* refers to administration of a fixed dosage of radioiodine as used for many decades[6–16] based typically on physician experience and modified by the physician weighting of various factors, such as (1) whether the dose is being given for ablation, adjuvant therapy, or treatment; (2) extent of tumor; (3) grade of histology; (4) patient age; (5) presence of distant metastases; and (6) whether the patient is a child or adult (**Box 1**). Several empiric approaches for the selection of dosages of 131-I for the treatment of metastatic WDTC[6–12] are described in **Fig. 2**.

Advantages of a fixed empiric dose include (1) ease of dosage selection, (2) a long history of use, and (3) a reasonably acceptable frequency and severity of complications. When the dose is given without a pretherapy diagnostic scan, an additional potential advantage is that the potential for stunning secondary to the diagnostic use of 131-I is avoided. Both the concept of stunning and the value of a preablation or pretreatment scans, however, in altering management prior to the administration of empiric fixed dosages are controversial. Although a complete discussion of these controversies is beyond the scope of this article, suffice it to say that the risk of stunning can be eliminated or reduced by using 123-I or by lowering the dosage of 131-I activity to 1 mCi to 2 mCi (0.037–0.074 GBq).[17] In the authors' view, the major disadvantage of the empiric approach is its failure to allow determination of whether or not the dose administered may (1) have a therapeutic effect and/or (2) may exceed the threshold radiation dose to a critical organ, such as the bone marrow. In other words, empiric fixed dosages by their nature make no attempt to determine either the minimal amount of radioiodine that delivers a lethal dose to the tumor or the maximum allowable safe dose. When a given empiric dose is not sufficiently effective and 1 or more subsequent doses is required, an additional potential limitation is that such multiple empiric fixed doses over time may not be equivalent to the same total dosimetrically determined radioiodine dosage given at 1 time. This may be the case for 2 reasons. First, dose rates (rad/h) may be important because fractionated dosages give lower dose rates. Secondly, previous nonlethal dosages may reduce the effectiveness of subsequent dosages.

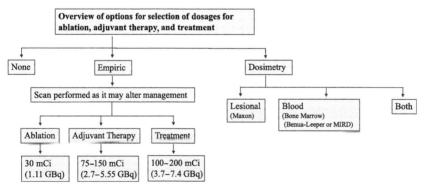

Fig. 1. This figure demonstrates an overview of various approaches for the selection of a dosage of 131-I for ablation, adjuvant therapy, or treatment. (*Adapted from* Van Nostrand D. 131-I treatment for distant metastases. In: Wartofsky L, Van Nostrand D, editors. Thyroid cancer: a comprehensive guide to clinical management. 3rd edition. New York: Springer; 2016. p. 618; with permission.)

Box 1
Various factors affecting selection of radioiodine dosages for ablation, adjuvant therapy, and treatment

- Stage (or risk)
- Convenience
- Cost
- Facilities
- Governmental regulations
- Age
- Histology
- Extent of surgery
- Percent uptake of radioiodine in residual thyroid tissue
- Volume of residual thyroid tissue
- Effective half-life of 131-I in the residual thyroid tissue
- Geometric shape of residual thyroid tissue
- Patient's compliance with low iodine diet
- Level of TSH
- Location of metastases (eg, lung vs bone vs brain)
- Number of metastases
- Size of metastasis(es)
- Number of organs involved
- Patient signs and symptoms secondary to metastases
- Uptake of radioiodine
- Radiological evidence of disease (eg, macronodular vs micronodular pulmonary disease on chest radiograph and/or CT)
- Potential for surgical excision
- Response of metastases to any previous radioiodine treatment (such as indicated by physical examination, radioiodine scan, chest radiograph, CT, MRI, ultrasound, and/or serum Tg levels)
- Total accumulative dosage of radioiodine
- Baseline complete blood cell count and differential pretreatment with special attention to granulocytes, lymphocytes, and platelets
- Response of absolute neutrophil and platelet count during the 3 weeks to 6 weeks after the previous treatment
- Change in baseline absolute neutrophil and platelet count after previous treatment
- Pulmonary function tests pretreatment
- Change in pulmonary function tests since previous treatment
- Bone marrow biopsy for assessment—not of metastases—but percent cellularity and adipose tissue in the bone marrow
- Concomitant disease(s)
- Patient desire(s)

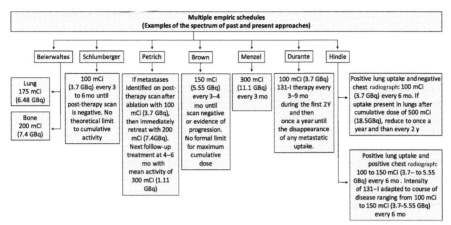

Fig. 2. This figure demonstrates various physicians' empiric approaches to the selection of 131-I activity for the treatment of patients with WDTC. (*Adapted from* Nostrand D. 131-I treatment for distant metastases. In: Wartofsky L, Van Nostrand D, editors. Thyroid cancer: a comprehensive guide to clinical management. 3rd edition. New York: Springer; 2016. p. 619; with permission.)

The *dosimetric approach* may be determined by either lesional and/or whole-body dosimetry (WBD). Lesional dosimetry as described by Maxon and colleagues[18] and Thomas and colleagues[19] determines the dosage of radioiodine to be administered on the basis of the radiation-absorbed dose (rads or grays) required to destroy a metastasis. The advantages of lesional dosimetry are (1) potentially improved outcomes by selecting and administering higher radioiodine dosages with greater chance of a tumoricidal effect and (2) administration of lower and safer radioiodine dosages that has a tumoricidal effect with reduced side effects, or (3) avoiding unnecessary costs and untoward effects in patients in whom tumoricidal doses cannot be achieved. The disadvantages of the lesional dosimetric approach include (1) increased cost and inconvenience to perform the dosimetry and (2) the limited number of facilities performing dosimetry.

WBD as described by Benua and Leeper[20] attempts to determine the maximum allowable activity (MTA) that delivers a maximum tolerable dose (MTD) to a critical organ to prevent or minimize unacceptable untoward events. The MTD is typically 200 rad (2 Gy) to blood, which serves as a surrogate for bone marrow. Using the medical internal radiation dose approach, 300 rad (3 Gy) to the blood has been proposed as the MTD.[21] The advantages of WBD are (1) ability to determine in each patient the MTA of radioiodine based on an MTD, (2) identification of up to 20% of patients whose MTA is less than the empiric fixed dosage that might have otherwise been given,[22,23] (3) safety of the administration of a 1-time higher radiation absorbed dose to metastases instead of multiple lower fractionated empiric dosages, (4) a long history of use, and (5) reasonable risk of complications relative to sites and severity of extent of distant metastatic disease. Limitations of the WBD approach are (1) increased cost and inconvenience; (2) failure to accurately estimate the radiation dose to the metastasis, thereby administering an MTA without therapeutic effect; (3) potential for stunning from the diagnostic dosage of 131-I; (4) failure to measure MTD to organs other than the blood, for example, salivary glands; and (5) the limited number of facilities performing dosimetry. To increase the number of nuclear centers that perform dosimetry, simplified dosimetry methods have been proposed.[24–27]

Whether dosimetry offers better outcomes compared with empiric therapy is still unclear. When only ablation is the goal, empiric doses should satisfactorily destroy the remnant thyroid tissue. When adjuvant therapy or treatment is indicated, however, whether the empiric or dosimetric approach provides better outcomes is controversial. Klubo-Gwiezdzinska and colleagues[28] have demonstrated in patients with locoregional disease a higher complete response rate in those treated by the dosimetric approach compared with patients receiving empiric therapy. On the other hand, Deandreis and colleagues[29] concluded that routine use of whole-body/blood clearance dosimetry without lesional dosimetry provided no difference in overall survival compared with empiric therapy. Limitations of both studies preclude any definitive conclusion. Existing ATA and SNMMI guidelines do not support one method over the other.[2,30] In conditions, such as reduced bone marrow reserve or impaired renal function, however, the SNMMI suggests dosimetry to ensure achieving the highest 131-I dose needed while delivering less than 2 Sv (200 rem) to bone marrow.[30] SNMMI also suggests dosimetry when prescribing high doses of 131-I exceeding 200 mCi (7.4 GBq) and in patients older than 55 years old.[30]

Unfortunately, well-controlled prospective outcome trials of patients with WDTC comparing empiric and dosimetric approaches are difficult to perform. Until further data are available, physicians should appreciate the benefits and disadvantages of both approaches and select the one most appropriate for a given patient.

THE OBJECTIVES OF RADIOIODINE ABLATION, ADJUVANT THERAPY, AND TREATMENT

Multiple objectives for radioiodine ablation have been proposed and include (1) ablating residual thyroid tissue to increase the sensitivity of detecting metastatic disease on subsequent follow-up radioiodine scans, (2) ablating residual thyroid tissue to facilitate interpretation of follow-up Tg levels, (3) potentially treating residual postoperative microscopic tumor, (4) decreasing rate of recurrence, (5) increasing survival, and (6) a means to obtain postablation whole-body scans that have higher sensitivity than diagnostic scans. The ATA guidelines state that ablation is "to facilitate detection of recurrent disease and initial staging by tests such as Tg and whole-body RAI scans." The objective of adjuvant therapy is "to improve disease-free survival by theoretically destroying suspected, but unproven residual disease, especially in patients at increased risk of disease recurrence."[2] The objective as noted by the SNMMI is "to eliminate residual normal tissue and presumed remaining cancerous tissue detected after thyroidectomy."[30] The objective of 131-I treatment remains "to improve disease-specific and disease-free survival by treating persistent disease in higher risk patients."[2] A clear distinction between ablation and adjuvant therapy is endorsed by the European Association of Nuclear Medicine.[31]

INDICATIONS FOR RADIOIODINE ABLATION AND ADJUVANT THERAPY

The ATA and the SNMMI have published their respective guidelines regarding the indications for ablation and adjuvant therapy.[2,30] The ATA recommendations are based on the AJCC TNM staging system and risk of stratification, and the SNMMI recommendations are based on staging, and both societies' recommendations are compared in **Table 1**.

In summary, the ATA guidelines make a clear distinction between ablation and adjuvant therapy, suggesting using ablation in low-risk patients only when adverse features are present and using adjuvant therapy in cases of intermediate-risk and high-risk patients. The SNMMI not having a distinction between ablation and adjuvant

Table 1
Indications of American Thyroid Association and Society of Nuclear Medicine and Molecular Imaging guidelines regarding radioiodine ablation and adjuvant therapy

Stage/Risk Stratification	Recommendations
ATA guidelines	
ATA low-risk differentiated thyroid cancer patients	RAI ablation is not routinely recommended after thyroidectomy[a] (weak recommendation, low-quality evidence).
Unifocal papillary microcarcinoma in absence of other adverse features	RAI ablation is not routinely recommended (strong recommendation, moderate-quality evidence).
Multifocal papillary microcarcinoma in absence of other adverse features	RAI ablation is not routinely recommended[a] (weak recommendation, low-quality evidence).
ATA intermediate-risk level differentiated thyroid cancer	RAI adjuvant therapy should be considered (weak recommendation, low-quality evidence).
ATA high-risk patients	RAI adjuvant therapy is routinely recommended (strong recommendation, moderate-quality evidence).
Society of Nuclear Medicine and Molecular Imaging guidelines	
Patient with a maximum tumor diameter >1 cm	RAI ablation is recommended.
Patients with maximum tumor diameter <1 cm in presence of high-risk features[b]	RAI ablation is recommended.
Very-low-risk and low-risk thyroid cancer	RAI treatment is controversial.

[a] Features that could modulate recurrence risk, disease follow-up, and patient preferences are relevant to RAI decision.
[b] Aggressive histology (Hurthle cell, insular, diffuse sclerosing, tall cell, columnar cell, trabecular, solid, and poorly differentiated subtypes of papillary carcinoma), lymphatic or vascular invasion, lymph node or distant metastases, multifocal disease, capsular invasion or penetration, perithyroidal soft-tissue involvement, or an elevated antithyroglobulin antibody level after thyroidectomy (so that scintigraphy can be used for surveillance).
Adapted from Haugen BR, Alexander EK, Bible KC, et al. 2015 American Thyroid Association management guidelines for adult patients with thyroid nodules and differentiated thyroid cancer: the American Thyroid Association guidelines task force on thyroid nodules and differentiated thyroid cancer. Thyroid 2016;26(1):1–133; and Silberstein EB, Alavi A, Balon HR, et al. The SNMMI practice guideline for therapy of thyroid disease with 131I 3.0. J Nucl Med 2012;53(10):1633–51, with permission.

therapy suggests ablation in tumors less than 1 cm with high-risk features and in all tumors larger than 1 cm.

INDICATIONS OF RADIOIODINE TREATMENT

ATA and SNMMI guidelines for 131-I treatment of locoregional disease, pulmonary metastases, bone metastases, and brain metastases are compared in **Table 2**.

RADIOIODINE DOSAGE SELECTION FOR ABLATION, ADJUVANT THERAPY, AND TREATMENT

Dosage recommendations and guidelines by the ATA and SNMMI for ablation, adjuvant therapy, and treatment are discussed later (**Table 3**). ATA guidelines suggest

Table 2
Indications from American Thyroid Association and Society of Nuclear Medicine and Molecular Imaging guidelines regarding radioiodine treatment

Locoregional disease	
ATA	RAI may be used in patients with low-volume disease or in combination with surgery in case of bulky disease.
SNMMI	Advanced local or regional disease may be treated first with surgical debulking, then with 131-I. In general 131-I therapy is less effective in bulky disease with a diameter greater than 1–2 cm.

Distant metastasis		
ATA		
	Pulmonary	(1) Pulmonary micrometastases: RAI treatment is recommended every 6–12 mo as long as disease continues to concentrate RAI and respond clinically (strong recommendation, moderate-quality evidence). (2) Macronodular metastases: may be treated with RAI and treatment repeated when objective benefit is demonstrated (decrease in the size of the lesions, decreasing Tg) (weak recommendation, low-quality evidence).
	Bone metastases	In iodine-avid bone metastases, RAI therapy should be used, although rarely curative (strong recommendation, moderate-quality evidence).
	Brain metastases	Surgical resection and EBRT are the mainstays of therapy for CNS metastases. RAI therapy can be considered in case of RAI-avid CNS metastases; in that case, stereotactic EBRT and concomitant glucocorticoid therapy are recommended prior to RAI therapy (weak recommendation, low-quality evidence).
SNMMI		RAI therapy is recommended for treatment of distant metastases. The radiation dose to the bone marrow is typically the limiting factor. Dosimetry is indicated in case of a high activity 131-I, in patients over 50–55 y old, especially in the presence of a reduced glomerular filtration rate and when lung metastases may concentrate a large amount of 131-I.

Absence of structurally evident disease	
ATA	In absence of structurally evident disease, stimulated serum Tg <10 ng/mL with thyroid hormone withdrawal or <5 ng/mL with rhTSH, the patient can be followed without empiric RAI therapy (weak recommendation, low-quality evidence). RAI therapy may be considered in patients with significantly elevated serum Tg levels, rapidly rising serum Tg levels, or rising ant-Tg antibody levels, in whom imaging (anatomic neck/chest imaging and/or fludeoxyglucose F 18–PET/CT) has failed to reveal a tumor source that is, amenable to directed therapy. If empiric RAI therapy is given and the post-therapy scan is negative, the patient should be considered to have RAI-refractory disease and no further RAI therapy should be administered (weak recommendation, low-quality evidence).
SNMMI	In the absence of anti-TG antibodies, an elevated or rising serum TG level may be an indication for empiric RAI therapy.

Abbreviations: CNS, Central Nervous System; SNMMI, Society of Nuclear Medicine and Molecular Images.

Adapted from Haugen BR, Alexander EK, Bible KC, et al. 2015 American thyroid association management guidelines for adult patients with thyroid nodules and differentiated thyroid cancer: The American thyroid association guidelines task force on thyroid nodules and differentiated thyroid cancer. Thyroid 2016;26(1):1–133; and Silberstein EB, Alavi A, Balon HR, et al. The SNMMI practice guideline for therapy of thyroid disease with 131I 3.0. J Nucl Med 2012;53(10):1633–51, with permission

Table 3
Comparison of recommendations from American Thyroid Association and Society of Nuclear Medicine and Molecular Imaging regarding radioiodine usage

	Recommendations
Ablation and adjuvant therapy	
ATA—ablation	1. If RAI remnant ablation is performed, a low administered activity of 30 mCi (1.11 GBq) is favored (strong recommendation, high-quality evidence).
	2. Higher administered activities may need to be considered for patients receiving near-total thyroidectomy in which a larger remnant is suspected (weak recommendation, low-quality evidence).
ATA—adjuvant therapy	RAI dosages up to 150 mCi (5.55 GBq) are generally recommended (weak recommendation, low-quality evidence).
SNMMI	For postoperative ablation of thyroid bed remnants, activity in the range of 30–100 mCi (1.11–3.7 GBq) is typically prescribed, depending on the radioiodine uptake measurement and amount of residual functioning tissue present.
Locoregional disease	
ATA	(1) No recommendation can be made about the superiority of 1 method of RAI administration over another (empiric high activity vs blood and/or body dosimetry vs lesional dosimetry) (no recommendation, insufficient evidence).
	(2) Empirically dosages of 131-I exceeding 150 mCi (5.55 GBq) that often potentially exceed the maximum tolerable tissue dose should be avoided in patients over age 70 y (strong recommendation, moderate-quality evidence).
SNMMI	For treatment of thyroid cancer in the cervical or mediastinal lymph nodes, RAI activity in the range of 150–200 mCi (5.55–7.4 GBq) is administered.
Distant metastasis	
ATA	
Pulmonary	Micrometastasis
	• Empiric RAI activity of 100–200 mCi (3.7–7.4 GBq) or 100–150 mCi (3.7–5.55 GBq) for patients >70 y old) or
	• Determined by dosimetry[a]
	Macrometastasis
	• Empiric dosage: 100–200 mCi (3.7–7.4 GBq) or
	• Lesional dosimetry or WBD[a]
Bone metastases	• RAI empiric dosage of 100–200 mCi (3.7–7.4 GBq) or
	• Determined by dosimetry (weak recommendation, low-quality evidence)
SNMMI	For treatment of distant metastases, an activity of 200 mCi (7.4 GBq) or more is suggested.
	To reduce the risk of significant myelosuppression, retention of 131-I in the body at 48 h should be <120 mCi (4.44 GBq), or <80 mCi (2.96 GBq) if diffuse lung metastases are present, to reduce the risk of radiation pneumonitis as well.
Absence of structurally evident disease	
ATA	RAI empiric activity of 100–200 mCi (3.7–7.4 GBq) or dosimetry (Weak recommendation, low-quality evidence)
SNMMI	Empiric RAI activity of 150–200 mCi (5.55–7.4 GBq) with marrow dosimetry if indicated

[a] Dosimetry, should limit whole-body retention to 80 mCi (2.96 GBq) at 48 h and 200 cGy to the bone marrow.

Adapted from Haugen BR, Alexander EK, Bible KC, et al. 2015 American thyroid association management guidelines for adult patients with thyroid nodules and differentiated thyroid cancer: The American thyroid association guidelines task force on thyroid nodules and differentiated thyroid cancer. Thyroid 2016;26(1):1–133; and Silberstein EB, Alavi A, Balon HR, et al. The SNMMI Practice Guideline for Therapy of Thyroid Disease with 131I 3.0. J Nucl Med 2012;53(10):1633–51, with permission.)

activity in the range of 30 mCi (1.11 GBq) for postoperative remnant ablation, although ablation could be waived for low-risk patients with no evidence of adverse features. For intermediate-risk or high-risk patients, adjuvant therapy dosage can range from 75 mCi to 150 mCi (2.77–5.55 GBq) based on individual risk factors for residual disease. For recurrence or distant metastases, 131-I empiric treatment dosage of 100 mCi to 200 mCi (3.7–7.4 GBq) is suggested or an activity estimated by dosimetry. The SNMMI guidelines differ slightly and suggest a postoperative ablation activity of 30 mCi to 100 mCi (1.11–3.7 GBq) and up to 200 mCi (7.4 GBq) for 131-I treatment given either on empiric or dosimetric basis.

USE OF RECOMBINANT HUMAN THYROID-STIMULATING HORMONE FOR RADIOIODINE ABLATION, ADJUVANT TREATMENT, OR TREATMENT

As described previously, virtually all traditional methods and approaches for radioiodine ablation, adjuvant therapy, or treatment require patients to be hypothyroid with elevated endogenous TSH levels either after thyroidectomy or after levothyroxine withdrawal. As a consequence, they undergo a period of hypothyroidism ranging from 3 weeks to 6 weeks with many unpleasant symptoms associated with thyroid hormone deficiency. With the development of rhTSH (thyrotropin alfa for injection [Thyrogen, Genzyme, Cambridge, MA]) physicians could offer patients an alternative option to achieve serum TSH elevations essential for scan and therapy.[32] Use of rhTSH has improved cancer diagnostic sensitivity by facilitating measurements of Tg to detect residual cancer while permitting radioiodine scans comparable to scans performed after thyroxine withdrawal.[33] Consequently, use of rhTSH has become a safe and effective alternative to thyroid hormone withdrawal in the detection of recurrent or residual thyroid cancer and for facilitation of radioiodine ablation.

The most common procedure is as follows:

Monday	Blood drawn for Tg
	Thyrogen injection 0.9 mg (intramuscular injection)
Tuesday	Thyrogen injection 0.9 mg (intramuscular injection)
Wednesday	4 mCi (0.148GBq) dose of 131-I
Thursday	No procedures
Friday	Blood drawn for Tg
	Whole-body scan

It was inevitable that its use would be extended to examine the efficacy of rhTSH as an alternative to thyroxine withdrawal for preparation prior to radioiodine treatment of either or both the initial ablation and for subsequent therapies for persistent disease.

Ablation and Adjuvant Therapy with Recombinant Human Thyroid-stimulating Hormone Preparation

The Memorial Sloan Kettering Cancer Center group pioneered the use of rhTSH for ablation therapy and reported comparable efficacy in achieving resolution of visible thyroid bed uptake with rhTSH ablation versus ablation after thyroxine withdrawal.[34] A recent report by Bartenstein and colleagues[35] described no differences in the ablation rate comparing rhTSH with withdrawal preparation in 144 high-risk patients with a T4 primary tumor. And a meta-analysis, including 1535 patients, comparing the 2 preparation methods indicated similar ablation rates. Patients prepared with rhTSH enjoyed a better quality of life at the time of ablation.[36] Although long-term follow-up data are lacking, recent retrospective studies suggest that final clinical outcomes (recurrence rates and likelihood of achieving no evidence of disease status at final follow-up) over 5 years to 10 years of follow-up are very similar with either method of preparation.[37] Nevertheless, physicians using rhTSH off-label for patients with metastatic disease should inform their patients that long-term outcomes are unknown. Currently, rhTSH is approved in Europe for preparation for 131-I treatment of patients with metastatic disease but is not Food and Drug Administration approved in the United States except for ablation.

Although it is common practice to place patients on a low iodine diet prior to ablation by either method, serum and urine iodine levels re higher when ablation is done with rhTSH stimulation due to iodine derived from the thyroxine being taken by the patient. Although the higher iodine milieu might theoretically reduce therapeutic efficacy of radioiodine, the comparable results for satisfactory ablation, described previously, seem to render this moot.

ATA guidelines suggest that preparation with rhTSH stimulation: (1) is acceptable in case of patients with ATA low-risk and ATA intermediate-risk differentiated thyroid cancer without extensive lymph node involvement (ie, T1–T3, N0/Nx/N1a, M0), in whom RAI remnant ablation or adjuvant therapy is planned; (2) is considered prior to adjuvant 131-I therapy in patients with ATA intermediate-risk differentiated thyroid cancer with extensive lymph node disease in the absence of distant metastases. The protocol for adjuvant therapy is similar to that described previously, with 0.9 mg rhTSH given intramuscularly on 2 consecutive days with the radioiodine dosage given 24 hours after the second injection.

Radioiodine-131 Treatment after Recombinant Human Thyroid-stimulating Hormone Preparation

Use of rhTSH preparation in lieu of thyroxine withdrawal for subsequent therapy for residual or metastatic thyroid cancer clearly represents an off-label use, and few studies have been published to support such use. Klubo-Gwiezdzinska and colleagues[38] retrospectively studied 56 patients with distant metastasis prepared by rhTSH or THW, showing comparable benefits from treatment based on survival rate, progression-free survival, biochemical and structural responses, and side effects in both methods. From a more technical perspective, Plyku and colleagues[39] studied 4 patients prepared with both THW and rhTSH and observed a higher absorbed dose per unit administered activity of 131-I after withdrawal compared with rhTSH, but the limited study does not permit definitive conclusions. The ATA guidelines indicate that insufficient outcome data exist to recommend this practice although rhTSH use might be justified in selected patients with comorbidities, making withdrawal and the attendant hypothyroidism of significant risk to the patient. Another indication for rhTSH is in the rare circumstance of patients with coincidental hypopituitarism who cannot raise their endogenous TSH after withdrawal or patients with such extensive metastatic disease that tumor production of thyroid hormone continues to suppress pituitary secretion of TSH after thyroxine withdrawal.

MedStar WASHINGTON HOSPITAL CENTER APPROACH

For those patients to be ablated with 131-I, the authors' facility typically uses an empiric dose of 30 mCi (1.11 GBq). Ablation, however, often may be deferred for low-risk patients with absent adverse features. If adjuvant therapy is required, an empiric or a dosimetrically determined dosage is recommended depending on clinical circumstances. If evidence of metastases prior to the 123-I preablation scan is lacking and if that scan demonstrates none of the findings in **Box 2**, then the adult patient is given an empiric dosage of 75 mCi to 150 mCi (2.78–5.55 GBq). For pediatric patients, based on body weight and body surface, the Reynolds modification factors of prescribed 131-I activity shown in **Table 4** are followed.[40] Empiric dosages for children or adults may be further modified, however, on an individual basis by 1 or more factors noted in **Box 1**. For children with diffuse lung uptake, significant distant metastasis, or limited bone marrow reserve, it is important to use WBD to calculate the largest activity of 131-I that could safely be administered so that the absorbed activity to the blood does not exceed 200 rad (2 Gy) and the whole-body retention 48 hours after administration does not exceed 120 mCi (4.44 GBq) in the absence, or 80 mCi (2.96 BGq) in the presence, of iodine-avid diffuse lung metastasis, respectively.[41] Adult dosage may also be modified based on the degree of thyroid bed uptake and the number and size of the area(s) of residual thyroid tissue seen on the diagnostic scan (**Fig. 3**). This has been discussed in more detail elsewhere.[42]

When a patient preablation scan demonstrates 1 of the findings in **Box 2**, then either (1) the empiric dosage may be increased, (2) WBD may be performed with the dosage selected, as discussed previously, or (3) the ablation or treatment may be postponed until further evaluation or treatment is performed. Further evaluation typically starts with imaging by ultrasound and/or MRI of the neck, CT of the chest, fluorodeoxyglucose-PET scanning, and fine-needle aspiration for cytologic examination of any lesions imaged that seem suspicious. With positive cytology for cancer, additional surgical intervention may be recommended.

Box 2
Utility of a preablation scan

- Pattern and the percent uptake of iodine in the thyroid bed or neck area that could alter the management or ablative/treatment dosage
  - A single area of 5% to 30% uptake, which suggests considering additional surgery or modifying the dosage activity of RAI
  - A single area of low uptake less than 1%, which suggest modifying the empiric dosage of RAI
  - A pattern of RAI uptake consistent with cervical metastasis suggesting (1) further evaluation with MR or high-resolution ultrasound; (2) additional fine needle aspiration, surgery, or both; and/or (3) the use a larger empiric prescribed activity of 131-I

- Distant metastasis that may alter the evaluation and/or the management of the patient prior to RAI therapy
  - Focal or diffuse uptake in lung that may warrant further evaluation with CT without contrast, pulmonary function tests, and dosimetry to determine the maximum tolerated prescribed activity without exceeding 48-h retained body weight. The latter may increase or decrease dosage relative to an empiric dosage and may help minimize the potential for acute radiation pneumonitis and pulmonary fibrosis.
  - Focal area suggesting bone metastasis that may warrant further evaluation with CT, surgery, larger empiric prescribed activity, dosimetry, and/or coordination of other treatment modalities, such as metastasectomy, subsequent external radiotherapy, or radiofrequency ablation, to name a few
  - Focal uptake in the head that may warrant an MR Em of the brain. If the focal area is a brain metastasis, then consideration of surgery. If external radiation therapy (ie, gamma knife) radioiodine is administered, then a reduction of the empiric prescribed activity, and/or treatment with steroids, glycerol, and/or mannitol prior to treatment with 131-I.

Adapted from Atkins F, Van Nostrand D. Radioiodine whole body imaging. In: Wartofsky L, Van Nostrand D, editors. Thyroid cancer: a comprehensive guide to clinical management. 3rd edition. New York: Springer; 2016. p. 145; with permission.

Table 4
Reynolds modifications factors of prescribed activity for treatment of children

Factor	Body Weight (kg)	Body Surface Area (m^2)
0.2	10	0.4
0.4	25	0.8
0.6	40	1.2
0.8	55	1.4
1.0	77	1.7

Body surface area = 0.1 × (weight in kg)$^{0.67}$.
Adapted from Van Nostrand D. Radioiodine treatment for distant metastases. In Wartofsky L, Van Nostrand D, editors: Thyroid cancer: a comprehensive guide to clinical management. 3rd edition. New York: Springer; 2016. p. 620; with permission.

For patients with known metastases prior to the first pretreatment scan or for follow-up of patients with elevated Tg levels, known or strongly suspected locoregional recurrence or distant metastatic disease, the authors perform WBD. Administered dosage does not exceed 80 mCi (2.96 GBq) whole-body retention at 48 hours in patients with pulmonary metastases or 120 mCi (4.44 GBq) whole-body retention at

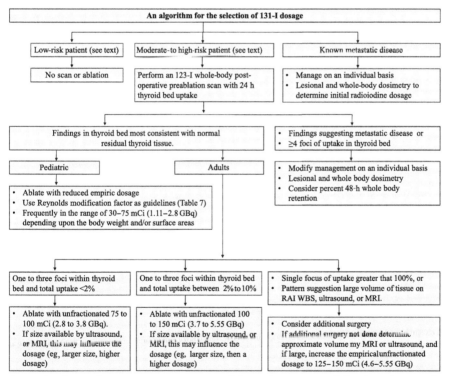

Fig. 3. This figure demonstrates an overview of the author's approach for the selection of a dosage of 131-I for ablation, adjuvant therapy, or treatment of patients with WDTC at MedStar Washington Hospital Center. WBS, whole body scan. (*Adapted from* Van Nostrand D. Radioiodine ablation. In: Wartofsky L, Van Nostrand D, editors. Thyroid cancer: a comprehensive guide to clinical management. 2nd edition. Totowa (NJ): Humana Press; 2006. p. 611–2; with permission.)

48 hours in all other patients. A low diagnostic dosage of 131-I in the range of 1 mCi to 2 mCi (0.037–0.074 GBq) is used to avoid any significant stunning. The final treatment dosage of 131-I is selected to not exceed the MTA and threshold for whole-body retention. The selected dosage may be individualized and decreased based on 1 or more of the factors listed in **Box 1**.

SUMMARY

Radioiodine ablation, adjuvant therapy, and treatment remain indispensable components in the armamentarium for the management of patients with WDTC, whether the dosages of 131-I are selected by either empiric or dosimetric approaches. With a thorough understanding of the various approaches along with consideration of the many factors that may alter the dosage of radioiodine, the health care team should optimally develop an appropriate personalized treatment plan.

Footnote

As an adjunct to this review on ablation and therapy, an understanding of the value of preablation scans is related insofar as they offer significant information that may (1) modify the management of a patient before rather than after the administration of the preablation dosage of radioiodine (**Box 2**) and (2) potentially improve outcomes. Although preablation scans do not provide unexpected important information in all cases, the potential that the information gained will alter management is worth the reasonable cost and minimal inconvenience.[13]

REFERENCES

1. Seidin SM, Marinelli LD, Oshry E. Radioactive iodine therapy effect on functioning metastases of adenocarcinoma of the thyroid. JAMA 1946;132:838–47.
2. Haugen BR, Alexander EK, Bible KC, et al. 2015 American thyroid association management guidelines for adult patients with thyroid nodules and differentiated thyroid cancer: the American thyroid association guidelines task force on thyroid nodules and differentiated thyroid cancer. Thyroid 2016;26(1):1–133.
3. Van Nostrand D. The benefits and risks of I-131 therapy in patients with well-differentiated thyroid cancer. Thyroid 2009;19(12):1381–91.
4. Tuttle RM, Haugen B, Perrier ND. Updated American Joint Committee on Cancer/tumor-node-metastasis staging system for differentiated and anaplastic thyroid cancer (eighth edition): what changed and why? Thyroid 2017;27(6):751–6.
5. Amin MB, Edge S, Greene F, et al, editors. AJCC cancer staging manual. New York: Springer; 2017.
6. Beierwaltes WH, Rabbani R, Dmuchowski C, et al. An analysis of ablation of thyroid remnants" with I-131 in 511 patients from 1947-1984: experience at University of Michigan. J Nucl Med 1984;25:1287–93.
7. Schlumberger M, Challeton C, De Vathaire F, et al. Radioactive iodine treatment and external radiotherapy for lung and bone metastases from thyroid carcinoma. J Nucl Med 1996;37:598–605.
8. Petrich T, Widjaja A, Musholt TJ, et al. Outcome after radioiodine therapy in 107 patients with differentiated thyroid carcinoma and initial bone metastases: side effects and influence of age. Eur J Nucl Med 2001;28:203–8.
9. Brown AP, Greening WP, McCready VR, et al. Radioiodine treatment of metastatic thyroid carcinoma: The Royal Marsden hospital experience. Br J Radiol 1984;57:323–7.

10. Menzel C, Grunwald F, Schomburg A, et al. "High-Dose" Radioiodine therapy in advanced differentiated thyroid carcinoma. J Nucl Med 1996;37:1496–503.
11. Hindié E, Melliere D, Lange F, et al. Functioning pulmonary metastases of thyroid cancer: does radioiodine influence the prognosis? Eur J Nucl Med Mol Imaging 2003;30:974–81.
12. Durante C, Haddy N, Baudin E, et al. Long-term outcome of 444 patients with distant metastases from papillary and follicular thyroid carcinoma: benefits and limits of radioiodine therapy. J Clin Endocrinol Metab 2006;91(8):2892–9.
13. Castagna MG, Cevenini G, Theodoropoulou A, et al. Post-surgical thyroid ablation with low or high radioiodine activities results in similar outcomes in intermediate risk differentiated thyroid cancer patients. Eur J Endocrinol 2013;169(1): 23–9.
14. Mallick U, Harmer C, Yap B, et al. Ablation with low-dose radioiodine and thyrotropin alfa in thyroid cancer. N Engl J Med 2012;366(18):1674–85.
15. Verburg FA, Mäder U, Reiners C, et al. Long-term survival in differentiated thyroid cancer is worse after low-activity initial post-surgical 131I therapy in both high- and low-risk patients. J Clin Endocrinol Metab 2014;99(12):4487–96.
16. Schlumberger M, Leboulleux S, Catargi B, et al. Outcome after ablation in patients with low-risk thyroid cancer (ESTIMABL1): 5-year follow-up results of a randomized, phase 3, equivalence trial. Lancet Diabetes Endocrinol 2018;6(8): 618–26.
17. Van Nostrand D. Stunning: does it exist? a commentary. In: Wartofsky L, Van Nostrand D, editors. Thyroid cancer: a comprehensive guide to clinical management. New York: Springer; 2016. p. 243–5.
18. Maxon HR, Thomas SR, Hertzbert VS, et al. Relation between effective radiation dose and outcome of radioiodine therapy for thyroid cancer. N Engl J Med 1983; 309:937–41.
19. Thomas SR, Maxon HR, Kereiakes JG. In vivo quantitation of lesion radioactivity using external counting methods. Med Phys 1976;3:253–5.
20. Benua RS, Leeper RD. A method and rationale for treating metastatic thyroid carcinoma with the largest safe dose of I-131. In: Medeiros-Neto G, Gaitan E, editors. Frontiers in thyroidology. Vol. 2. New York: Plenum Medical Book Co; 1986. p. 1317–21.
21. Dorn R, Kopp J, Vogt H, et al. Dosimetry-guided radioactive iodine treatment in patients with metastatic differentiated thyroid cancer: largest safe dose using a risk-based approach. J Nucl Med 2003;44:451–6.
22. Kulkarni K, Van Nostrand D, Atkins FB, et al. The frequency with which empiric amounts of radioiodine "over-" or "under-" treat patients with metastatic well-differentiated thyroid cancer. Thyroid 2006;16:1019–23.
23. Tuttle RM, Leboeuf R, Robbins RJ, et al. Empiric radioactive iodine dosing regimens frequently exceed maximum tolerated activity levels in elderly patients with thyroid cancer. J Nucl Med 2006;47:1587–91.
24. Hanscheid H, Lassmann M, Luster M, et al. Blood dosimetry from a single measurement of the whole body radioiodine retention in patients with differentiated thyroid carcinoma. Endocr Relat Cancer 2009;16:1283–9.
25. Van Nostrand D, Atkins F, Moreau S, et al. Utility of the radioiodine whole-body retention at 48 hours for modifying empiric activity of 131-iodine for the treatment of metastatic well-differentiated thyroid carcinoma. Thyroid 2009;19:1093–8.
26. Jentzen W, Bockisch A, Ruhlmann M. Assessment of simplified blood dose protocols for the estimation of the maximum tolerable activity in thyroid cancer patients undergoing radioiodine therapy using 124I. J Nucl Med 2015;56:832–8.

27. Atkins F, Van Nostrand D, Moreau S, et al. Validation of a simple thyroid cancer dosimetry model based on the fractional whole-body retention at 48 hours post-administration of (131)I. Thyroid 2015;25(12):1347–50.

28. Klubo-Gwiezdzinska J, Van Nostrand D, Atkins F, et al. Efficacy of dosimetric versus empiric prescribed activity of 131I for therapy of differentiated thyroid cancer. J Clin Endocrinol Metab 2011;96(10):3217–25.

29. Deandreis D, Rubino C, Tala H, et al. Comparison of empiric versus whole-body/blood clearance dosimetry-based approach to radioactive iodine treatment in patients with metastases from differentiated thyroid cancer. J Nucl Med 2017;58(5): 717–22.

30. Silberstein EB, Alavi A, Balon HR, et al. The SNMMI practice guideline for therapy of thyroid disease with 131I 3.0. J Nucl Med 2012;53(10):1633–51.

31. Verburg FA, Aktolun C, Chiti A, et al, EANM and the EANM Thyroid Committee. Why the European Association of Nuclear Medicine has declined to endorse the 2015 American Thyroid Association management guidelines for adult patients with thyroid nodules and differentiated thyroid cancer. Eur J Nucl Med Mol Imaging 2016 Jun;43(6):1001–5.

32. Ringel MD, Burgun SJ. Recombinant human thyrotropin. In: Wartofsky L, Van Nostrand D, editors. Thyroid cancer: a comprehensive guide to clinical management. New York: Springer; 2016. p. 119–29.

33. Ladenson PW. Recombinant thyrotropin for detection of recurrent thyroid cancer. Trans Am Clin Climatol Assoc 2002;113:21–30.

34. Robbins RJ, Larson SM, Sinha N, et al. A retrospective review of the effectiveness of recombinant human TSH as a preparation for radioiodine thyroid remnant ablation. J Nucl Med 2002;43(11):1482–8.

35. Bartenstein P, Calabuig EC, Maini CL, et al. High-risk patients with differentiated thyroid cancer T4 primary tumors achieve remnant ablation equally well using rhTSH or thyroid hormone withdrawal. Thyroid 2014;24(3):480–7.

36. Tu J, Wang S, Huo Z, et al. Recombinant human thyrotropin-aided versus thyroid hormone withdrawal-aided radioiodine treatment for differentiated thyroid cancer after total thyroidectomy: a meta-analysis. Radiother Oncol 2014;110(1):25–30.

37. Sabra MM, Tuttle RM. Recombinant human thyroid-stimulating hormone to stimulate 131-I uptake for remnant ablation and adjuvant therapy. Endocr Pract 2013;19(1):149–56.

38. Klubo-Gwiezdzinska J, Burman KD, Van Nostrand D, et al. Radioiodine treatment of metastatic thyroid cancer: relative efficacy and side effect profile of preparation by thyroid hormone withdrawal versus recombinant human thyrotropin. Thyroid 2012;22(3):310–7.

39. Plyku D, Hobbs RF, Huang K, et al. Recombinant human thyroid-stimulating hormone versus thyroid hormone withdrawal in 124I PET/CT-based dosimetry for 131I therapy of metastatic differentiated thyroid cancer. J Nucl Med 2017; 58(7):1146–54.

40. Reynolds JC. Comparison of I-131 absorbed radiation doses in children and adults; a tool for estimating therapeutic I-131 doses in children. In: Robbins J, editor. Treatment of thyroid cancer in children, DOE/EH-0406, US Department of Commerce Technology Administration, National Technical Information Service. Springfield, Virginia; 1994. p. 127–35.

41. Francis G, Waguespsk SG, Bauer AJ, et al. Management Guidelines for the Children with thyroid nodules and differentiated thyroid cancer. Thyroid 2015;25(7): 716–59.

42. Van Nostrand D. Remnant ablation, adjuvant and treatment of locoregional metastasis with I^{131}. In: Wartofsky L, Van Nostrand D, editors. Thyroid cancer: a comprehensive guide to clinical management. 3rd edition. New York: Springer; 2016. p. 611–2.
43. Van Nostrand D. To perform or not to perform radioiodine scans prior to 131 Remnant Ablation? PRO. In: Wartofsky L, Van Nostrand D, editors. Thyroid cancer: a comprehensive guide to clinical management. New York: Springer; 2016. p. 245–54.

Management of Papillary Thyroid Microcarcinoma

Juan P. Brito, MD, MSc[a,b,*], Ian D. Hay, MD, PhD, FRCP[c]

KEYWORDS

- Papillary thyroid cancer • Microcarcinoma • Management • Shared decision-making

KEY POINTS

- The incidence of thyroid cancer has increased, mainly due to the incidental finding of papillary thyroid microcarcinomas (PTM).
- Patients with PMC should be offered individualized treatment options according to the biology of the tumor and the patient's context and values.
- Shared decision making is an approach of care that helps clinician individualize the care of patients with PTM.

EPIDEMIOLOGY

The incidence of thyroid cancer has increased worldwide. In the United States, thyroid cancer incidence has tripled over the last 3 decades from 4.9 to 14.7 per 100,000 people in 2011.[1] The increase has been mostly caused by papillary thyroid cancer (PTC), particularly thyroid cancers 1 cm or less in size, so-called papillary thyroid microcarcinomas (PTMs).[2] **Fig. 1** illustrates the changing frequency of small tumors confined to the thyroid diagnosed annually at the Mayo Clinic in Rochester, Minnesota, during 1936 to 2015.[3] In the United States, between 1974 and 2013, the annual percentage change for thyroid cancer less than or equal to 1 cm (9%) was, on average, higher than that for tumors greater than 1 cm to less than or equal to 2 cm (5%), greater than 2 cm to less than or equal to 4 cm (4.5%), and greater than 4 cm (6%). In fact, it is estimated that 39% of all thyroid cancers are PTM.[4] **Fig. 2** demonstrates the proportion of PTCs

Disclosure: J.P. Brito is supported by the Karl-Erivan Haub Family Career Development Award in Cancer Research at Mayo Clinic in Rochester, honoring Richard F. Emslander, MD. I.D. Hay is funded by the Richard F. Emslander Professorship in Endocrine Research, the William Stamps Farrish Fund, and the Colin and Brenda Reed Family Foundation.

[a] Division of Diabetes, Endocrinology, Metabolism, and Nutrition, Department of Medicine, Mayo Clinic, 200 First Street Southwest, Rochester, MN 55905, USA; [b] Knowledge and Evaluation Research Unit, Mayo Clinic, 200 First Street Southwest, Rochester, MN 55905, USA; [c] Division of Diabetes, Endocrinology, Metabolism, and Nutrition, Department of Medicine, Mayo Clinic, 200 First Street Southwest, Rochester, MN 55905, USA
* Corresponding author. 200 First Street Southwest, Rochester, MN 55905.
E-mail address: brito.juan@mayo.edu

Endocrinol Metab Clin N Am 48 (2019) 199–213
https://doi.org/10.1016/j.ecl.2018.10.006
0889-8529/19/© 2018 Elsevier Inc. All rights reserved.

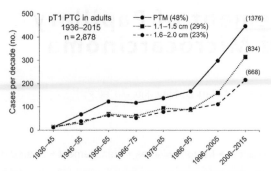

Fig. 1. Changing frequency of various sizes (maximum tumor diameter) of adult pT1 (small tumors confined to the thyroid) PTC tumors seen in 2878 adults managed at the Mayo Clinic in Rochester, Minnesota, during 8 decades (1936–2015). (*Data from* Hay ID, Johnson TR, Kaggal S, et al. Papillary Thyroid Carcinoma (PTC) in children and adults: comparison of initial presentation and long-term postoperative outcome in 4432 patients consecutively treated at the Mayo Clinic during eight decades (1936–2015). World J Surg 2018;42(2):329–42.)

by tumor size seen at the Mayo Clinic from 1936 to 2015. These PTMs have been found in 5% to 10% of thyroid glands removed for benign thyroid conditions or examined at autopsy in patients who died of unrelated causes.[5,6] Because of the increased detection of tiny thyroid tumors in older patients, the most common presentation of thyroid cancer in the United States is now a PTM in a patient older than 45 years old.[7]

Recent changes suggested by the American Thyroid Association (ATA) guidelines for the management of thyroid nodules might affect current thyroid cancer incidence trends.[8] The guideline recommends that thyroid nodules less than or equal to 1 cm should not undergo biopsy unless there are ultrasonographic and clinical symptoms of potentially aggressive malignant behavior (eg, clear evidence of extrathyroid extension, vocal cord paralysis), features that are not typically found in patients with PTM.[8] As a result, it is possible that more thyroid nodules harboring PTM will not undergo biopsy, thereby decreasing the incidence of thyroid cancer. Although there is as yet no clear evidence of an impact of the new guideline recommendations on the frequency of PTM diagnosis, a recent analysis of thyroid cancer trends suggests that the annual

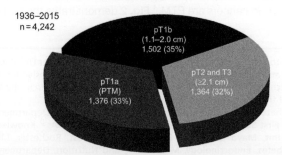

Fig. 2. Proportions of 4242 adult PTC tumors treated from 1936 to 2015 at the Mayo Clinic divided by tumor size, demonstrating that 33% of tumors seen during those 8 decades were microcancers (≤1 cm). (*Data from* Hay ID, Johnson TR, Kaggal S, et al. Papillary Thyroid Carcinoma (PTC) in children and adults: comparison of initial presentation and long-term postoperative outcome in 4432 patients consecutively treated at the Mayo Clinic during eight decades (1936–2015). World J Surg 2018;42(2):329–42.)

percentage change of thyroid cancer incidence has decreased over the last few years.[9,10]

SYMPTOMS AND PRESENTATION

Given the size of PTMs, these tumors often do not cause symptoms and are incidentally found in patients through the use of non–thyroid-dedicated imaging such as neck MRI or through the histologic examination of thyroid glands removed for non–cancer-related reasons. A recent study also suggested that thyroid cancer, including PTM, can be found through screening asymptomatic individuals simply with neck palpation. Palpation often did not actually identify the PTM but the discovery of another nodule had triggered the use of thyroid ultrasound. Finally, in countries where thyroid cancer screening is widespread, the most common method of detection of PTM is by screening with thyroid ultrasound.[11]

CONVENTIONAL TREATMENT OPTIONS
Thyroid Surgery

Surgical treatment has been the traditional cornerstone for treatment of patients with PTM. Surgical intervention includes either bilateral lobar resection (BLR), which could involve, as an extreme, removing the whole thyroid gland (total thyroidectomy) or sometimes, at the other end of the spectrum, just 1 affected lobe (unilateral lobectomy) (**Fig. 3**). Although no clinical trials have been conducted comparing these surgical interventions, the very low mortality for PTM (**Fig. 4**) strongly argues that there would not likely be a comparative mortality benefit. Indeed, at the Mayo Clinic, in an 83-year period, only 4 PTM patients died from their disease. Accordingly, the main differences between both interventions are related to the risk of thyroid recurrence, monitoring, surgical adverse effects, and the need for thyroid hormone replacement therapy. Proponents of total thyroidectomy as the treatment of choice for PTM argue that the multifocality (often microfoci)[12] of thyroid cancer (~30%) and postoperative follow-up (including thyroglobulin tumor marker measurement) are better addressed and facilitated by removing the whole thyroid gland.[13] On the other hand, proponents of thyroid lobectomy argue that the presence of tumor focality does not carry an additional risk of clinically relevant disease. This argument is supported because the risk of

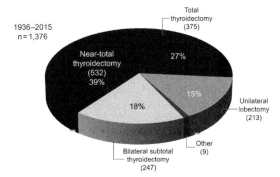

Fig. 3. Extent of thyroid resection in primary operations performed at the Mayo clinic for 1376 PTM adult patients from 1936 to 2015, demonstrating that only 15% underwent unilateral lobectomy. (*Data from* Hay ID, Johnson TR, Kaggal S, et al. Papillary Thyroid Carcinoma (PTC) in children and adults: comparison of initial presentation and long-term postoperative outcome in 4432 patients consecutively treated at the Mayo Clinic during eight decades (1936–2015). World J Surg 2018;42(2):329–42.)

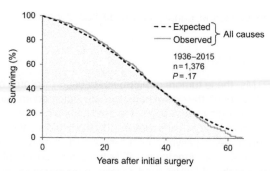

Fig. 4. Expected and observed all-causes survival for 1376 adult PTM patients having definitive surgical treatment (see **Fig. 3**) at the Mayo Clinic during 8 decades and demonstrating no significant difference (*P* = .17). (*Data from* Hay ID, Johnson TR, Kaggal S, et al. Papillary Thyroid Carcinoma (PTC) in children and adults: comparison of initial presentation and long-term postoperative outcome in 4432 patients consecutively treated at the Mayo Clinic during eight decades (1936–2015). World J Surg 2018;42(2):329–42.)

recurrence for both interventions is very low (<5%) and similar in both groups.[14] Lobectomy may provide the additional benefit of sparing approximately 50% to 60% of patients the need for thyroxine replacement therapy (TRT): a treatment burden that includes taking a pill daily for the rest of the patient's life and frequent monitoring. Finally, the most important argument in favor of thyroid lobectomy as the surgical treatment of choice for patients with PTM is the possible lack of access to experienced thyroid surgeons. Two of the most important surgical adverse effects (vocal cord paresis and hypoparathyroidism) are directly associated with the extent of surgery and the experience of surgeons. Total thyroidectomy carries a risk of temporary or persistent vocal cord damage and hypoparathyroidism between 1% and 2%, whereas the risk for partial surgery is often temporary and in the range of 0% and 1%.[15] These estimates are based on reports from tertiary care centers where experienced surgeons perform the operation; recent population-based studies now suggest that those estimates are significantly higher for centers without adequate surgical experience.[11] At the Mayo Clinic, a recent analysis of 1376 PTM patients treated from 1936 to 2015 demonstrated that 20-year locoregional recurrence rates after unilateral lobectomy were not significantly different from those achieved after either BLR or near-total or total thyroidectomy (**Fig. 5**).

Radioiodine Remnant Ablation

For patients undergoing total thyroidectomy, radioactive iodine (RAI) is an option to treat remnant thyroid tissue (to facilitate monitoring) or as an approach to reduce the risk of thyroid cancer recurrence.[16] RAI is commonly used in patients at higher risk of recurrence, yet the use of radioiodine remnant ablation (RRA) for PTM is controversial given the low risk for mortality and morbidity of these tumors.[17] Several systematic reviews have been conducted to understand the benefit of RAI. Despite the significant heterogeneity of included studies, it was noted that the relative risk (RR) reduction for thyroid cancer recurrence was between 5% and 20%.[18] Thus, for a high-risk thyroid cancer with a risk of recurrence of 50% in 10 years, the use of RAI will decrease this risk to 40%. On the other hand, for a very-low-risk thyroid cancer in which the risk of thyroid cancer recurrence is less than 5% in 10 years, the absolute risk reduction will be only 1% or less. This small benefit in comparison with costs and logistical burden of RAI treatment (ie, the need for imaging, low-iodine diet in preparation for the treatment,

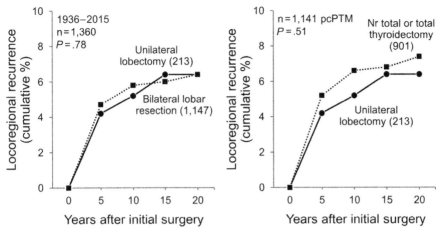

Fig. 5. Comparison of locoregional recurrence rates during 20 postoperative years in potentially curable (pc) adult PTM patients treated at Mayo during 1936 to 2015 and demonstrating no significant differences between rates seen in 213 patients undergoing lobectomy versus those having (*left*) BLR or (*right*) near (Nr)-total or total thyroidectomy. (*Data from* Hay ID, Johnson TR, Kaggal S, et al. Papillary Thyroid Carcinoma (PTC) in children and adults: comparison of initial presentation and long-term postoperative outcome in 4432 patients consecutively treated at the Mayo Clinic during eight decades (1936–2015). World J Surg 2018;42(2):329–42.)

possible need for withdrawal protocol with associated hypothyroid symptoms, and posttreatment restriction) has resulted in some clinical guidelines that suggest against its use for patients with PTM.[19] At the Mayo Clinic, RRA for PTM was selectively used in only 15% of 1287 subjects treated from 1956 to 2015 (**Fig. 6**). Twenty-year locoregional recurrence rates (**Fig. 7**) were not improved with RRA after either BLR or near-total or total thyroidectomy in 375 node-positive PTM patients.

Thyrotropin Suppression Therapy

The main goal of thyrotropin supression therapy (TST) is to prevent and treat symptoms of hypothyroidism. Yet, doses higher than replacement doses are often given

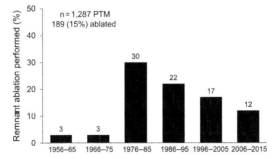

Fig. 6. Percentage of 1287 adult PTM patients managed at the Mayo Clinic during 6 decades (1956–2015) who underwent RRA, demonstrating increasingly selective use of RRA from 1976 through 2015. (*Data from* Hay ID, Johnson TR, Kaggal S, et al. Papillary Thyroid Carcinoma (PTC) in children and adults: comparison of initial presentation and long-term postoperative outcome in 4432 patients consecutively treated at the Mayo Clinic during eight decades (1936–2015). World J Surg 2018;42(2):329–42.)

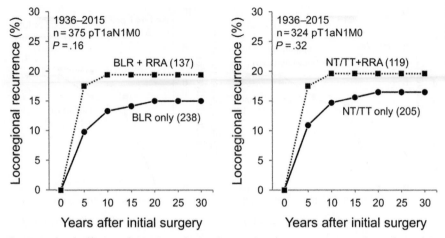

Fig. 7. Lack of efficacy of RRA in reducing locoregional recurrence rates in node-positive adult PTM patients treated during 1936 to 2015 and undergoing (*left panel*) either BLR or (*right panel*) near-total or total thyroidectomy (NT/TT). (*Data from* Hay ID, Johnson TR, Kaggal S, et al. Papillary Thyroid Carcinoma (PTC) in children and adults: comparison of initial presentation and long-term postoperative outcome in 4432 patients consecutively treated at the Mayo Clinic during eight decades (1936–2015). World J Surg 2018;42(2):329–42.)

to patients with thyroid as TST to potentially prevent the growth of tumors that might retain responsiveness to thyroid-stimulating hormone (TSH).[20] In support of this practice, a meta-analysis of 4174 subjects with well-differentiated thyroid cancer showed that TST reduced the risk of disease progression or recurrence and death (RR 0.73, CI 0.6–0.88).[21] Yet, this benefit has been mostly seen in patients with greater risk of mortality and recurrence than in patients with PTM.[22] Prospective data from a large multicenter thyroid cancer registry involving 2936 patients found that TST, suppressing to very low concentrations (<0.1 mU/L) for patients with low-risk thyroid cancer, including PTM, did not improve the overall survival.[23] Similarly, a small randomized clinical trial comparing TST versus no TST in mostly low-risk PTCs found no difference in rates of recurrence or mortality after a mean follow-up of 6.9 years.[24] Given concerns of limited effectiveness, possible adverse effects of TSH suppressive therapy (iatrogenic thyrotoxicosis, atrial fibrillation, or fracture[25]), and burden of treatment (frequent monitoring and titration), ATA guidelines have recommended against TSH suppressive therapy for PTM patients.[8] Instead, it has been suggested that PTM patients should receive only TST to maintain low normal TSH values (TSH 0.5–2.0 mU/L).

NEWER MANAGEMENT OPTIONS
Active Surveillance

Over the last decade, as with indolent prostate cancers, active surveillance (close monitoring of symptoms and tumor ultrasound characteristics with later selective surgical intervention) has been applied to PTM patients.[15] Three observational studies have shown that active surveillance is safe and may be desirable for many PTM patients[26–28] In 2015, the ATA guidelines[8] recognized active surveillance as an alternative to immediate surgery in patients with PTM. The evidence behind active surveillance, its implementation, barriers, and future research is beyond the scope of this article. (See Akira Miyauchi and Yasuhiro Ito's article, "Conservative Surveillance Management of Low-Risk Papillary Thyroid Microcarcinoma," in this issue.) This article only explores the option of active surveillance in the decision-making process for the management of PTM (see later discussion).

Ultrasound-Guided Percutaneous Ethanol Ablation

Ultrasound-guided percutaneous ethanol ablation (UPEA) involves the direct intratumoral injection of 95% ethanol under ultrasound guidance and local anesthesia.[29] This technique has been used effectively at the Mayo Clinic since 1991 for managing postoperative neck nodal metastases in papillary, Hurthle cell, and medullary thyroid carcinoma. In a long-term follow-up study of locally advanced papillary macrocancers (tumor size greater than 1 cm maximal diameter) published in 2013, Hay and colleagues[30] reported that the technique was found safe, effective, and considerably less expensive than operative management. Since 2010, this group has used UPEA to control and often eliminate the primary tumor of PTM (cT1aN0M0) in an outpatient local anesthetic approach adapted from the neck nodal ablative technique. As recently reported to the 2018 meetings of the European Thyroid Association and the ATA, 16 biopsy-proven tumor foci in 14 PTM subjects have been treated to date. Neck tenderness was minor and lasted hours; no subjects experienced hoarseness due to vocal cord paralysis. Follow-up ranged from 15 to 95 months (mean 4.2 years); no subjects developed a neck nodal metastasis. All tumor foci shrunk in dimensions and tumor-associated Doppler blood flow was eliminated. Median tumor volume reduction in 16 tumor foci was 82% (range 48%–100%). At the latest assessment, 10 tumors (62%) were still identifiable and, in these cases, median volume decrease was 76%. Six foci (38%) in 5 subjects were no longer seen on repeated ultrasound neck scans. Serum thyroglobulin levels did not significantly change after the UPEA procedure. The authors believe that this ongoing pilot study has demonstrated that UPEA could become a cheap, safe, and well-tolerated definitive minimally invasive alternative for PTM patients who do not wish to have surgery and are uncomfortable with active surveillance.[31]

Radiofrequency and Laser Ablation

Radiofrequency and laser ablation are percutaneous, image-guided procedures that use thermal energy to ablate in situ tumors. This procedure is said to provide a more predictable and well-defined area of tumor necrosis than that caused by ethanol ablation.[32] Radiofrequency ablation has historically been used for large benign thyroid nodules, as well as for locoregional recurrence of thyroid cancer.[33] Given that it has been shown to be safe and effective for these thyroid-related indications, this procedure has been recently applied to managing some patients with PTM. Zhang and colleagues[34] reported that, in 92 subjects with 98 PTMs, radiofrequency ablation effectively reduced tumor volume (mean volume reduction ratio) to 0.47, 0.19, 0.08, at 6, 12, and 18 months, respectively. Of all nodules, 10 resolved in 6 months and 23 resolved in 12 months. No suspicious metastatic lymph nodes were detected on follow-up and no major complications were encountered, although 1 subject had moderate pain and 1 had transient hoarseness.

Percutaneous laser ablation (PLA) has also been tested in patients with PTM. Zhou and colleagues[35] used PLA in 30 subjects. In 1 case the ablation was incomplete and a second ablation was performed. PLA effectively reduced tumor volume from 44 mm^3 preablation to 9.1 mm^3 at 12 months postablation. At the last follow-up (mean 13.2 months, range, 12–24 months) 10 (33.3%) ablation zones had disappeared and 20 (66.67%) ablation zones remained as scar-like lesions. No regrowth of treated tumors, local recurrence, or distant metastases were detected. Similar to UPEA, ablation procedures may only apply to a selected number of patients with so-called ideal tumors and all such ablative techniques should be done at centers with considerable expertise in such technically demanding procedures.

CURRENT CONTROVERSIES
Papillary Thyroid Microcarcinoma Overtreatment

Over the last few decades, given the rapid increase in the incidence of thyroid cancer, there is a growing concern that many patients with PTM are receiving treatments with a risk of morbidity that is not justified by the very low risks of mortality and recurrence. Recent observational studies have shown that the frequency of total thyroidectomy has increased in the United States despite most incident cases being patients with small thyroid cancers who might also benefit from lobectomy.[36] **Fig. 8** demonstrates changes in the extent of surgery for PTM at the Mayo Clinic during 1936 to 2015. During the most recent 2 decades (1996–2015) the most frequently performed primary surgical procedure was a total thyroidectomy, accounting for 27% of all definitive surgical procedures for PTM performed during 1936 to 2015. By contrast, the frequency of lobectomy (at the Mayo Clinic, over 8 decades, only 15% of the total number of operations) has remained fairly steady over the last 3 decades in the United States.

Unfortunately, many of these thyroid surgeries are performed by less experienced thyroid surgeons. A population-based study noted that the frequency of surgical adverse effects is correlated with the number of thyroid surgeries performed every year, noting that perhaps surgeons who perform more than 25 thyroid procedures a year have better outcomes (less surgical complications and fewer hospital days) than those with fewer than 25 yearly procedures. The rate of complications was 68% when surgeons conducted 2 to 5 cases, 42% for 6 to 10 cases, 22% for 11 to 15 cases, 10% for 16 to 20 cases, and 3% for 21 to 25 cases per year. This study also noted that, among approximately 17,000 patients undergoing total thyroidectomy between 1998 and 2009, the median annual surgical volume was 7 cases (51% of surgeons performed 1 case per year) demonstrating that most patients with thyroid cancer, including PTM patients, undergo surgery at centers with a high risk of adverse complications due to their low volume.[37]

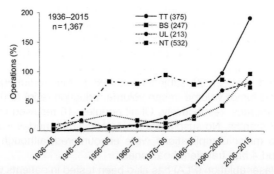

Fig. 8. Changing frequencies of definitive surgical procedures performed in 1367 adult PTM patients treated at the Mayo Clinic during 8 decades and demonstrating that TT was the most common procedure performed for adult PTM during the 2 decades of 1996 to 2005 and 2006 to 2015. BS, bilateral subtotal thyroidectomy; NT, near-total thyroidectomy; TT, total thyroidectomy; UL, unilateral lobectomy. (*Data from* Hay ID, Johnson TR, Kaggal S, et al. Papillary Thyroid Carcinoma (PTC) in children and adults: comparison of initial presentation and long-term postoperative outcome in 4432 patients consecutively treated at the Mayo Clinic during eight decades (1936–2015). World J Surg 2018;42(2):329–42.)

Similar to the increased use of thyroidectomy, the use of RAI for low-risk thyroid cancers has increased over the last decade in the United States.[38] Between 1983 and 2009, the proportion of US patients receiving RAI for PTM increased from 8% to 42%,[39] a trend not mirrored in the Mayo Clinic practice (see **Fig. 6**). A higher use of RAI for PTM and other low-risk thyroid cancer lesions was correlated with socioeconomic indices of lower health care access (eg, uninsured, poverty, unemployment[38]), specialty of the primary decision-maker (nuclear medicine physicians were more likely than endocrinologists or surgeons to administer RAI[40]), and practice setting (RAI was used more often in nonacademic settings than in academic settings).[41] In 2009, the ATA for the first time explicitly recommended against postoperative RAI for PTM, and this recommendation marginally affected the use of RAI in the United States.[8] The proportion of patients with tumors of PTM receiving RAI dropped from 42% before 2009 to 32% after 2009, a decrease of 10 percentage points compared with tumors greater than 1.1 cm, which dropped from 69% to 68%, a decrease of 2 percentage points.[38] These findings suggest that RAI use for PTM is still widely practiced in the United States despite guideline recommendations.

The excessive use of surgery and RAI for patients with PTM may reflect a continuation of the 1-size-fits-all style of thyroid cancer practice. This approach treats patients the same, regardless of risk of recurrence or mortality. With the advent of research clarifying the risk of recurrence, harms of surgery, and the rapid increase in incidence of PTM, it has become evident that a 1-size-fits-all approach is no longer needed nor desirable. Instead, an individualized approach in which the treatment fits the threat and respects patients' biology, values, and context is necessary.

THE NEED TO INDIVIDUALIZE TREATMENT DECISIONS

Clinicians and patients with PTM have several management options. No comparative effectiveness research exists between treatment options, yet each offers a set of attributes that makes the choice of best the treatment of each individual patient quite difficult. Preferably, what is technically possible and how both patients and clinicians value these different attributes, should guide actual decision-making.

What Is Technically Possible?

Not all PTM lesions are the same and lesion characteristics will determine which options are available for a patient. The most important tool for understanding which options are available to a patient is a reliable and high-quality ultrasound assessment of the patient's neck. During this assessment, clinicians need to pay attention to the location of the tumor foci, diameter, multicentricity, and proximity to the thyroid capsule, trachea, and esophagus. An ideal tumor[42] for all available options is a thyroid tumor with a diameter no larger than 10 mm, no sonographic evidence of multicentricity, and at least 3 to 5 mm from the thyroid capsule. Unfortunately, these ideal tumors are not frequently found. A retrospective analysis led by Griffin and colleagues[15] investigated a total of 243 subjects with thyroid cancer who underwent surgery for PTC from 2003 to 2012 at Duke University Medical Center. From this cohort, 27 subjects had PTM and none had with ideal tumors. They noted that, very often, tumors were located in the periphery of the thyroid. Similarly, Tuttle and colleagues[28] followed 291 subjects with PTC less than or equal to 1.5 cm with active surveillance during a median follow-up of 25 months. They noticed that only 4.5% of these tumors had features that could fit the ideal tumor. These findings suggest that often PTM presents in a way in which treatment options are limited.

How to Individualize Treatment Options

When discussing available and possible treatment options for patients with PTM, it is important to understand what the patient wants and needs, and what is most appropriate in the individual context. A young patient with PTM might highly value avoiding the long-term monitoring needed in active surveillance and choose lobectomy as the best treatment option. A 76-year-old man on dialysis might place a lower value in removing the thyroid and a higher value on a more conservative treatment such as UPEA or active surveillance. To have these meaningful conversations, patients need to navigate the benefits, harms, costs, and impact on daily life that is associated with each option; and clinicians need to communicate this complex information and elicit patients' preferences within the limited time of a clinical encounter. This is a daunting task for both parties. To facilitate this process, clinicians are encouraged to make use of shared decision-making (SDM) methods.

SDM is an approach of care that involves the clinician using the best available evidence to discuss the attributes of different treatment options with patients, and finding a method that makes intellectual and practical sense.[43] This SDM process could be supported by the use of encounter tools or decision aids (**Figs. 9** and **10**). These tools help clinicians present balanced information with the use of ordered icon arrays or pictograms to represent the risks and attributes of the treatment options.[43] Brito and colleagues[44] developed an encounter tool to help clinicians and patients with PTM make treatment decisions. The Thyroid Cancer Choice (TCC) tool, developed with the input of thyroid cancer experts, patients with PTM, and clinicians includes (1) an estimate of the frequency of thyroid cancer in the population; (2) the management options, active surveillance, and thyroid surgery (lobectomy vs total thyroidectomy); (3) the risk of death, metastasis, tumor growth, and adverse effects with

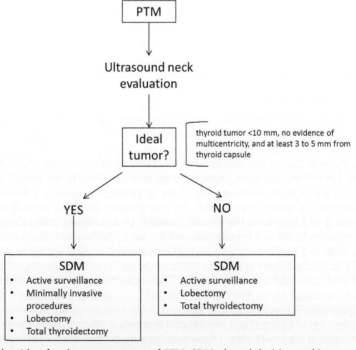

Fig. 9. Algorithm for the management of PTM. SDM, shared decision making.

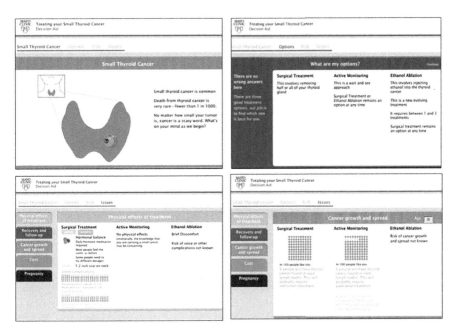

Fig. 10. Screenshots of the electronic decision aid *Thyroid Cancer Treatment Choice.*

each option; (4) the planned type and frequency of follow-up; (5) the out-of-pocket costs with each choice; and (6) the interaction of pregnancy and each management option. A paper version of this tool was adapted for use in South Korea and tested in a prospective observational study to assess its effect on treatment choice. Researchers found that among the 220 subjects with PTM, clinicians and patients using TCC during the encounter were more likely to choose active surveillance than the patients and clinicians who did not use TCC during the encounter (RR 1.16, 95% CI 1.04–1.29). Although this result suggests that this tool increases acceptance of active surveillance, additional and more rigorous studies are needed to confirm this finding.

Ideally, individualization of treatment decisions should not only be based on the context and values of the patient but also on the biology of the tumor. Several genetic studies have been conducted or are ongoing to establish if any specific mutation carries any prognostic value, and thus help patients and clinicians in decision-making. Among all known genetic mutations in patients with PTC, the genetic duet of BRAF V600 E plus telomerase reverse transcriptase (TERT) have been associated with aggressive clinicopathologic outcomes, including tumor recurrence and mortality.[45] In a cohort of 1051 subjects, 30 subjects died. Of all 1051 subjects, 6% (n = 66) had the genetic duet of BRAF V600 E plus TERT, and 25% (n = 15) of these 66 subjects died, accounting for half of the thyroid cancer specific deaths in this cohort. The risk of mortality for patients with this duet mutation remained strongly significant after adjustment for clinical factors.[46] Whether these findings in a cohort of PTC could be extrapolated to PTM is not clear. However, it seems unlikely that these highly mutated tumors will be PTMs at presentation,[47] thereby limiting its prognostic value. Therefore, current evidence does not support the use of these genetic markers to help decision-making. However, it is possible that future studies in molecular profiling will help distinguish those PTMs that are more likely to grow and metastasize from those PTMs destined to remain biologically silent within the thyroid.

Monitoring

The goal of thyroid cancer monitoring is to detect clinically relevant thyroid recurrences, and minimize the burden of treatment and tests. The 2 tests most frequently used to achieve this goal are the neck ultrasound and the serum thyroglobulin tumor markers. The frequency of these tests, however, will vary depending on the management options used. For patients treated with thyroidectomy, initial follow-up in 6 weeks to 3 months after the procedure includes assessment of thyroid hormone and thyroglobulin tumor marker levels. For patients treated with lobectomy, the use of thyroglobulin has not been found to be helpful. A recent study of 208 subjects with low-risk thyroid cancer, including patients with PTM, treated with lobectomy and followed up with thyroglobulin found that serum thyroglobulin levels increased gradually after lobectomy in patients with and without recurrences, without any significant differences. After initial follow-up for thyroid surgery, an ultrasound of the neck is needed within 6 and 12 months. If there is no evidence of disease during the first 2 years of treatment, the likelihood of thyroid recurrence is less than 1%, and future follow-up could be sparser and based on clinical examination and laboratory tests.[48] For patients undergoing active surveillance, the monitoring is long-term and every 6 months with neck ultrasound. For patients treated with minimally invasive procedures, the follow-up should be dictated by local protocols; however, it is likely to mimic active surveillance follow-up for the first 5 years. Given the low risk of recurrence in patients with PTM, there is limited or no role for recombinant human thyrotropin-stimulated thyroglobulin testing, whole body RAI scans, or fluorodeoxyglucose (FDG)-PET scanning.[8]

REFERENCES

1. Davies L, Welch HG. Current thyroid cancer trends in the United States. JAMA Otolaryngol Head Neck Surg 2014;140(4):317.
2. Davies L, Morris LG, Haymart M, et al, on behalf of the AACE Endocrine Surgery Scientific Committee. American Association of Clinical Endocrinologists and American College of Endocrinology disease state clinical review : the increasing incidence of thyroid cancer. Endocr Pract 2016;21(6):686–96.
3. Hay ID, Johnson TR, Kaggal S, et al. Papillary Thyroid Carcinoma (PTC) in children and adults: comparison of initial presentation and long-term postoperative outcome in 4432 patients consecutively treated at the Mayo Clinic during eight decades (1936–2015). World J Surg 2018;42(2):329–42.
4. Lim H, Devesa SS, Sosa JA, et al. Trends in thyroid cancer incidence and mortality in the United States, 1974-2013. JAMA 2017;317(13):1338.
5. Harach HR, Franssila KO, Wasenius VM. Occult papillary carcinoma of the thyroid. A "normal" finding in Finland. A systematic autopsy study. Cancer 1985; 56(3):531–8.
6. Martinez-Tello FJ, Martinez-Cabruja R, Fernandez-Martin J, et al. Occult carcinoma of the thyroid. A systematic autopsy study from Spain of two series performed with two different methods. Cancer 1993;71(12):4022–9.
7. Hughes DT, Haymart MR, Miller BS, et al. The most commonly occurring papillary thyroid cancer in the United States is now a microcarcinoma in a patient older than 45 years. Thyroid 2011;21(3):231–6.
8. Haugen BR, Alexander EK, Bible KC, et al. 2015 American Thyroid Association management guidelines for adult patients with thyroid nodules and differentiated thyroid cancer: the American Thyroid Association guidelines task force on thyroid nodules and differentiated thyroid cancer. Thyroid 2016;26(1):1–133.

9. Morris LG, Tuttle RM, Davies L. Changing trends in the incidence of thyroid cancer in the United States. JAMA Otolaryngol Head Neck Surg 2015;91(2):165–71.
10. Haymart MR, Davies L. South Korean thyroid cancer trends: good news and bad. Thyroid 2018;28(9):1081–2.
11. Brito JP, Al Nofal A, Montori VM, et al. The impact of subclinical disease and mechanism of detection on the rise in thyroid cancer incidence: a population-based study in Olmsted County, Minnesota during 1935 through 2012. Thyroid 2015; 25(9):999–1007.
12. Wu AW, Nguyen C, Wang MB. What is the best treatment for papillary thyroid microcarcinoma? Laryngoscope 2011;121(9):1828–9.
13. Merdad M, Eskander A, De Almeida J, et al. Current management of papillary thyroid microcarcinoma in Canada. J Otolaryngol Head Neck Surg 2014;43:32.
14. Sung MW, Park B, An SY, et al. Increasing thyroid cancer rate and the extent of thyroid surgery in Korea. PLoS One 2014;9(12):1–10.
15. Griffin A, Brito JP, Bahl M, et al. Applying criteria of active surveillance to low-risk papillary thyroid cancer over a decade: how many surgeries and complications can be avoided? Thyroid 2017;27(4):518–23.
16. R Michael Tuttle M. Controversial issues in thyroid cancer management. J Nucl Med 2017;008748:1–31.
17. Tulchinsky M, Binse I, Campenn A, et al. Radioactive iodine therapy for differentiated thyroid cancer : lessons from confronting controversial literature on risks for secondary malignancy. J Nucl Med 2018;59(5):723–5.
18. Hu G, Zhu W, Yang W, et al. The effectiveness of radioactive iodine remnant ablation for papillary thyroid microcarcinoma: a systematic review and meta-analysis. World J Surg 2016;40(1):100–9.
19. Schvartz C, Bonnetain F, Dabakuyo S, et al. Impact on overall survival of radioactive iodine in low-risk differentiated thyroid cancer patients. J Clin Endocrinol Metab 2012;97(5):1526–35.
20. Brabant G. Thyrotropin suppressive therapy in thyroid carcinoma: what are the targets? J Clin Endocrinol Metab 2008;93(4):1167–9.
21. Brito JP, Hay ID, Morris JC. Low risk papillary thyroid cancer. BMJ 2014;348: g3045.
22. Biondi B, Cooper DS. Benefits of thyrotropin suppression versus the risks of adverse effects in differentiated thyroid cancer. Thyroid 2010;20(2):135–46.
23. Diessl S, Holzberger B, Mäder U, et al. Impact of moderate vs stringent TSH suppression on survival in advanced differentiated thyroid carcinoma. Clin Endocrinol (Oxf) 2012;76(4):586–92.
24. Sugitani I, Fujimoto Y. Does postoperative thyrotropin suppression therapy truly decrease recurrence in papillary thyroid carcinoma? A randomized controlled trial. J Clin Endocrinol Metab 2010;95(10):4576–83.
25. Papaleontiou M, Hawley ST, Haymart MR. Effect of thyrotropin suppression therapy on bone in thyroid cancer patients. Oncologist 2016;21(2):165–71.
26. Ito Y, Miyauchi A, Kihara M, et al. Patient age is significantly related to the progression of papillary microcarcinoma of the thyroid under observation. Thyroid 2014;24(1):27–34.
27. Sugitani I, Toda K, Yamada K, et al. Three distinctly different kinds of papillary thyroid microcarcinoma should be recognized: our treatment strategies and outcomes. World J Surg 2010;34(6):1222–31.
28. Tuttle RM, Fagin JA, Minkowitz G, et al. Natural history and tumor volume kinetics of papillary thyroid cancers during active surveillance. JAMA Otolaryngol Head Neck Surg 2017;10065(10):1015–20.

29. Hay ID, Charboneau JW, Reading CC. Percutaneous ethanol injection for treatment of cervical lymph node papillary thyroid carcinoma. AJR Am J Roentgenol 2002;178(3):699–704.

30. Hay ID, Lee RA, Davidge-Pitts C, et al. Long-term outcome of ultrasound-guided percutaneous ethanol ablation of selected "recurrent" neck nodal metastases in 25 patients with TNM stages III or IVA papillary thyroid carcinoma previously treated by surgery and131I therapy. Surgery 2013;154(6):1448–55.

31. Hay ID, Lee R, Morris J, et al. Ultrasound-guided percutaneous ethanol ablation for selected patients with papillary thyroid microcarcinoma: a novel, effective and well tolerated alternative to neck surgery or observation; 87th Annual Meeting of the American Thyroid Association. Victoria (BC), October 18–22, 2017.

32. Cervelli R, Mazzeo S, De Napoli L, et al. Radiofrequency ablation in the treatment of benign thyroid nodules: an efficient and safe alternative to surgery. J Vasc Interv Radiol 2017;28(10):1400–8.

33. Chung SR, Suh CH, Baek JH, et al. Safety of radiofrequency ablation of benign thyroid nodules and recurrent thyroid cancers: a systematic review and meta-analysis. Int J Hyperthermia 2017;33(8):920–30.

34. Zhang M, Luo Y, Zhang Y, et al. Efficacy and safety of ultrasound-guided radiofrequency ablation for treating low-risk papillary thyroid microcarcinoma: a prospective study. Thyroid 2016;26(11):1581–7.

35. Zhou W, Jiang S, Zhan W, et al. Ultrasound-guided percutaneous laser ablation of unifocal T1N0M0 papillary thyroid microcarcinoma: preliminary results. Eur Radiol 2017;27(7):2934–40.

36. Welch HG, Doherty GM. Saving thyroids — overtreatment of small papillary cancers. N Engl J Med 2018;379(4):308–10.

37. Adam MA, Thomas S, Youngwirth L, et al. Is there a minimum number of thyroidectomies a surgeon should perform to optimize patient outcomes? Ann Surg 2017;265(2):402–7.

38. Marti JL, Davies L, Haymart MR, et al. Inappropriate use of radioactive iodine for low-risk papillary thyroid cancer is most common in regions with poor access to healthcare. Thyroid 2015;25(7):865–6.

39. Roman BR, Feingold JH, Patel SG, et al. The 2009 American Thyroid Association guidelines modestly reduced radioactive iodine use for thyroid cancers less than 1 cm. Thyroid 2014;24(10):1549–50.

40. Haymart MR, Banerjee M, Yang D, et al. The role of clinicians in determining radioactive iodine use for low-risk thyroid cancer. Cancer 2013;119(2):259–65.

41. Haymart MR, Banerjee M, Yang D, et al. Variation in the management of thyroid cancer. J Clin Endocrinol Metab 2013;98(5):2001–8.

42. Brito JP, Ito Y, Miyauchi A, et al. A clinical framework to facilitate risk stratification when considering an active surveillance alternative to immediate biopsy and surgery in papillary microcarcinoma. Thyroid 2016;26(1):144–9.

43. Kunneman M, Montori VM, Castaneda-Guarderas A, et al. What is shared decision making? (and what it is not). Acad Emerg Med 2016;23(12):1320–4.

44. Brito JP, Moon JH, Zeuren R, et al. Thyroid cancer treatment choice: a pilot study of a tool to facilitate conversations with patients with papillary microcarcinomas considering treatment options. Thyroid 2018;28(10):1325–31.

45. Xing M, Liu R, Liu X, et al. BRAF V600E and TERT promoter mutations cooperatively identify the most aggressive papillary thyroid cancer with highest recurrence. J Clin Oncol 2014;32(25):2718–26.

46. Liu R, Bishop J, Zhu G, et al. Mortality risk stratification by combining *BRAF* V600E and *TERT* promoter mutations in papillary thyroid cancer. JAMA Oncol 2017;3(2):202.
47. Melo M, Da Rocha AG, Vinagre J, et al. TERT promoter mutations are a major indicator of poor outcome in differentiated thyroid carcinomas. J Clin Endocrinol Metab 2014;99(5):754–65.
48. Momesso DP, Vaisman F, Yang SP, et al. Dynamic risk stratification in patients with differentiated thyroid cancer treated without radioactive iodine. J Clin Endocrinol Metab 2016;101(7):2692–700.

Conservative Surveillance Management of Low-Risk Papillary Thyroid Microcarcinoma

Akira Miyauchi, MD, PhD*, Yasuhiro Ito, MD, PhD

KEYWORDS

- Papillary thyroid microcarcinoma • Active surveillance • Guidelines
- Unfavorable events • Medical cost • Lifetime probability of disease progression

KEY POINTS

- Most low-risk papillary thyroid microcarcinomas remain small.
- Ten years of active surveillance at Kuma Hospital revealed that 8.0% of patients showed tumor enlargement greater than or equal to 3 mm, and 3.8% developed novel node metastases.
- None of the patients, including those who underwent rescue surgery, showed life-threatening recurrence or distant metastasis, and none died of thyroid carcinoma.
- The incidences of unfavorable events and medical costs were significantly higher in patients who underwent immediate surgery than in those who had active surveillance.
- Active surveillance should be the first-line management method for low-risk papillary thyroid microcarcinoma.

BACKGROUND

Papillary thyroid microcarcinoma (PTMC) refers to papillary thyroid carcinomas (PTCs) less than or equal to 10 mm. Many autopsy studies reported high incidences of latent PTC in adults who died of other causes. Furthermore, the incidence of ultrasonography-detectable latent carcinomas measuring 3 to 10 mm ranges from 0.5% to 5.2%.[1] A screening study by Takebe and colleagues[2] discovered thyroid carcinoma in 3.5% of Japanese adult women who underwent ultrasonography and ultrasound-guided fine-needle aspiration cytology (FNAC). This incidence rate was consistent with that of latent PTMC in autopsy studies and was more than 1000-fold greater than that of clinical thyroid carcinoma in Japanese women reported at that time (3.1 per 100,000). This study was a herald of the recent increase in the

Disclosure Statement: The authors have nothing to disclose.
Department of Surgery, Kuma Hospital, 8-2-35 Shimoyamate-dori, Chuo-ku, Kobe 650-0011, Japan
* Corresponding author.
E-mail address: miyauchi@kuma-h.or.jp

Endocrinol Metab Clin N Am 48 (2019) 215–226
https://doi.org/10.1016/j.ecl.2018.10.007   endo.theclinics.com
0889-8529/19/© 2018 The Author(s). Published by Elsevier Inc. This is an open access article under the CC BY-NC-ND license (http://creativecommons.org/licenses/by-nc-nd/4.0/).

incidences of thyroid cancer in many countries.[3–6] In the United States, the incidence of thyroid carcinoma increased between 2.4-fold and 2.9-fold between 1973 and 2009.[3,4] This increase was mostly due to improved detection of small PTCs. In Korea, the incidence of thyroid carcinoma increased 15-fold between 1993 and 2011 owing to the introduction of a national thyroid cancer screening program.[5] In all of these countries, mortality due to thyroid cancer did not change despite the increase in disease incidence. These results strongly suggest that small PTCs are overdiagnosis and overtreated.

INITIATION OF ACTIVE SURVEILLANCE FOR LOW-RISK PAPILLARY THYROID MICROCARCINOMA IN JAPAN

The aforementioned studies imply that many people are living with PTMC asymptomatically and are unaware of their disease. The large difference between the incidences of PTMCs on autopsy and screening studies, and the prevalence of clinical thyroid carcinoma, led Miyauchi and colleagues[7] to hypothesize that most PTMCs remain small, only a small proportion progress, and surgery after the detection of progression is still feasible. It was also posited that indicating immediate surgery for all PTMCs would produce more harm than good and, in 1993, proposed an observational clinical trial of patients forgoing immediate surgery; the trial commenced that same year. In 1995, the Cancer Institute Hospital in Tokyo started a similar trial.[8] The knowledge acquired from the active surveillance for low-risk papillary microcarcinoma of the thyroid in these Japanese institutes is briefly summarized in **Box 1**.

CONTRAINDICATIONS FOR ACTIVE SURVEILLANCE

Although active surveillance is an excellent strategy, it cannot be applied to all patients with PTMCs. Contraindications for active surveillance can be divided into 2 categories (**Table 1**). One category is the presence of high-risk features such as clinical node

---

Box 1
Knowledge acquired from the active surveillance for low-risk papillary thyroid microcarcinoma in Japanese studies

1. Most low-risk PTMCs remain dormant or grow very slowly. Some PTMCs shrink over time.

2. None of the patients with low-risk PTMC showed distant metastasis or died of thyroid carcinoma during active surveillance to date.

3. None of the patients who underwent surgery after the detection of progression signs showed life-threatening recurrence or died of thyroid carcinoma.

4. In contrast to clinical PTC, low-risk PTMCs in older patients are less likely progress.

5. Although a small portion of PTMCs grow during pregnancy, it is not too late to perform surgery after delivery.

6. The incidences of adverse events such as recurrent laryngeal nerve paralysis and hypoparathyroidism are significantly higher in patients who undergo immediate surgery than in those who undergo active surveillance, even when expert thyroid surgeons perform the operations.

7. Medical costs for immediate surgery followed by 10 years of postoperative management are 4.1-fold higher than the total costs of active surveillance for 10 years.

8. The estimated lifetime probability of disease progression is inversely correlated with age at presentation.

Table 1
Contraindications for the active surveillance of papillary microcarcinoma

Categories	Contraindications
High-risk features	1. Presence of clinical node metastasis and/or clinical distant metastasis at diagnosis 2. Signs or symptoms of invasion to the recurrent laryngeal nerve or trachea 3. High-grade malignancy on cytology (eg, tall cell variant and poorly differentiated carcinoma)
Features rendering active surveillance unsuitable	1. Tumors attaching to the trachea 2. Tumors located in the pathway of the recurrent laryngeal nerve

metastasis, distant metastasis at diagnosis (very rare), vocal cord paralysis due to invasion of the recurrent laryngeal nerve, or high-grade malignancy on cytology. The other category includes PTMCs attached to the trachea or located along the path of the recurrent laryngeal nerve. Although PTMCs with these features are not necessarily biologically aggressive, active surveillance may not be appropriate. Ito and colleagues'[9] previous study highlighted the possibility of tracheal invasion being related to the angles formed by the tumor and tracheal surfaces (**Fig. 1**). In that study, 12 (24%) of 51 PTMCs greater than or equal to 7 mm that formed obtuse angles showed tracheal invasion requiring resection of the tracheal cartilage and mucosa (**Fig. 2A**), whereas none of the 286 PTMCs greater than or equal to 7 mm that formed acute or near-right angles showed significant tracheal invasion (**Fig. 2B**).

The possibility of recurrent laryngeal nerve invasion was associated with the absence of the normal rim of the thyroid between the tumor and thyroid surfaces in the direction of the nerve (**Fig. 3**). Nine percent of 98 PTMCs greater than or equal to 7 mm lacking the normal rim (**Fig. 4**) required partial layer or segmental resection of the recurrent laryngeal nerve, whereas none of the 776 PTMCs greater than or equal to 7 mm with normal rims invaded the recurrent laryngeal nerve. PTMCs less than 7 mm did not exhibit tracheal or recurrent laryngeal nerve invasion. Tumors located within the thyroid lobe (**Fig. 5A**) are ideal candidates for active surveillance; moreover, those with possible minimal extrathyroid extension at the anterior or lateral surface of the thyroid (**Fig. 5B, C**) were not considered contraindicated for active surveillance. Tumor multiplicity and family history of differentiated thyroid carcinoma were also not regarded as contraindications. Although these may be weak risk factors,

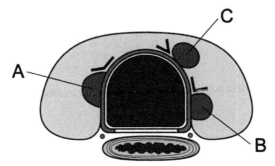

Fig. 1. The types of angles formed between the tumor surface and tracheal cartilage are related to the risk of tracheal invasion: (A) obtuse angle, (B) near-right angle, and (C) acute angle.

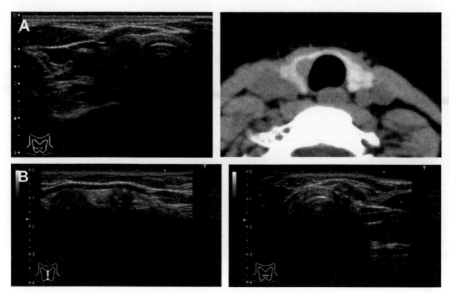

Fig. 2. (A) *Upper two*; A typical example of PTMC forming an obtuse angle (*right*, ultrasonography; *left*, computed tomography scan). This case required resection of the tracheal cartilage (B) *Lower two*; A typical example of a PTMC forming an acute angle. (Ultrasonography; right, sagittal scan. Head to the left; *left*, transverse scan). This tumor was excised according to the patients' wishes. There was no tracheal invasion.

performing total thyroidectomies in these patients might result in more harm (including vocal cord paralysis and hypoparathyroidism) than good.

PRACTICING ACTIVE SURVEILLANCE OF LOW-RISK PAPILLARY THYROID MICROCARCINOMAS

At Kuma Hospital, thyroid nodules greater than or equal to 5 mm with suspicious features on ultrasonography are evaluated with ultrasound-guided FNAC. In Japan, there were no guidelines for performing FNAC on thyroid nodules until the Japan Association of Breast and Thyroid Sonology guidebook was published in 2016, which stated that thyroid nodules greater than or equal to 5 mm with strongly suspicious features on

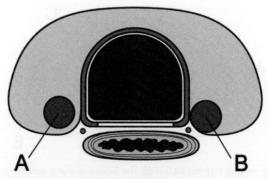

Fig. 3. The presence (A) or absence (B) of a normal tissue rim in the direction of the recurrent laryngeal nerve is related to the risk of invasion to the nerve.

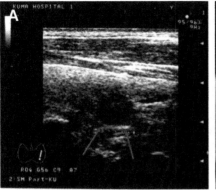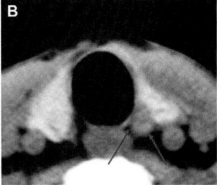

Fig. 4. (A) Ultrasonography showing a hypoechoic mass lesion extending from the dorsal surface of the left thyroid lobe in a patient presenting with left vocal cord paralysis. (B) A computed tomography scan of the same patient revealing a low-density mass without a normal tissue rim in the direction of the left recurrent laryngeal nerve. Arrows indicate a tumor extending from the dorsal surface of the thyroid lobe.

ultrasonography should be evaluated with FNAC.[10] Without FNAC, patients may visit other doctors who may recommend unnecessary surgery. Furthermore, without FNAC-based diagnosis, the results of the authors' trial would not have been considered reliable. Adopting the promising results of active surveillance trials from 2 Japanese institutes, Kuma Hospital,[1,7,9] and the Cancer Institute Hospital,[8] the American Thyroid Association (ATA) guidelines no longer recommend FNAC for suspicious tumors less than or equal to 1 cm, unless clinical symptoms or aggressive features are present, and endorse active surveillance for low-risk PTMCs.[11]

At Kuma Hospital, until recently, the authors proposed 2 options to the patients with the disease: active surveillance or immediate surgery. However, currently, active surveillance is recommended as first-line management following evidence of favorable outcomes in patients who underwent active surveillance (see later description). Some physicians favor prescribing levothyroxine to maintain patients' serum thyroid-stimulating hormone (TSH) levels in the low-normal range.

Patients who choose active surveillance undergo ultrasonography 6 months later and annually thereafter. A greater than or equal to 3 mm increase in the maximal diameter of a PTMC is deemed enlargement. Surgery is recommended for some patients,

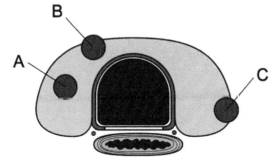

Fig. 5. (A) Tumor located within a thyroid lobe is an ideal tumor for active surveillance. Tumors located at the anterior (B) and lateral (C) capsules of the thyroid lobe, with possible minimal extrathyroid extension, are not ideal for active surveillance but are nevertheless included in such surveillance.

although others may continue active surveillance until the tumor reaches 13 mm. Suspicious lymph nodes undergo FNAC and thyroglobulin measurement of the needle wash-out is also performed to diagnose lymph node metastasis. Total thyroidectomy and therapeutic lymph node dissection are performed if metastasis is detected.

DISEASE PROGRESSION DURING THE ACTIVE SURVEILLANCE TRIALS FOR LOW-RISK PAPILLARY THYROID MICROCARCINOMA IN JAPAN

The results of the first active surveillance study at Kuma Hospital, published in 2003, demonstrated that more than 70% of PTMCs were stable during the surveillance period.[12] In 2010, Ito and colleagues[13] reported that incidences of tumor enlargement by greater than or equal to 3 mm and nodal metastasis appearance at 10 years were 15.9% and 3.4%, respectively. If these patients were treated at diagnosis, the most likely surgery was hemithyroidectomy with or without paratracheal dissection. This procedure is unlikely to prevent nodal metastases in the lateral compartment and such patients would require a second surgery. However, the authors advocate for 1 surgery instead of 2 because the final outcome is equally favorable.[14] The most recent report, which included 1235 patients and was published in 2014, showed tumor enlargement in 8.0% of patients, as well as metastatic node appearance in 3.8% at 10 years.[15] Unexpectedly, this study showed an inverse relationship between disease progression and patient age. Multivariate analyses for disease progression revealed that only young age (≤40 years) was a significant prognostic factor, whereas family history of differentiated thyroid carcinoma and multiple foci were not. The inverse relationship between disease progression and age in patients with PTMCs is in sharp contrast to larger PTCs, in which old age is a very strong prognostic factor.[16] Multiplicity and family history of differentiated thyroid carcinoma are not included in the contraindication of active surveillance in the authors' protocol, which is consistent with the abovementioned data. Notably, none of the patients at Kuma Hospital and the Cancer Institute Hospital who underwent rescue surgery after slight progression of their PTMCs showed life-threatening recurrence or died of thyroid carcinoma.

The Cancer Institute Hospital also commenced an active surveillance program in 1995. During the active surveillance of 230 patients with 300 PTMCs, only 7% showed enlargement and 1% showed the development of nodal metastasis.[8] Moreover, rich vascularity in the tumor and a lack of strong calcification on ultrasonography was associated with PTMC growth.[17]

Active surveillance has been adopted as a management strategy for low-risk PTMCs in the first edition of the Japan Association of Endocrine Surgeons and Japanese Society of Thyroid Surgery guidelines[18]; the second edition published in 2018 maintains this recommendation.

ESTIMATION OF THE LIFETIME DISEASE PROGRESSION RATE DURING ACTIVE SURVEILLANCE

Although it can be argued that active surveillance merely delays surgery, Ito and colleagues[15] showed that the disease progression rate is inversely correlated with age. Hence, after 10 years of active surveillance during which time patients have aged, the probability of disease progression ought to decrease. Miyauchi and colleagues estimated the lifetime probability of disease progression during active surveillance for each age decade between the 20s and 70s was estimated.[19] First, disease progression (ie, tumor enlargement ≥3 mm and/or nodal metastasis) rates at year 10 of active surveillance for each age decade were calculated. Using these values, the lifetime probability of disease progression according to age at presentation was calculated under the following 3 hypotheses: hypothesis A, PTMCs progress according to the age decade-specific disease progression rates throughout the patient's lifetime; hypothesis B, patients who show disease progression during the initial 10-year period undergo surgical treatment, whereas the remaining patients only have non-progressing tumors; and hypothesis C, the actual probability of disease progression lies between the values estimated using hypotheses A and B. Hypothesis C was considered the most likely estimate. The estimated lifetime probabilities of PTMC progression in patients in their 20s, 30s, 40s, 50s, 60s, and 70s were 48.6%, 25.3%, 20.9%, 10.3%, 8.2%, and 3.5%, respectively.[19] Thus, nearly half of the patients who are in their 20s at presentation will have disease progression requiring surgery, whereas the remaining half will likely not require surgery during their lifetimes. In this series, none of the patients who underwent rescue surgery after the detection of progression showed life-threatening recurrence or died of thyroid carcinoma. Therefore, although PTMCs in young patients are more likely to progress, the authors propose that they can still be candidates for active surveillance. Older patients are less likely to require surgery during their lifetime.

ADVERSE EVENTS DURING ACTIVE SURVEILLANCE VERSUS IMMEDIATE SURGERY

Surgery for low-risk PTMC may be perceived as easier than active surveillance for both physicians and patients. However, in Korea, where the thyroid cancer has become "epidemic" owing to the thyroid cancer-screening program, a considerable increase in patients experiencing surgical complications was reported, along with no decrease in thyroid cancer mortality rates.[5] In a study by Oda and colleagues of 2153 subjects with low-risk PTMCs treated at Kuma Hospital, it was found that 45% underwent immediate surgery, whereas 55% chose active surveillance.[20] The oncological outcomes were excellent in both groups. However, incidences of adverse events such as temporary and permanent vocal cord paralysis, temporary and permanent hypoparathyroidism, levothyroxine administration, and surgical scars were significantly higher in the immediate surgery group than in the active surveillance group, although all of the surgeries were performed by well-experienced endocrine surgeons at Kuma Hospital.[20] In the immediate surgery group, transient and permanent vocal cord paralysis occurred in 4.1% and 0.2% of subjects, respectively, whereas transient and permanent hypoparathyroidism occurred in 16.7% and 1.6%, respectively. Had they been treated by nonexperts, the incidences of these adverse events would be much higher. Levothyroxine administration was required in 66.1% of subjects after surgery. These data demonstrate that active surveillance is superior to immediate surgery for patients with low-risk PTMCs.

PREGNANCY DURING ACTIVE SURVEILLANCE

A large amount of human chorionic gonadotropin is secreted during pregnancy. This hormone shares a common alpha subunit with TSH and stimulates follicular cells; therefore, pregnancy might stimulate the progression of PTMCs. In a previous case series of 9 pregnant subjects, 4 experienced PTMC enlargement during pregnancy.[21] Ito and colleagues[22] then investigated hospital patients and found that only 4 (8%) of the 51 pregnancies or deliveries occurring in 50 patients were associated with PTMC enlargement. Two of the 4 patients underwent surgery after delivery without subsequent recurrence; the remaining 2 maintained active surveillance because their PTMCs stabilized after delivery. Surgery after delivery for patients whose PTMCs enlarge during pregnancy is still possible; thus, young women with PTMCs planning future pregnancies are categorized as appropriate rather than ideal or inappropriate in terms of risk stratification for active surveillance.[23]

THYROID-STIMULATING HORMONE SUPPRESSION DURING ACTIVE SURVEILLANCE

A recent study showed that PTMCs in young patients progress more frequently than those in middle-aged and elderly patients.[15] Although the number of subjects was small, none who underwent mild TSH suppression (low-normal serum TSH) showed disease progression.[15] Sugitani and colleagues[24] showed that patients' TSH levels were not related to their PTMC progression, whereas a study in Korea showed that sustained elevation of serum TSH levels was associated with PTMC progression.[25] To date, no studies have compared subjects with and without TSH suppression, and TSH suppressive management (especially in young patients) may be worth evaluating in future studies.

MEDICAL COSTS OF ACTIVE SURVEILLANCE VERSUS IMMEDIATE SURGERY

Medical cost is an important issue for individual patients and society. In Japan, almost all clinical interventions are performed under the Japanese Health Care Insurance System. Oda and colleagues[26] compared the total cost of immediate surgery plus postoperative management for 10 years to the total cost of active surveillance for a 10-year period. The total costs included costs at presentation, surgery, conversion surgery, surgery for local recurrence, examinations, and prescriptions. It was found that the total cost of immediate surgery was 4.1 times the total cost of active surveillance; similar results were also reported from Hong Kong.[27]

PATHOLOGIC STUDY

Hirokawa and colleagues'[28] histopathological study on surgical PTMC specimens that were resected owing to the appearance of nodal metastasis (11 cases), tumor enlargement (18 cases), and other nonprogression-related causes (160 cases) revealed intraglandular dissemination in 36.4%, 22.2%, and 2.5%; psammoma bodies in 18.2%, 5.6%, and 1.3%; and Ki-67 labeling index greater than 5% in 9.1%, 50.0%, and 5.0%, respectively. Thus, intraglandular dissemination and psammoma bodies were associated with the appearance of nodal metastasis, whereas a high Ki-67 labeling index was associated with tumor enlargement.

BRAF AND *TERT* MUTATIONS

Xing and colleagues[29] reported that the combination of *BRAF* and telomerase reverse transcriptase (*TERT*) mutations were associated with poor prognoses in patients with PTC. However, Yabuta and colleagues'[30] study on selected PTMC surgical specimens resected following the appearance of nodal metastasis (5 cases), tumor enlargement (10 cases), and other nonprogression-related reasons (11 cases) revealed similar incidences of *BRAF* mutation (80%, 70%, and 64%, respectively), whereas none had detectable *TERT* mutations. Thus, analyses of these mutations on fine-needle aspirates from PTMCs are unlikely to predict future disease progression.

ACTIVE SURVEILLANCE FOR LOW-RISK PAPILLARY THYROID MICROCARCINOMA OUTSIDE JAPAN

In 2012, soon after visiting Kuma Hospital and observing the active surveillance practices, Michael Tuttle commenced active surveillance at Memorial Sloan Kettering

Cancer Center, NY, USA. It was the first such trial outside Japan. His associates, Brito and colleagues,[23] proposed a clinical framework for active surveillance risk stratification in collaboration with the authors' group. The framework classified patients as ideal, appropriate, and inappropriate for active surveillance based on tumor and patient characteristics, as well as the medical team's prerogative.

In 2017, Tuttle and colleagues[31] published the first prospective study of active surveillance in the United States. They confirmed the authors' findings that young age at diagnosis was independently related to tumor growth. Of their 284 subjects who underwent active surveillance, 12.7% showed tumor volume increases by greater than 50%, 80.2% had stable disease, and 6.7% experienced volume decreases greater than 50%. They also reported that increases in tumor diameter greater than or equal to 3 mm were detected in only 3.8% of their subjects and concluded that tumor volume evaluation detected its growth sooner.

Recently, a Memorial Sloan Kettering Cancer Center group developed the Thyroid Cancer Treatment Choice study, in collaboration with Korean teams, involving 2 PTMC management options (surgery vs active surveillance) in subjects who were either engaged in conversations regarding their options with their physicians or who were not.[32] They showed that subjects who used the conversation aid were more likely to choose active surveillance than those who did not.

Two Australian studies based on querying physicians regarding active surveillance found that many hesitated to accept this type of management.[33,34] However, these studies were performed before the publication of Oda and colleagues paper on the incidences of adverse events,[20] which convinced Kuma Hospital physicians of the superiority of active surveillance over immediate surgery.

A retrospective study in Korea investigated subjects with small PTCs who did not undergo surgery for reasons such as refusal, other associated malignancies, or high-risk comorbidities. Of their 192 subjects, 27 (14%) showed a tumor volume increase by 50% at a median follow-up of 30 months; 24 of these patients (13%) delayed surgery.[35]

DISCUSSION

Active surveillance for low-risk PTMC commenced at Kuma Hospital in 1993; it is now approved as an alternative management method in Japanese and American guidelines.[11,18] At Kuma Hospital, it is currently recommended that active surveillance be used as the first-line management for patients with low-risk PTMCs. However, adopting this directive required approximately 20 years and was not universally accepted by all physicians at Kuma Hospital. Between 1993 and 1997, the proportion of patients who chose active surveillance was 30%, which increased gradually over time and reached 88% after 2014.[36] There were also marked differences in the proportions of patients who chose active surveillance based on who their attending physicians were. These phenomena may be expected when an institute initiates a new management strategy, especially when convincing evidence of its superiority is lacking early in a trial. However, the authors expect a much faster adoption rate for active surveillance given the accumulated evidence of its safety and superiority.

Some important clinical questions remain. One is how to evaluate the enlargement of PTMC tumors. At Kuma Hospital, 3 dimensions of each PTMC tumor are measured using ultrasonography; however, the depth of the tumor may not be evaluable because of coarse calcification that causes a strong echoic shadow. As such, the change is simply evaluated in its maximum diameter; an increase that is greater than or equal to 3 mm is deemed enlargement. Surgery is recommended for patients with enlarged PTMCs but they are allowed to pursue active surveillance until the tumor size reaches 13 mm if they desire. Tuttle and colleagues[31] claimed that a 50% increase in the tumor volume, as calculated with 3-dimensional measurements, allowed earlier identification of tumor growth than evaluation based on a greater than or equal to 3 mm increase in the maximum diameter. They reported that the cumulative incidences of tumor enlargement greater than or equal to 3 mm were 2.5% in 2 years and 3.8% in 5 years, whereas cumulative incidences of 50% increases were 11.5% in 2 years and 24.8% in 5 years. However, the enlargement of a tumor (from $6 \times 6 \times 6$ mm to $7 \times 7 \times 7$ mm) represents a 59% increase in volume; hence, this criterion may be too sensitive. Furthermore, the authors often observed fluctuations in tumor size and volume during active surveillance. Therefore, the most appropriate criteria or timing for deciding on rescue surgery remains unclear. However, none of the patients who underwent active surveillance at Kuma Hospital and the Cancer Institute Hospital, where a greater than or equal to 3 mm increase in the maximum diameter is considered tumor enlargement, showed distant metastases or died of thyroid carcinoma.

It is important to reduce patients' psychological burdens when they are diagnosed with PTMC. This could be among the reasons that the ATA 2015 guidelines do not recommend FNAC for nodules less than or equal to 10 mm with suspicious features on ultrasonography if they lack symptoms or aggressive features.[11] The Thyroid Cancer Treatment Choice program was created to promote conversations between patients with PTMCs and their physicians regarding the management of their disease,[32] and more patients who experienced this conversation aid chose active surveillance. Although the patients' emotional states were not investigated, the approach using the conversation aid may possibly reduce anxiety related to keeping PTMCs untreated. Of course, conveying all relevant information to patients is critical when deciding on a treatment strategy for any disease. However, good physician communication skills are essential and physicians should, therefore, have deep knowledge of this very common disease to provide appropriate guidance to patients.

Finally, the authors wish to highlight a simple and easy tactic: creating a brochure on PTMCs to provide to patients, with a short explanation of its implications, before performing FNAC. This simple approach has clearly helped patients in their decision-making regarding management if they are found to have low-risk PTMCs. Recently, the proportion of the authors' patients who chose active surveillance has increased to approximately 95%. Another brochure has also been prepared for patients who are undergoing active surveillance to reassure them regarding the safety and superiority of this management modality over immediate surgery, with the intention of reducing anxiety as much as possible.

SUMMARY

Data accumulated over 25 years have clearly demonstrated the safety and superiority of active surveillance over immediate surgery for patients with low-risk PTMC. Because most PTMCs remain small and rescue surgery after the detection of progression is still feasible, active surveillance should be first-line management for low-risk PTMCs.

REFERENCES

1. Ito Y, Miyauchi A. A therapeutic strategy for incidentally detected papillary microcarcinoma of the thyroid. Nat Clin Pract Endocrinol Metab 2007;3:240–8.

2. Takebe K, Date M, Yamamoto N, et al. Mass screening for thyroid cancer with ultrasonography. KARKINOS 1994;7:309–17 [in Japanese].

3. Davies L, Welch HG. Increasing incidence of thyroid cancer in the United States, 1973-2002. JAMA 2006;295:2164–7.

4. Davies L, Welch HG. Current thyroid cancer trends in the United States. JAMA Otolaryngol Head Neck Surg 2014;140:217–22.

5. Ahn HS, Kim HJ, Welch HG. Korea's thyroid-cancer "epidemic" – screening and overdiagnosis. N Engl J Med 2014;371:1765–7.

6. Vaccarella S, Franceschi S, Bray F, et al. Worldwide thyroid-cancer epidemic? The increasing impact at overdiagnosis. N Engl J Med 2016;375:614–7.

7. Miyauchi A, Ito Y, Oda H. Insights into the management of papillary microcarcinoma of the thyroid. Thyroid 2018;28:23–31.

8. Sugitani I, Toda K, Yamada K, et al. Three distinctly different kinds of papillary thyroid microcarcinoma should be recognized our treatment strategies and outcomes. World J Surg 2010;34:1222–31.

9. Ito Y, Miyauchi A, Oda H, et al. Revisiting low-risk thyroid papillary microcarcinomas resected without observation: was immediate surgery necessary? World J Surg 2016;40:523–8.

10. Ver 3. In: Japan Association of Breast and Thyroid Sonology, editor. Guidebook on ultrasound diagnosis of the thyroid. Tokyo: Nankodo; 2016. p. 50 [in Japanese].

11. Haugen BR, Alexander EK, Bible KC, et al. 2015 American Thyroid Association management guidelines for adult patients with thyroid nodules and differentiated thyroid cancer: The American Thyroid Association Guidelines Task Force on thyroid nodules and differentiated thyroid cancer. Thyroid 2016;26:1–133.

12. Ito Y, Uruno T, Nakano K, et al. An observation trial without surgical treatment in patients with papillary microcarcinoma of the thyroid. Thyroid 2003;13:381–7.

13. Ito Y, Miyauchi A, Inoue H, et al. An observation trial for papillary thyroid microcarcinoma in Japanese patients. World J Surg 2010;34:28–35.

14. Miyauchi A. Clinical trials of active surveillance of papillary microcarcinoma of the thyroid. World J Surg 2016;40:516–22.

15. Ito Y, Miyauchi A, Kihara M, et al. Patient age is significantly related to the progression of papillary microcarcinoma of the thyroid under observation. Thyroid 2014;24:27–34.

16. Ito Y, Miyauchi A, Kihara M, et al. Overall survival of papillary thyroid carcinoma patients: a single-institution long-term follow-up of 5897 patients. World J Surg 2018;42:615–22.

17. Fukuoka O, Sugitani I, Ebina A, et al. Natural history of asymptomatic papillary thyroid microcarcinoma: time-dependent changes in calcification and vascularity during active surveillance. World J Surg 2016;40:529–37.

18. Takami H, Ito Y, Okamoto T, et al. Therapeutic strategy for differentiated thyroid carcinoma in Japan based on a newly established guideline managed by Japanese Society of Thyroid Surgeons and Japanese Association of Endocrine Surgeons. World J Surg 2011;35:111–21.

19. Miyauchi A, Kudo T, Ito Y, et al. Estimation of the lifetime probability of disease progression of papillary microcarcinoma of the thyroid during active surveillance. Surgery 2018;163:48–52.

20. Oda H, Miyauchi A, Ito Y, et al. Incidences of unfavorable events in the management of low-risk papillary microcarcinoma of the thyroid by active surveillance versus immediate surgery. Thyroid 2016;26:150–8.

21. Shindo H, Amino N, Ito Y, et al. 2014 Papillary thyroid microcarcinoma might progress during pregnancy. Thyroid 2014;24:840–4.
22. Ito Y, Miyauchi A, Kudo T, et al. Effects of pregnancy on papillary microcarcinoma of the thyroid re-evaluated in the entire patients series at Kuma Hospital. Thyroid 2016;26:156–60.
23. Brito JP, Ito Y, Miyauchi A, et al. A clinical framework to facilitate risk stratification when considering an active surveillance alternative to immediate biopsy and surgery in papillary microcarcinoma. Thyroid 2016;26:144–9.
24. Sugitani I, Fujimoto Y, Yamada K. Association between serum thyrotropin concentration and growth of asymptomatic papillary thyroid microcarcinoma. World J Surg 2014;38:673–8.
25. Kim HI, Jang HW, Ahn HS, et al. High serum TSH level is associated with progression of papillary thyroid microcarcinoma during active surveillance. J Clin Endocrinol Metab 2018;103:446–51.
26. Oda H, Miyauchi A, Ito Y, et al. Comparison of the costs of active surveillance and immediate surgery in the management of low-risk papillary microcarcinoma of the thyroid. Endocr J 2017;64:59–64.
27. Lang BH, Wong CK. A cost-effectiveness comparison between early surgery and non-surgical approach for incidental papillary thyroid microcarcinoma. Eur J Endocrinol 2015;173:367–75.
28. Hirokawa M, Kudo T, Ota H, et al. Pathological characteristics of low-risk papillary thyroid microcarcinoma with progression during active surveillance. Endocr J 2016;63:805–10.
29. Xing A, Liu R, Liu X, et al. BRAF V600E and TERT promoter mutations cooperatively identify the most aggressive papillary thyroid cancer with highest recurrence. J Clin Oncol 2014;32:2718–26.
30. Yabuta T, Matsuse M, Hirokawa M, et al. TERT promoter mutations were not found in papillary thyroid microcarcinomas that showed disease progression on active surveillance. Thyroid 2017;27:1206–7.
31. Tuttle RM, Fagin JA, Minkowitz G, et al. Natural history and tumor volume kinetics of papillary thyroid cancers during active surveillance. JAMA Otolaryngol Head Neck Surg 2017;143:1015–20.
32. Brito JP, Moon JH, Zeuren R, et al. Thyroid Cancer Treatment Choice: a pilot study of a tool to facilitate conversations with patients with papillary microcarcinomas considering treatment choice. Thyroid 2018. https://doi.org/10.1089/thy.2018.0105.
33. Nickel B, Brito JP, Barratt A, et al. Clinicians' view on management and terminology for papillary thyroid microcarcinoma: a qualitative study. Thyroid 2017;27:661–71.
34. Nickel B, Brito JP, Moynihan R, et al. Patients' experiences of diagnosis and management of papillary thyroid microcarcinoma: a qualitative study. BMC Cancer 2018;18:242.
35. Kwon H, Oh HS, Kim M, et al. Active surveillance for patients with papillary thyroid microcarcinoma: a single center's experience in Korea. J Clin Endocrinol Metab 2017;102:1917–25.
36. Ito Y, Miyauchi A, Kudo T, et al. Trends in the implementation of active surveillance for low-risk papillary thyroid microcarcinomas at Kuma Hospital: Gradual increase and heterogeneity in the acceptance of this new management option. Thyroid 2018;28:488–95.

Thyroid Hormone Suppression Therapy

Bernadette Biondi, MD[a], David S. Cooper, MD[b],*

KEYWORDS

- Thyroid cancer • Levothyroxine • Thyrotropin • Cardiovascular system • Bone
- Mortality

KEY POINTS

- Thyroid hormone suppression therapy is a strategy to lower serum thyroid-stimulating hormone (TSH) levels in patients with differentiated thyroid cancer in the hope that it will improve outcomes.
- Evidence for improved outcomes with TSH suppression is lacking, except in patients with the most advanced disease.
- Iatrogenic hyperthyroidism produced by thyroid hormone suppression therapy can lead to adverse outcomes such as osteoporosis, fractures, and cardiovascular disease, including atrial fibrillation.
- The use of thyroid hormone suppression should be based on initial risk of disease and ongoing risk assessment of disease status. The lowest amount of thyroid hormone should be used whenever possible.

INTRODUCTION

The rationale behind thyroid hormone suppression therapy is the knowledge that thyroid-stimulating hormone (TSH), secreted by the pituitary, affects growth and proliferation of thyroid cancer cells.[1] Several epidemiologic studies suggest that higher serum TSH levels, even within the normal range, are associated with an increase in the frequency of differentiated thyroid cancer (DTC) in patients with thyroid nodules, as well as a more aggressive course in those patients with a thyroid cancer diagnosis.[2–5] This theory is supported by a mutant mouse model in which there is altered thyroid hormone receptor signaling, resulting in chronically elevated serum TSH levels, with such mice developing a high frequency of metastatic thyroid cancer.[6] In another mouse model, in which thyroid cancer was induced by knock-in of the oncogenic

The authors have nothing to disclose.
[a] Department of Clinical Medicine and Surgery, University of Naples Federico II, Via Pansini 5, Naples 80131, Italy; [b] Division of Endocrinology, Diabetes, and Metabolism, Johns Hopkins University School of Medicine, 1830 East Monument Street, Suite 333, Baltimore, MD 21287, USA
* Corresponding author.
E-mail address: dscooper@jhmi.edu

0889-8529/19/© 2018 Elsevier Inc. All rights reserved.

V600E BRAF mutation, the development of thyroid cancer was slowed considerably in mice whose genome had the TSH receptor gene knocked out.[7] Because of absence of TSH receptor expression, these animals also have very high serum TSH levels. Although thyroid cancer occurred, it was less aggressive than in animals that expressed the wild-type TSH receptor. This suggests that, although TSH may not be necessary for the initiation of thyroid cancer, TSH signaling is important for its maintenance and progression. On the other hand, suppression of TSH levels in animals with the V600E mutation did not prevent the spread of thyroid cancer after it had been established, possibly due to subsequent tumor-related alterations in TSH receptor expression.[8] This observation may support the idea that TSH suppression may be of limited value in patients with more advanced thyroid cancer (see later discussion).

CLINICAL STUDIES

All patients undergoing total thyroidectomy, as well as the very few patients who undergo lobectomy, require thyroid hormone therapy to maintain normal serum TSH levels. In contrast, the concept behind TSH suppressive therapy is that, at least theoretically, a subnormal serum TSH may lead to slower growth and spread of existing DTC. In support of this idea, a 2002 meta-analysis of 10 studies published from the 1970s to the 1990s concluded that thyroid hormone suppression therapy was efficacious in decreasing thyroid cancer morbidity and mortality (relative risk 0.71, P<.05) for adverse events (combined disease progression/recurrence and death)[9] However, these older studies did not necessarily distinguish replacement from suppression therapy, and lacked modern technology (eg, ultrasound and thyroglobulin measurement) to adequately detect small-volume recurrences. However, 2 subsequent studies published more recently[10,11] also concluded that aggressive serum TSH suppression led to a survival benefit in patients with distant metastases, although the difference in cause-specific survival did not reach statistical significance in 1 of the studies.[10] Importantly, in the other study,[11] no further survival benefit was noted in patients with metastatic disease with serum TSH levels that were fully suppressed (<0.03 mU/L) compared with patients with serum TSH levels that were only suppressed to less than 0.1 mU/L.

Studies from the National Thyroid Cancer Treatment Cooperative Study Group, a thyroid cancer registry consortium in the United States, have concluded that the most aggressive TSH suppression therapy was of no value in patients at low risk for recurrence but was of benefit in high-risk patients.[12,13] In the most recent analysis from this prospective cohort involving almost 5000 subjects followed for a median of 6 years, moderate degrees of TSH suppression, meaning serum TSH levels that were consistently maintained in the subnormal (0.1–0.4 mU/L) to normal ranges (0.4–4 mU/L) led to better outcomes in patients at all stages of disease, compared with subjects whose serum TSH levels were in the normal to elevated ranges.[14] However, benefits of TSH suppression were no longer observed after 5 years of follow-up. This is consistent with an earlier Dutch study showing very low recurrence and mortality rates in subjects whose serum TSH levels were maintained at a median of less than 2 mU/l over a 9 year follow-up compared with subjects whose median serum TSH levels were greater than 2 mU/L.[15] In the only randomized prospective study of TSH suppression in thyroid cancer, 400 Japanese subjects were randomized to receive levothyroxine (L-T4) therapy to maintain serum TSH levels within the reference range versus serum TSH levels less than 0.01 mU/L.[16] After a mean follow-up of almost 7 years, there were no differences in disease-free survival between the 2 groups, even when high-risk subjects were analyzed separately.[16]

Recent American Thyroid Association (ATA) Guidelines recommend either total thyroidectomy or lobectomy for low-risk patients with DTC.[17] Many patients undergoing lobectomy will not require thyroid hormone replacement therapy to maintain serum TSH levels within the reference range. A recent retrospective analysis by Park and colleagues[18] of subjects with thyroid cancer who had undergone lobectomy showed that the use of thyroid hormone to maintain serum TSH levels less than or equal to 2.0 mU/L was of no benefit in terms of recurrence-free survival. Furthermore, even in those subjects who did not receive L-T4 therapy, there was no difference in recurrence-free survival in those subjects whose TSH levels were less than 2 mU/L compared with subjects whose serum TSH levels were between 2 and 4.5 mU/L. However, there were differences in dynamic risk stratification, with more subjects not receiving thyroid hormone having biochemically indeterminate responses compared with those lobectomized subjects who were receiving thyroid hormone treatment to maintain their TSH levels at less than 2 mU/L (17.2% vs 9.4%).[18] The study should be interpreted with caution, however, because all subjects who underwent lobectomy also underwent prophylactic ipsilateral central neck dissections, a procedure not generally performed in the United States.

In general, daily L-T4 doses of 1.6 to 1.8 µg/kg are required to achieve a normal TSH level in athyreotic individuals, whereas doses of 2.0 to 2.2 µg/kg are needed to suppress the serum TSH. However, the dose requirements in individual patients are highly variable and depend on multiple factors, including body mass index, the use of concomitant medications, and drug bioavailability, among others.

ADVERSE EFFECTS OF THYROID-STIMULATING HORMONE-SUPPRESSIVE THERAPY WITH LEVOTHYROXINE

For many years, all patients with DTC likely received excessive L-T4 doses after thyroid surgery and radioiodine (RAI) ablation to intentionally suppress serum TSH at undetectable levels (TSH levels <0.01 mU/L with a third-generation sensitive assay).[19,20] In these patients, serum free thyroxine (FT4) concentrations were often at the upper limit of the reference range or frankly elevated.[21–23] This condition, termed exogenous (Exo) subclinical hyperthyroidism (SHyper), may be associated with symptoms and signs of hyperthyroidism; impaired psychological, social, and physical quality of life[20,24–28]; and adverse effects on the heart and skeleton, including increased cardiovascular (CV) morbidity and mortality, and increased risk of osteoporosis and fractures.[19]

CARDIOVASCULAR MORBIDITY AND MORTALITY

Several retrospective studies reported that long-term TSH-suppressive therapy increases heart rate and left ventricular mass (LVM)[20,29–31]; leads to myocardial strain[30] and impaired diastolic function[32–34]; and reduces arterial elasticity,[35] cardiac reserve, and exercise capacity.[36,37] Although none of these studies stratified the assessment of CV morphology and function according to the level of TSH suppression, the increase in LVM was related to the duration of TSH suppression more than to the thyroid hormone levels in the circulation. These results suggest that the chronic hemodynamic overload and persistent hyperkinetic CV state due to the slight thyroid hormone excess was the main determinant of this concentric cardiac remodeling.[19,38] The negative alterations in CV morphology and function were reversible after beta-blockade[30,39] or the restoration of euthyroidism.[38] Atrial fibrillation (AF) and a prothrombotic state were the most important adverse events in DTC patients with Exo SHyper and were responsible for the greater risk of hospitalization for CV disease

(CVD).[40] One population-based study in subjects receiving long-term TSH-suppressive therapy reported that the risk of CVD and dysrhythmias increased with age.[41] Similarly, in 2 retrospective studies among 136[42] and 518[43] DTC subjects, a higher prevalence of AF was found in the older group (18% vs 8% older than the age of 60 years vs younger than 60 years).[42] The risk of AF was 17.5%, significantly higher that the predicted sex-and age adjusted risks.[42]

In contrast, a prospective study reported that the risk of AF was comparable in 756 subjects with low risk and intermediate risk when serum TSH levels were less than or equal to 0.4 mU/L or greater than 0.4 mU/L.[44] Similarly, no correlation was found between the level of TSH and the occurrence of AF in 2 other studies.[43,44] Interestingly, the risk of AF was independent from the traditional risk factors,[43] whereas it was correlated with the cumulative dose of RAI.[43] These data suggest a potential role of RAI on cardiac inflammation, oxidative stress, or fibrosis because the sodium-iodine symporter gene is expressed in cardiac tissue.[45] All of these data could suggest that advanced age, duration of TSH suppression, and coexistence of associated morbidities are probably the main factors correlated with the negative CV prognosis of patients with Exo SHyper.

There are conflicting data on CV and all-cause mortality in DTC patients.[40,46–49] In 1 large retrospective study, the risk of CV mortality increased 3.3-fold and the risk of all-cause mortality increased 4.4-fold in subjects with DTC compared with controls.[46] These risks were independent of age, sex, and CV risk factors. For each fold decrease in geometric mean, TSH was independently linked with a 3.1-fold increased risk of CV mortality.[46] Regarding RAI therapy, no correlation with the cumulative RAI dose was observed for the risk of all-cause mortality in patients treated with RAI ablation (cumulative RAI dose 100 MCi), despite an increased risk of CVD morbidity compared with the control group and to untreated patients.[40] Therefore, the potential role of a different degree of TSH suppression and the effects of RAI therapy on CV morbidity and mortality remain to be established.

RISK OF OSTEOPOROSIS

Thyroid hormone excess exerts important effects on bone remodeling by shortening bone remodeling cycle and accelerating bone turnover.[50] On the other hand, TSH is a negative regulator of bone turnover and has a specific inhibitory effect on bone resorption.[51,52] Cross-sectional and longitudinal studies report conflicting findings on the effects of Exo SHyper on bone turnover. Two overviews assessing the effects of TSH suppressive therapy on bone mineral density (BMD) in patients with DTC suggested that TSH suppression did not affect BMD in men or in premenopausal women, whereas postmenopausal women were at risk of bone loss.[53,54]

Similarly, 2 meta-analyses[55,56] on postmenopausal women with Exo SHyper found a decrease in BMD with an annual bone mass loss of 0.91%.[55] Some studies reported that TSH suppressive therapy can affect trabecular bone microstructure as detected by trabecular bone score measurement,[57] peripheral high-resolution quantitative computed tomography,[58,59] or radiological vertebral fractures,[60] which were found in about one-third of women with DTC and was linked with the duration of treatment, degree of TSH suppression, and age of patient.[60]

A prospective study in DTC subjects with low or intermediate risk suggested that subjects with TSH suppression less than 0.4 mU/L had a higher incidence of osteoporosis compared with nonsuppressed subjects (hazard ratio 2.1, $P = .05$), and that prolonged TSH suppression with L-T4 increased the risk of postoperative osteoporosis in DTC subjects.[44] The duration of TSH suppression is an important factor to be considered. A randomized controlled trial in female subjects randomly assigned to receive TSH suppressive or no therapy reported that subjects with TSH suppressive therapy had a significant deterioration in BMD from 1 year after surgery. Moreover, a significant decrease in BMD was observed in older subjects (>50 years) but not in younger subjects (<50 years). A marked deterioration in BMD was reported in subjects who continued TSH suppression for 5 years, especially in those with older age and lower preoperative BMD.[61] Subjects who did not receive TSH suppression did not show any significant decrease in T-score until 5 years postoperatively.[61] All of these results suggest that a long-term TSH suppressive therapy is associated with bone loss, especially in elderly patients and postmenopausal women.

FRACTURE RISK

Postmenopausal women with serum TSH levels lower than 0.1 mU/L during L-T4 treatment had a 2-fold to 4-fold greater risk of osteoporotic fracture compared with the general population. The risk of fracture was associated with a strong dose-response relation among adults aged 70 years or more.[62] Several studies and meta-analyses, including prospective studies, have confirmed the association between subclinical thyroid hormone excess and the risk of fractures, mainly in postmenopausal women.[41,62–68] Most of these studies confirmed the associated between duration of TSH suppression and increased fracture risk. The negative effects of the slight thyroid hormone excess in SHyper on muscle strength, weight, and lean body mass loss, as well as the possible association with a cognitive decline in elderly patients, could contribute to the increased risk of fractures in patients during TSH suppressive therapy.[69]

EFFECTS OF HIGHER FREE THYROXINE LEVELS AND CARDIOVASCULAR RISK

Total T3 or FT3 levels are usually in the middle or lower part of the reference range in Exo SHyper, with a consequent increased T4/T3 ratio.[13–16] Therefore, endogenous and Exo SHyper (caused by Graves' disease or toxic nodular goiter) are not comparable biochemically due to differences in severity and in the pattern of circulating thyroid hormone levels.[69] This could suggest that a different mechanism of action may explain the adverse effects of endogenous and Exo SHyper on the CV system and bone structure. Some studies reported that high serum FT4 levels within the reference range might be associated with negative health outcomes in elderly patients in terms of AF and CV mortality.[70–73] Elderly subjects with serum FT4 in the highest quartile of their reference range can have an increased risk of AF and CV morbidity and mortality.[70–73] Moreover, lower TSH and higher FT4 within the reference range were associated with 22% to 25% increased risk of hip fractures in euthyroid postmenopausal women.[74] Prospective studies are needed to assess the role of increased T4/T3 ratio on the CV and bone risk in patients with DTC.

TREATMENT OF EXOGENOUS SUBCLINICAL HYPERTHYROIDISM

Large randomized controlled studies are required to prove causality in the cardiac and skeletal effects, and to assess the efficacy of TSH normalization on CV risk and fractures. No study has evaluated the effects of beta-blocking drugs on CV mortality, even though these drugs can improve CV parameters associated with increased morbidity in the general population. Treatment with alendronate could prevent trabecular bone loss in patients with thyroid cancer receiving thyroxine replacement.[75] However, the potential risk of AF should be considered and a risk-benefit assessment made.[76]

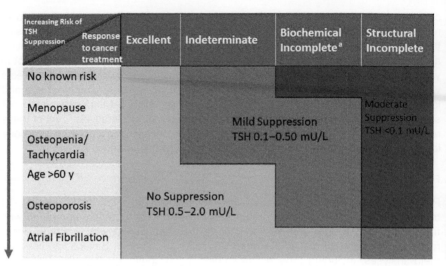

Fig. 1. 2015 ATA Thyroid Guidelines: long-term TSH suppression. [a] TSH target for patients with a biochemical incomplete response can be quite different based on original ATA risk, thyroglobulin (Tg) level, Tg trend over time, and risk of TSH suppression.

RECOMMENDATIONS FOR THYROID HORMONE THERAPY

Given the evidence that aggressive TSH suppression is of little to no benefit to almost all patients with thyroid cancer who are at low risk of recurrence and death, the ATA recommends a graded algorithm, considering that the potential benefits of such therapy must be balanced against CV and skeletal risks (**Fig. 1**).[17] Using the concept of ongoing risk stratification, the ATA recommends maintaining serum TSH levels between 0.5 and 2 mU/L in low-risk and intermediate-risk patients with an excellent response to treatment but using mild TSH suppression (TSH 0.1–0.5 mU/L) in high-risk patients who have had an excellent response (negative imaging and undetectable suppressed thyroglobulin). Mild TSH suppression is also recommended in patients with a biochemically incomplete response. More significant TSH suppression (ie, serum TSH <0.1 but not necessarily undetectable) is recommended in patients with residual structural disease or a biochemically incomplete response if they are young or at low risk of complications from Exo SHyper. Ongoing assessment of the patient's clinical disease status, as well as the temporal development of risk factors such as advanced age, postmenopausal state, and the development of osteoporosis and/or CVD are essential to prevent the treatment from becoming worse for the patient than the disease being treated.

REFERENCES

1. McLeod DS. Thyrotropin in the development and management of differentiated thyroid cancer. Endocrinol Metab Clin North Am 2014;43:367–83.
2. Boelaert K, Horacek J, Holder RL, et al. Serum thyrotropin concentration as a novel predictor of malignancy in thyroid nodules investigated by fine-needle aspiration. J Clin Endocrinol Metab 2006;91:4295–301.
3. Haymart MR, Repplinger DJ, Leverson GE, et al. Higher serum thyroid stimulating hormone level in thyroid nodule patients is associated with greater risks of differentiated thyroid cancer and advanced tumor stage. J Clin Endocrinol Metab 2008;93:809–14.

4. McLeod DS, Watters KF, Carpenter AD, et al. Thyrotropin and thyroid cancer diagnosis: a systematic review and dose-response meta-analysis. J Clin Endocrinol Metab 2012;97:2682–92.
5. McLeod DS, Cooper DS, Ladenson PW, et al. Prognosis of differentiated thyroid cancer in relation to serum thyrotropin and thyroglobulin antibody status at time of diagnosis. Thyroid 2014;24:35–42.
6. Suzuki H, Willingham MC, Cheng SY. Mice with a mutation in the thyroid hormone receptor beta gene spontaneously develop thyroid carcinoma: a mouse model of thyroid carcinogenesis. Thyroid 2002;12:963–9.
7. Franco AT, Malaguarnera R, Refetoff S, et al. Thyrotrophin receptor signaling dependence of Braf-induced thyroid tumor initiation in mice. Proc Natl Acad Sci U S A 2011;108:1615–20.
8. Xing M, Usadel H, Cohen Y, et al. Methylation of the thyroid-stimulating hormone receptor gene in epithelial thyroid tumors: a marker of malignancy and a cause of gene silencing. Cancer Res 2003;63:2316–21.
9. McGriff NJ, Csako G, Gourgiotis L, et al. Effects of thyroid hormone suppression therapy on adverse clinical outcomes in thyroid cancer. Ann Med 2002;34:554–664.
10. Ito Y, Masuoka H, Fukushima M, et al. Prognosis and prognostic factors of patients with papillary carcinoma showing distant metastasis at surgery (M1 patients) in Japan. Endocr J 2010;57:523–31.
11. Diessl S, Holzberger B, Mäder U, et al. Impact of moderate vs stringent TSH suppression on survival in advanced differentiated thyroid carcinoma. Clin Endocrinol (Oxf) 2012;76:586–92.
12. Cooper DS, Specker B, Ho M, et al. Thyrotropin suppression and disease progression in patients with differentiated thyroid cancer: results from the National Thyroid Cancer Treatment Cooperative Registry. Thyroid 1998;8:737–44.
13. Jonklaas J, Sarlis NJ, Litofsky D, et al. Outcomes of patients with differentiated thyroid carcinoma following initial therapy. Thyroid 2006;16:1229–42.
14. Carhill AA, Litofsky DR, Ross DS, et al. Long-term outcomes following therapy in differentiated thyroid carcinoma: NTCTCS Registry Analysis 1987-2012. J Clin Endocrinol Metab 2015;100:3270–9.
15. Hovens GC, Stokkel MP, Kievit J, et al. Associations of serum thyrotropin concentrations with recurrence and death in differentiated thyroid cancer. J Clin Endocrinol Metab 2007;92:2610–5.
16. Sugitani I, Fujimoto Y. Does postoperative thyrotropin suppression therapy truly decrease recurrence in papillary thyroid carcinoma? A randomized controlled trial. J Clin Endocrinol Metab 2010;95:4576–83.
17. Haugen BR, Alexander EK, Bible KC, et al. 2015 American Thyroid Association management guidelines for adult patients with thyroid nodules and differentiated thyroid cancer. Thyroid 2016;26:1–133.
18. Park S, Kim WG, Han M, et al. Thyrotropin suppressive therapy for low-risk small thyroid cancer: a propensity score-matched cohort study. Thyroid 2017;27:1164–70.
19. Biondi B, Cooper DS. Benefits of thyrotropin suppression versus the risks of adverse effects in differentiated thyroid cancer. Thyroid 2010;20:135–46.
20. Biondi B, Fazio S, Carella C, et al. Cardiac effects of long term thyrotropin-suppressive therapy with levothyroxine. J Clin Endocrinol Metab 1993;77:334–8.
21. Jonklaas J, Davidson B, Bhagat S, et al. Triiodothyronine levels in athyreotic individuals during Levothyroxine therapy. JAMA 2008;299:769–77.

22. Gullo D, Latina A, Frasca F, et al. Levothyroxine monotherapy cannot guarantee euthyroidism in all athyreotic patients. PLoS One 2011;6:e2255.
23. Ito M, Miyauchi A, Morita S, et al. TSH-suppressive doses of levothyroxine are required to achieve preoperative native serum triiodothyronine levels in patients who have undergone total thyroidectomy. Eur J Endocrinol 2012;167:373–8.
24. Botella-Carretero JI, Galan JM, Caballero C, et al. Quality of life and psychometric functionality in patients with differentiated thyroid carcinoma. Endocr Relat Cancer 2003;10(4):601–10.
25. Eustatia-Rutten CF, Corssmit EP, Pereira AM, et al. Quality of life in long-term exogenous subclinical hyperthyroidism and the effects of restoration of euthyroidism, a randomized controlled trial. Clin Endocrinol 2006;64:284–91.
26. Hoftijzer HC, Heemstra KA, Corssmit EP, et al. Quality of life in cured patients with differentiated thyroid carcinoma. J Clin Endocrinol Metab 2008;93:200–3.
27. Tagay S, Herpertz S, Langkafel M, et al. Health-related quality of life, anxiety and depression in thyroid cancer patients under short-term hypothyroidism and TSH-suppressive levothyroxine treatment. Eur J Endocrinol 2005;153:755–63.
28. Vigario Pdos S, Chachamovitz DS, Cordeiro MF, et al. Effects of physical activity on body composition and fatigue perception in patients on thyrotropin-suppressive therapy for differentiated thyroid carcinoma. Thyroid 2011;21:695–700.
29. Ching G, Franklyn J, Stallard TJ, et al. Cardiac hypertrophy as a result of long-term thyroxine therapy and thyrotoxicosis. Heart 1996;75:363–8.
30. Gullu S, Altuntas F, Dincer I, et al. Effects of TSH-suppressive therapy on cardiac morphology and function: beneficial effects of the addition of beta-blockade on diastolic dysfunction. Eur J Endocrinol 2004;150:655–61.
31. Abdulrahman RM, Delgado V, Hoftijzer HC, et al. Both exogenous subclinical hyperthyroidism and short-term overt hypothyroidism affect myocardial strain in patients with differentiated thyroid carcinoma. Thyroid 2011;21:471–6.
32. Fazio S, Biondi B, Carella C, et al. Diastolic dysfunction in patients on thyroid-stimulating hormone suppressive therapy with levothyroxine: beneficial effect of beta-blockade. J Clin Endocrinol Metab 1995;80:2222–6.
33. Abdulrahman RM, Delgado V, Ng A, et al. Abnormal cardiac contractility in long term exogenous subclinical hyperthyroid patients as demonstrated by two-dimensional echocardiography speckle tracking imaging. Eur J Endocrinol 2010;163:435–41.
34. Smit JW, Eustatia-Rutten CF, Corssmit EP, et al. Reversible diastolic dysfunction after long-term exogenous subclinical hyperthyroidism: a randomized, placebo-controlled study. J Clin Endocrinol Metab 2005;90:6041–7.
35. Shargorodsky M, Serov S, Gavish D, et al. Long-term thyrotropin-suppressive therapy with Levothyroxine impairs small and large artery elasticity and increases left ventricular mass in patients with thyroid carcinoma. Thyroid 2006;16:381–6.
36. Biondi B, Fazio S, Cuocolo A, et al. Impaired cardiac reserve and exercise capacity in patients receiving long-term thyrotropin suppressive therapy with Levothyroxine. J Clin Endocrinol Metab 1996;81:4224–8.
37. Mercuro G, Panzuto MG, Bina A, et al. Cardiac function, physical exercise capacity, and quality of life during long-term thyrotropin mild thyrotropin-suppressive therapy with levothyroxine: effect of individual dose tailoring. J Clin Endocrinol Metab 2000;85:159–64.
38. Taillard V, Sardinoux M, Oudot C, et al. Early detection of isolated left ventricular diastolic dysfunction in high-risk differentiated thyroid carcinoma patients on TSH-suppressive therapy. Clin Endocrinol (Oxf) 2011;75:709–14.

39. Biondi B, Fazio S, Carella C, et al. Control of adrenergic overactivity by β-blockade improves the quality of life in patients receiving long term suppressive therapy with levothyroxine. J Clin Endocrinol Metab 1994;78:1028–33.
40. Pajamäki N, Metso S, Hakala T1, et al. Long-term cardiovascular morbidity and mortality in patients treated for differentiated thyroid cancer. Clin Endocrinol (Oxf) 2018;88:303–10.
41. Flynn RW, Bonellie SR, Jung RT, et al. Serum thyroid-stimulating hormone concentration and morbidity from cardiovascular disease and fractures in patients on long-term thyroxine therapy. J Clin Endocrinol Metab 2010;95:186–93.
42. Abonowara A, Quraishi A, Sapp JL, et al. Prevalence of atrial fibrillation in patients taking TSH suppression therapy for management of thyroid cancer. Clin Invest Med 2012;35:152–6.
43. Klein Hesselink EN, Lefrandt JD, Schuurmans EP, et al. Increased risk of atrial fibrillation after treatment for differentiated thyroid carcinoma. J Clin Endocrinol Metab 2015;100:4563–9.
44. Wang LY, Smith AW, Palmer FL, et al. Thyrotropin suppression increases the risk of osteoporosis without decreasing recurrence in ATA low-and intermediate-risk patients with differentiated thyroid carcinoma. Thyroid 2015;25:300–7.
45. Spitzweg C, Joba W, Eisenmenger W, et al. Analysis of human sodium iodide symporter gene expression in extrathyroidal tissues and cloning of its complementary deoxyribonucleic acids from salivary gland, mammary gland, and gastric mucosa. J Clin Endocrinol Metab 1998;83:1746–51.
46. Klein Hesselink EN, Klein Hesselink MS, de Bock GH, et al. Long-term cardiovascular mortality in patients with differentiated thyroid carcinoma: an observational study. J Clin Oncol 2013;31:4046–53.
47. Eustatia-Rutten CFA, Corssmit EPM, Biermasz NR, et al. Survival and death causes in differentiated thyroid carcinoma. J Clin Endocrinol Metab 2006;91:313–9.
48. Links TP, van Tol KM, Jager PL, et al. Life expectancy in differentiated thyroid cancer: a novel approach to survival analysis. Endocr Relat Cancer 2005;12:273–80.
49. Zoltek M, Andersson TML, Hedman C, et al. Cardiovascular mortality in 6900 patients with differentiated thyroid cancer: a Swedish population-based study. Clin Surg 2017;2:1–6.
50. Bassett JH, Williams GR. Role of thyroid hormones in skeletal development and bone maintenance. Endocr Rev 2016;37:135–87.
51. Abe E, Marians RC, Yu W, et al. TSH is a negative regulator of skeletal remodeling. Cell 2003;115:151–62.
52. Mazziotti G, Sorvillo F, Piscopo M, et al. Recombinant human TSH modulates in vivo C-telopeptides of type-1 collagen and bone alkaline phosphatase, but not osteoprotegerin production in postmenopausal women monitored for differentiated thyroid carcinoma. J Bone Miner Res 2005;20:480–6.
53. Quan ML, Pasieka JL, Rorstad O. Bone mineral density in well-differentiated thyroid cancer patients treated with suppressive thyroxine: a systematic overview of the literature. J Surg Oncol 2002;79:62–9.
54. Heemstra KA, Hamdy NA, Romijn JA, et al. The effects of thyrotropin-suppressive therapy on bone metabolism in patients with well-differentiated thyroid carcinoma. Thyroid 2006;16:583–91.
55. Faber J, Galloc AM. Changes in bone mass during prolonged subclinical hyperthyroidism due to L-thyroxine treatment: a meta-analysis. Eur J Endocrinol 1994;130:350–6.

56. Uzzan B, Campos J, Cucherat M, et al. Effect on bone mass of long term treatment with thyroid hormones: a meta analysis. J Clin Endocrinol Metab 1996;81: 4278–489.
57. Moon JH, Kim KM, Oh TJ, et al. The effect of TSH suppression on vertebral trabecular bone scores in patients with differentiated thyroid carcinoma. J Clin Endocrinol Metab 2017;102:78–85.
58. Tournis S, Antoniou JD, Liakou CG, et al. Volumetric bone mineral density and bone geometry assessed by peripheral quantitative computed tomography in women with differentiated thyroid cancer under TSH suppression. Clin Endocrinol (Oxf) 2015;82:197–204.
59. Kim K, Kim IJ, Pak K, et al. Evaluation of bone mineral density using DXA and central QCT in postmenopausal patients under thyrotropin suppressive therapy. Evaluation of bone mineral density using DXA and central QCT in postmenopausal patients under thyrotropin suppressive therapy. J Clin Endocrinol Metab 2018. https://doi.org/10.1210/jc.2017-02704.
60. Mazziotti G, Formenti AM, Frara S, et al. High prevalence of radiological vertebral fractures in women on thyroid-stimulating hormone-suppressive therapy for thyroid carcinoma. J Clin Endocrinol Metab 2018;103:956–64.
61. Sugitani I, Fujimoto Y. Effect of postoperative thyrotropin suppressive therapy on bone mineral density in patients with papillary thyroid carcinoma: a prospective controlled study. Surgery 2011;150:1250–7.
62. Turner MR, Camacho X, Fischer HD, et al. Levothyroxine dose and risk of fractures in older adults: nested case-control study. BMJ 2011;342:d2238.
63. Bauer DC, Ettinger B, Nevitt MC, et al, Study of Osteoporotic Fractures Research Group. Risk for fracture in women with low serum levels of thyroid-stimulating hormone. Ann Intern Med 2001;134:561–8.
64. Lee JS, Buzková P, Fink HA, et al. Subclinical thyroid dysfunction and incident hip fracture in older adults. Arch Intern Med 2010;170:1876–83.
65. Blum MR, Bauer DC, Collet TH, et al. Subclinical thyroid dysfunction and fracture risk: a meta-analysis. JAMA 2015;313:2055–65.
66. Wirth CD, Blum MR, da Costa BR, et al. Subclinical thyroid dysfunction and the risk for fractures: a systematic review and meta-analysis. Ann Intern Med 2014; 161:189–99.
67. Yan Z, Huang H, Li J, et al. Relationship between subclinical thyroid dysfunction and the risk of fracture: a meta-analysis of prospective cohort studies. Osteoporos Int 2016;27:115–25.
68. Yang R, Yao L, Fang Y, et al. The relationship between subclinical thyroid dysfunction and the risk of fracture or low bone mineral density: a systematic review and metaanalysis of cohort studies. J Bone Miner Metab 2018;36(2):209–20.
69. Biondi B, Cooper DS. Subclinical hyperthyroidism. N Engl J Med 2018;378: 2411–9.
70. Gammage MD, Parle JV, Holder RL, et al. Association between free thyroxine concentration and atrial fibrillation. Arch Intern Med 2007;167:928–34.
71. Heeringa J, Hoogendoorn EH, van der Deure WM, et al. High normal thyroid function and risk of atrial fibrillation. Arch Intern Med 2008;168:2219–24.
72. Chaker L, Heeringa J, Dehghan A, et al. Normal thyroid function and the risk of atrial fibrillation: the Rotterdam Study. J Clin Endocrinol Metab 2015;100: 3718–24.
73. Yeap BB, Alfonso H, Hankey GJ, et al. Higher free thyroxine levels are associated with all-cause mortality in euthyroid older men: the Health In Men Study. Eur J Endocrinol 2013;169:401–8.

74. Aubert CE, Floriani C, Bauer DC, et al. Thyroid function tests in the reference range and fracture: individual participant analysis of prospective cohorts. J Clin Endocrinol Metab 2017;102:2719–28.
75. Panebianco P, Rosso D, Destro G, et al. Use of disphosphonates in the treatment of osteoporosis in thyroidectomized patients on levothyroxin replacement therapy. Arch Gerontol Geriatr 1997;25:219–25.
76. Sharma A, Einstein AJ, Vallakati A, et al. Risk of atrial fibrillation with use of oral and intravenous bisphosphonates. Am J Cardiol 2014;113:1815–21.

Surveillance for Differentiated Thyroid Cancer Recurrence

Prasanna Santhanam, MBBS, MD[a],*, Paul W. Ladenson, MD[b]

KEYWORDS

- Differentiated thyroid cancer • Cancer recurrence • Serum thyroglobulin monitoring
- Thyroid cancer imaging

KEY POINTS

- Serum thyroglobulin monitoring along with anatomic and functional imaging play key roles in the surveillance of patients with differentiated thyroid cancer after initial treatment.
- Among patients with a disease stage justifying thyroid remnant ablation or with suspected metastatic disease, radioiodine whole-body scans are vital in the months after surgery.
- For patients with low to moderate-risk cancers, ultrasonography of the neck (with measurement of serum thyroglobulin on thyroid hormone replacement) are the best initial diagnostic modalities, and are often the only tests required.
- In individuals suspected of having distant metastases, CT, MRI, and 18F-FDG PET can make important contributions in localizing residual disease and monitoring its progression and responses to therapy, provided they are used in the appropriate setting.

INTRODUCTION

Recurrence of differentiated (epithelial) thyroid cancer is common, occurring in 3% to 13% of low-risk, 21% to 36% of intermediate-risk, and approximately 68% of high-risk patients based on the American Thyroid Association's (ATA) risk classification.[1,2] In almost all cases, these thyroid cancer recurrences arise from residual disease that escaped detection and treatment by primary surgical treatment with or without postoperative radioiodine. Serum thyroglobulin monitoring plays the frontline role in raising suspicion that residual disease is present, but it lacks specificity in the presence of remaining thyroid gland tissue, fails to identify residual thyroid cancer in a minority of poorly differentiated cancers, and provides only a general clue by its level to the

The authors have nothing to disclose.

[a] Division of Endocrinology, Metabolism and Diabetes, Johns Hopkins University School of Medicine, 5501 Hopkins Bayview Circle, Suite 3 B 73, Baltimore, MD 21224, USA; [b] Division of Endocrinology, Diabetes, and Metabolism, Johns Hopkins University School of Medicine, 1830 East Monument Street, Suite 333, Baltimore, MD 21287, USA
* Corresponding author.
E-mail address: psantha1@jhmi.edu

site(s) of residual disease.[3–5] Consequently, anatomic and functional imaging techniques for surveillance, localization, therapeutic decision making, and assessing treatment responses are essential in patients whose thyroid cancer has recurred. The anatomic imaging modalities covered in this review include ultrasonography, computed tomography (CT), and MRI; and functional imaging with radioiodine and PET.

There are important limitations to this highly sensitive surveillance approach to patients with treated thyroid cancers. The thyroglobulin, as a tumor marker, not infrequently identifies clinically irrelevant residual normal thyroid or tumor tissue. In almost two-thirds of patients with detectable serum thyroglobulin after surgery, there will be no structural disease localized, no treatment possible or required, and, nonetheless, a generally excellent prognosis. One study, in patients 6 months after thyroidectomy and radioiodine remnant ablation, showed that among those with a levothyroxine-suppressed thyroglobulin level 1 to 5 ng/mL, 54% eventually achieved a thyroglobulin of less than 1 ng/mL with no further therapy.[6] In another study of patients with a biochemically incomplete response (ie, detectable thyroglobulin), 34% had the spontaneous remission of "disease," whereas only 20% went on to develop clinical manifestation of their residual disease.[1,2,7]

There also can be many false-positive imaging findings. Ultrasonography often demonstrates benign cervical adenopathy with indeterminate features, such as rounding or lack of a fatty hilum. CT imaging not infrequently shows incidental unrelated lung, liver, or bone findings. Even radioiodine diagnostic and posttreatment scans can be misleading because of physiologic uptake in breast and thymus, tissue inflammation (eg, bronchitis and sarcoidosis), skin contamination, and retention in anomalous structures (eg, esophageal and tracheal diverticula).[8,9]

Consequently, use of combined thyroglobulin and imaging must be thoughtfully applied, especially keeping in mind the patient's pretest probability of having residual disease, based on the patient's age and tumor surgical pathology findings. We here review current techniques for detecting residual disease and propose an effective and cost-effective algorithm to localize such lesions.

SERUM THYROGLOBULIN IN THYROID CANCER SURVEILLANCE: ROLE AND LIMITATIONS

The exclusively thyroid-derived circulating protein thyroglobulin is a highly specific and sensitive marker for residual thyroid tissue after initial treatments for thyroid cancer.[10] In 1973, Van Herle and colleagues[11] described the earliest specific and reproducible double antibody radioimmunoassay for measurement of thyroglobulin in human serum; it had an analytical sensitivity of 1.6 ng/mL. The same group later showed that patients with untreated differentiated thyroid cancer had a mean thyroglobulin of 144 ng/mL, which after treatment fell to a mean 6 ng/mL; but in patients with documented metastasis remained elevated at a mean of 465 ng/mL.[12] Spencer and colleagues[13] aptly described serum thyroglobulin as a circulating marker integrating the mass of the benign and/or malignant thyroid tissue remaining, degree of thyroid-stimulating hormone (TSH) receptor stimulation, and the ability of the tumor tissue to synthesize and release the protein.

The responsiveness of thyroglobulin to TSH seen in normal thyroid tissue and most tumors means that all serum thyroglobulin values need to be interpreted in light of with their simultaneous TSH levels. Thyroglobulin measured after recombinant TSH administration, which is usually done in the context of concurrent radioiodine scanning, adds to the sensitivity of thyroglobulin testing by doing so after intense short-term TSH stimulation. Thyroglobulin testing after recombinant TSH, 0.9 ng intramuscularly daily for 2 days, has been shown to be as accurate in detection of residual remnant and cancer tissue as when TSH elevation is produced by thyroid hormone withdrawal; and the highest thyroglobulin values are seen 72 hours after the second recombinant TSH dose.[14] The extent of thyroglobulin increase after recombinant TSH is typically approximately 10-fold in patients with well-differentiated thyroid cancer, whereas poorly differentiated tumors may show a less than 3-fold increase.[13] Recombinant TSH-stimulated testing is most helpful when the thyroglobulin assay being used has a detection limit of 1 to 2 ng/mL or more.[15,16] One selective literature review found that a thyroglobulin assay with a cutoff of 1 ng/mL would fail to detect 36% of cases with residual disease, whereas 91% would be identified if a cutoff of 2 ng/mL after recombinant TSH stimulation was used.[3] However, the availability of highly sensitive assays with detection limits as low as 0.1 ng/mL has reduced the need to use recombinant TSH before thyroglobulin testing.[17]

An important limitation of thyroglobulin surveillance occurs in the 20% of patients with differentiated thyroid cancer who have circulating thyroglobulin antibodies, which interfere with widely used immunometric ("sandwich") thyroglobulin assays, leading to falsely low reported values.[13,18] Two alternate thyroglobulin assay methods can sometimes circumvent this problem: a traditional 2-antibody immunoassay and liquid chromatography-tandem mass spectrometry.[19–21] In patients with thyroglobulin antibodies, serial monitoring of antibody levels in a single assay, can also sometimes be informative about the presence of residual disease and its progression or response to therapy.[22–24]

The ATA's 2015 clinical practice guideline uses the postoperative thyroglobulin level, which reaches its nadir 3 to 4 weeks after surgery, to (1) categorize patients' responses to primary treatment, and (2) guide decision making about the prognosis of patients with thyroid cancer and recommended monitoring regimen[7,25–27] (Table 1). A TSH-suppressed or TSH-stimulated serum thyroglobulin less than 1 ng/mL does not rule out entirely the possibility of detecting disease on a subsequent posttreatment 131-I scan, but the likelihood is extremely low, except in patients who presented with high-stage disease. Recurrence (presence of residual disease) risk increases as postoperative thyroglobulin values reach 5 to 10 ng/mL.[7]

In the course of following patients after their initial surgery and possible radioiodine (treatment), there are several ways in which serial thyroglobulin measurements are helpful. First, in most patients with low-stage disease at very low risk of recurrence, an undetectable or very low serum thyroglobulin can provide reassurance that there is less need for nonspecific imaging. Second, it can refute or corroborate the significance of radiological findings that might represent residual disease. Third, it designates patients with rising thyroglobulin levels who need periodic imaging for localization. Fourth, when cervical node disease is suspected, but cytology is negative, thyroglobulin measurement on the fine-needle aspirate can sometimes reveal disease.[28] Fifth, in patients with known local or distant metastatic disease, changes in serial thyroglobulin values can serve as a marker of therapeutic response and support decision making, about when to initiate or repeat 131-I treatments and/or chemotherapy. Finally, the proportionality of the serum thyroglobulin level to the known disease burden based on imaging speaks to the degree of tumor differentiation and its likelihood of responding to 131-I and other therapies.

CONVENTIONAL IMAGING MODALITIES FOR DETECTING RESIDUAL DISEASE
Ultrasonography of the Neck

Ultrasonography is a highly sensitive tool for the detection of residual thyroid cancer in cervical lymph nodes or soft tissues.[29,30] The European guidelines recommend at

Table 1
Thyroid cancer response categories after initial therapy

Category	Characteristics	Prognosis
Complete response	Negative imaging, suppressed Tg[a] <0.2 (and no interfering Tg antibodies), or stimulated Tg <1.0	1%–4% recurrence, <1% risk of death
Biochemically incomplete	Negative imaging, suppressed Tg ≥1 or stimulated Tg ≥10 or rising anti-Tg antibody levels	30% resolve spontaneously, 20% require additional therapy to achieve complete response, 20% progress to develop structural disease, <1% risk of death
Structurally incomplete	Structural disease With any Tg level	50%–85% have persistent disease, 11% risk of death with locoregional metastasis, 50% risk of death with distant metastasis
Indeterminate	Nonspecific imaging findings, suppressed Tg <1, stimulated Tg <10, anti-Tg antibodies declining or stable	15%–20% will develop disease, remainder will resolve spontaneously, <1% risk of death

[a] Thyroglobulin (abbreviated as Tg) values are all ng/mL.
Adapted from Haugen BR, Alexander EK, Bible KC, et al. 2015 American Thyroid Association Management guidelines for adult patients with thyroid nodules and differentiated thyroid cancer. the American Thyroid Association guidelines task force on thyroid nodules and differentiated thyroid cancer. Thyroid 2016;26(1):48; with permission.

least a 12-MHZ probe for grayscale imaging, examination of the thyroid bed and lymph nodes (LNs) located in levels II to VI bilaterally, and use of Doppler for assessment of flow.[31] The ATA recommends a cervical ultrasonography using a 10-MHZ frequency for detection of lymph node metastasis.[7] Higher-frequency transducer (>10 MHz or above) allows for better resolution for superficial lymph nodes but with poor penetration for deeper structures, whereas the lower frequencies (5 MHZ) allow for deeper penetration but lower resolution.[32] Its sensitivity for detection of residual disease can be as high as 94% compared with stimulated thyroglobulin and diagnostic radioiodine scanning, which have sensitivities close to 50%.[30]

However, ultrasonography of the neck is associated with false positives, especially in patients in the low and intermediate ATA risk categories.[33] After bilateral thyroidectomy, the surgical bed usually is a flat inverted triangular area representing fibrofatty connective tissue.[34] Small (<5 mm) thyroid bed nodules are common, but fewer than 10% of these increase in size over 5 years of follow-up, even though 60% or more of them display suspicious features, such as hypo echogenicity, taller than wide, microcalcifications, irregular margins, and/or increased vascularity on the initial sonogram.[35] Benign cervical LNs and scar tissue are often identified and of uncertain significance. Other normal structures within or adjacent to the thyroid bed that can mimic residual disease include a small normal thyroid remnant, cricoid and thyroid cartilages, cervical thymus, sympathetic ganglion, terminal aspect of thoracic duct, transverse process of the cervical spine, and nerve roots.[36] There also can be misleading findings due to chronic granulomatous lesions, surgical scarring, pharyngoesophageal diverticula (sometimes with calcifications), parathyroid adenoma, and thyroglossal duct cysts. In addition, in the lateral neck, traumatic neuromas, nerve sheath tumors, and paragangliomas may be seen.[36]

Cervical LNs are considered sonographically suspicious if they show one or more of the following: loss of fatty hilum, cystic regions, intranodal hyperechoic small punctuate lesions, and increased peripheral vascular flow[37]; however, these criteria are imperfect in identifying or excluding malignancy.[7] Absence of fatty hilum has the highest sensitivity of 100%, but a low specificity of 29%.[38] The presence of microcalcifications has the highest specificity of 100%, but poor sensitivity.[37] The presence of peripheral vascularity was a feature associated with sensitivity of 86% and specificity of 82%.[7] A long-to-short axis ratio less than 2 and a short axis diameter greater than 8 mm are both suspicious for metastatic disease.[31,39]

The ATA 2015 guidelines recommend cervical ultrasound to evaluate the central and lateral compartments depending on the risk and thyroglobulin status every 6 to 12 months.[7] We recommend follow-up cervical ultrasonography 6 months after radioiodine treatment and then 6 to 12 months thereafter for 1 to 3 years, especially in patients with high-risk tumors.[31] During subsequent years, annual ultrasound is recommended for high-risk patients, whereas for low-risk patients, clinical judgment should be exercised based on clinical findings and thyroglobulin values.[31] Further ultrasonography should generally not be done in patients with low-risk and very low risk thyroid cancers based on surgical findings, reassuringly negative cervical ultrasonography in the first 2 years after surgery, and serum thyroglobulin levels that are undetectable in patients who received radioiodine or less than 2 ng/mL levels that have been stable over time, in patients who did not undergo remnant ablation. In such patients, an indeterminate ultrasonographic finding is much more likely to be a false-positive than true-positive finding. However, in patients with serum thyroglobulin levels indicative of residual disease, in those with intermediate-risk or high-risk cancers, continued ultrasonography at 6-month to 12-month intervals may be appropriate and the imaging technique most likely to define the locations of recurrent disease.

Computed Tomography Scanning of the Neck, Chest, and Other Regions

CT has numerous applications in thyroid cancer preoperative staging, surveillance, restaging, metastatic disease localization and serial monitoring for progression and treatment responsiveness. CT scanning of the region from the skull base to the tracheal bifurcation with and without intravenous contrast can complement ultrasonography in localizing residual/recurrent disease in cervical LNs, particularly before surgery in the central neck and after surgery caudal to the sternal notch and in the posterior neck.[8–40] In CT-detected cervical adenopathy, metastatic disease is suspected if the lymph node has cystic components, calcifications, and/or enhancement. Sometimes, CT also may demonstrate hyperdensities reflecting hemorrhagic or proteinaceous content in metastatic lesions.[40]

CT scan is also key to delineate the extent of remaining disease and anatomic relationships of aggressive thyroid malignancies causing or threatening laryngeal or tracheal invasion, airway obstruction, or paraspinal or muscular invasion.[41] The ATA 2015 guideline recommends that CT scanning be performed in patients with a high serum thyroglobulin but negative neck ultrasound,[7] particularly when the serum thyroglobulin is greater than 10 ng/mL and/or rising while on TSH suppressive levothyroxine therapy.[42,43] Thyroid cancer also can infrequently cause a malignant pleural effusion for which CT is the investigation of choice.[44]

Consequently, although CT scanning is not a routinely recommended element of surveillance for all postoperative patients, it plays a key role in the localization of residual/recurrent disease not adequately revealed by ultrasonography. CT requires iodinated contrast for delineation of neck masses and so its use must be coordinated with planned future I-131 scanning and treatment.[45]

Role of the MRI

MRI has limited specific applications in thyroid cancer preoperative staging, surveillance, postoperative restaging, metastatic disease localization, and serial monitoring for progression and treatment responsiveness. The MRI protocol typically involves axial and coronal T1-weighted, fat-saturated T2-weighted images, followed by post-contrast axial and coronal T1-weighted images.[40] Both preoperatively and postoperatively, the finding of completely effaced fatty tissue predicts disease involvement of the recurrent laryngeal nerve (88%, 94% sensitivity and 82% specificity, n = 32).[46] The combination of cartilage soft tissue signal, presence of an intraluminal mass, and/or tumor abutting 180° of tracheal circumference predicts tracheal invasion by thyroid cancer with 90% accuracy.[47] Similarly, MRI can sometimes detect esophageal invasion.[48] MRI can be helpful in detection of lymph node involvement before surgery and nodal recurrences afterward; but its findings are, of course, less specific in distinguishing metastatic from benign reactive nodes than radioiodine whole-body scanning.[49] MRI as well as fludeoxyglucose (FDG)-PET/CT typically perform better than conventional CT scan for detection of bony metastatic disease with better sensitivities, especially in lesions involving the spine.[50]

Newer MRI diffusion-weighted imaging, which is based on the principle that water molecules exhibit lower diffusion coefficients in highly cellular tissues, are being evaluated for their ability to detect thyroid cancer–specific characteristics. In one small cohort of patients with thyroid cancer, the apparent diffusion coefficient values of papillary thyroid cancer with extrathyroidal extension were significantly lower than corresponding values for metastases without extrathyroidal extension.[51]

FUNCTIONAL IMAGING MODALITIES FOR DETECTING RESIDUAL DISEASE
Radioiodine Planar and Single-Photon Emission Computed Tomography/Computed Tomography Scanning

Radioiodine imaging exploits the thyrocyte's intrinsic iodine concentrating ability to (1) detect residual normal thyroid tissue for potential subsequent ^{131}I ablation or differential diagnosis of persistent circulating thyroglobulin; and (2) identify, localize, and monitor progression or treatment responses of iodine-avid metastases from differentiated thyroid cancer. Three radioiodine isotopes are used commonly (**Table 2**). In patients whose clinicopathological staging may justify postoperative ^{131}I therapy, whole-body scanning is typically performed 2 to 12 weeks postoperatively.[7] In most circumstances, ^{123}I has been the preferred radioisotope, because its emissions are suitable for planar and single-photon emission CT (SPECT)/CT imaging, but they do not "stun," that is, subtly injure, thyrocytes and limit their ability to concentrate the subsequent therapeutic ^{131}I dose.[52,53] [131]I imaging is used for the posttreatment scan, which is more sensitive for detection of metastatic disease due to its higher administered dose and longer physical half-life, which permits imaging at later time points when background activity has dissipated.[54] Tracer doses of ^{131}I are also used for therapeutic dosimetry because its slower decay permits quantitative prediction of delivered radiation doses to iodine-avid metastases and radiation-sensitive normal tissues (eg, bone marrow and lung) over longer periods of 5 to 10 days.

Radioiodine scanning requires TSH stimulation of iodine uptake by residual normal and malignant thyroid tissue. Traditionally, an endogenous rise in circulating TSH was induced postoperatively by withholding or withdrawing thyroid hormone therapy for

Table 2
Iodine radioisotopes used for differentiated thyroid cancer imaging

Isotope	Emissions	Physical T$_{1/2}$	Typical Scan Dose	Imaging Characteristics	Uses
[131]Iodine	Beta particle (606 keV), isometric transition emitting gamma rays (364 keV)	8.02 d	2–3 mCi (diagnostic scan) 30–200 mCi (post-treatment scan)	Normal uptake in nasal area, oropharynx and salivary glands, stomach and intestines; residual uptake in the thyroid bed may be due to either remnant tissue or residual disease	Diagnostic whole-body scans are typically imaged 48 h after tracer administration; posttreatment whole-body scans are typically imaged 5–7 d after treatment
[123]Iodine	Gamma rays (159 keV)	13.2 h	1.5–2.0 mCi	Normal uptake in nasal area, oropharynx and salivary glands, stomach and intestines; residual uptake may be seen in the thyroid bed that is difficult to distinguish between remnant tissue and residual disease	Diagnostic whole-body scan after thyroidectomy; follow-up diagnostic scan 9–12 mo later for detection of RAI avid residual disease
[124]Iodine	Multiple high-energy photons, gamma rays, positrons	4.18 d	1.5–1.7 mCi	As above, but with increased resolution due to high-energy photons	Investigational, 3-dimensional whole-body and lesion-based dosimetry

Abbreviations: mCi, millicurie; RAI, radioactive iodine.
Data from Refs.[82–84]

approximately 4 weeks. This approach is effective in most patients but has several disadvantages. First, it results almost universally in severe clinical hypothyroidism with diminished quality of life (physical and mental).[55] Second, prolonged and profound TSH stimulation can rarely provoke tumor growth with potentially severe consequences, especially when metastases are located at critical sites. Third, a minority of patients may be unable to surmount an endogenous TSH rise, including those with incidental pituitary or hypothalamic disease and some elderly patients.[56] Recombinant TSH (rTSH, thyrotropin alfa, Thyrogen) permits equivalently accurate scanning and stimulated thyroglobulin testing while avoiding clinical hypothyroidism.[14,57] However, rTSH administration has also rarely been associated with acute enlargement of metastatic lesions, causing upper airway obstruction, fractures, and neurologic complications.

Radioiodine imaging is more accurate when the patient has a low level of circulating stable iodine, which competes with diagnostic and therapeutic radioiodine for uptake by iodine-avid thyroid tissue. Consequently, patients are placed on a low-iodine diet (https://www.thyrogen.com/patients/Low-Iodine-Diet.aspx) for 1 week before planned imaging and potential therapy.[58] In patients who have received iodinated radiocontrast dye or iodine-containing medications within 6 to 8 weeks of planned radioiodine scanning, measurement of the urinary iodine level can provide reassurance that the iodine load has been cleared.

The sensitivity of diagnostic ^{123}I scans are less than posttreatment ^{131}I scans in revealing the extent of disease. Concordance rates are high between the 2 isotopes for thyroid bed recurrence and bone metastasis, but low for lymph node and pulmonary disease, approximately 60% and 40%, respectively.[59]

The specificity of positive findings in patients with thyroid cancer is imperfect, with both diagnostic ^{123}I and posttreatment ^{131}I whole-body scans. False-positive foci of activity can be due to skin and contamination, asymmetric salivary gland activity and breast uptake, tracheal and esophageal diverticula, inflammatory lung disease (eg, bronchitis and sarcoidosis), retained gastrointestinal tract contents in the appendix, endometriosis, ovarian dermoid cysts, healing fractures, spermatoceles, renal granulomas and cysts, and subcutaneous lipomas.[60–63]

Combining radioiodine scans with CT (SPECT/CT) better localizes foci of tracer concentration in one-fourth of cases when there is ambiguity on planar imaging alone.[64] Consequently, SPECT/CT imaging is often helpful in confirming spurious sites of activity described previously. Detection of additional lesions, changes in TNM staging, and improved disease prognostication have all been associated with use of SPECT/CT imaging, especially after the posttreatment scan.[65,66]

In practice then, postoperative ^{123}I whole-body scans are performed in patients whose disease stage may warrant subsequent ^{131}I therapy, and an ^{131}I posttreatment is performed several days thereafter. Typically, a second ^{123}I whole-body scan is recommended 9 to 12 months later to confirm eradication of remnant thyroid tissue and any iodine-avid residual disease. Once this follow-up scan is negative, radioiodine scanning has no role to play in the surveillance of most patients.[67] Exceptions are the patients with follicular and, less often, papillary thyroid cancers with iodine-avid metastatic disease requiring additional cycles of ^{131}I therapy.

18F-Fluorodeoxyglucose PET/Computed Tomography Scanning

18F-FDG PET imaging is based on the release of 2 high-energy 511 keV photons in opposite directions (termed coincidence detection) after a positron and an electron annihilate each other. Enhanced glucose uptake by hypermetabolic tumor tissue can localize many types of cancers with high spatial resolution, especially when coupled with CT.[68] 18F-FDG PET/CT imaging plays a secondary role in disease localization when patients are suspected of having additional, yet unidentified metastases based on their high-risk clinicopathological staging, serum thyroglobulin concentration, or clinical findings. When such suspected disease sites have escaped localization by ^{123}I/^{131}I scanning and ultrasonographic and CT imaging, residual disease has been variously reported to be detectable by 18F-FDG in 45% to 100% of patients, and can alter management in as many as 50% of patients.[69] Stimulation with recombinant TSH before PET/CT image acquisition improves the sensitivity and specificity of the imaging modality.[70]

In a meta-analysis including 515 patients, 18F-FDG PET/CT was found to have a pooled sensitivity of 0.84 (95% confidence interval [CI] 0.77–0.89) and a pooled specificity of 0.78 (95% CI 0.67–0.86) for detection of residual differentiated thyroid cancer.[71] The sensitivity of 18F-FDG PET/CT increases with higher thyroglobulin levels, which typically reflect the volume of residual disease. The sensitivity of 18F-FDG PET/CT was greater than 90% when the thyroglobulin level was greater than

4.6 ng/mL in one study.[72] The serum thyroglobulin levels at which 18F-FDG PET/CT achieves its maximum sensitivity and specificity ranges between 12 and 32 ng/mL.[73] When 18F-FDG PET/CT is added to ^{131}I imaging, PET detected additional lesions in 14% of patients with differentiated thyroid cancer.[74,75]

Quantitative 18F-FDG PET/CT has also been used to assess thyroid cancer recurrence. A standardized uptake value (SUV) at the 90th minute of greater than 2.75 and a change of maximum SUV between the 60th and 90th minute greater than −1.1% provides a sensitivity, specificity, and accuracy of 81%, 90%, and 83%, respectively, for detection of metastatic subcentimeter cervical LNs.[76] The presence of BRAF^{V600E} mutation in papillary thyroid cancer confers a higher likelihood of 18F-FDG PET/CT avidity and is associated with higher SUV uptake values compared with the wild-type papillary thyroid cancer.[77] Finally, detection of disease on FDG PET/CT is associated with poorer prognosis and lesser likelihood of responding to chemotherapy.[78] 18F-FDG PET also has been combined with MRI, which was shown in one study to alter management in approximately half of patients with differentiated thyroid cancer by providing additional information about the extent of the disease.[79]

The positron-emitting isotope [124]Iodine also can be used for whole-body and lesional dosimetry[80,81] (see **Table 2**); however, this modality remains investigational at this time.

SUMMARY

Serum thyroglobulin monitoring along with anatomic and functional imaging play leading roles in surveillance of patients with differentiated thyroid cancer after their initial treatment. Among patients with a disease stage justifying thyroid remnant ablation or with suspected metastatic disease, radioiodine whole-body scans are essential tools in the months after surgery. For patients with low-risk to moderate-risk papillary cancer, who are at greatest risk of cervical node or soft tissue recurrence, ultrasonography is the best initial imaging approach, and often the only modality required. In individuals suspected of having additional more distant metastases, CT, MRI, and 18F-FDG PET imaging can all make important contributions in localizing that residual disease and monitoring its progression and responses to therapy.

REFERENCES

1. Vaisman F, Momesso D, Bulzico DA, et al. Spontaneous remission in thyroid cancer patients after biochemical incomplete response to initial therapy. Clin Endocrinol 2012;77(1):132–8.

2. Tuttle RM, Tala H, Shah J, et al. Estimating risk of recurrence in differentiated thyroid cancer after total thyroidectomy and radioactive iodine remnant ablation: using response to therapy variables to modify the initial risk estimates predicted by the new American Thyroid Association staging system. Thyroid 2010;20(12): 1341–9.

3. Mazzaferri EL, Robbins RJ, Spencer CA, et al. A consensus report of the role of serum thyroglobulin as a monitoring method for low-risk patients with papillary thyroid carcinoma. J Clin Endocrinol Metab 2003;88(4):1433–41.

4. Torlontano M, Crocetti U, Augello G, et al. Comparative evaluation of recombinant human thyrotropin-stimulated thyroglobulin levels, 131I whole-body scintigraphy, and neck ultrasonography in the follow-up of patients with papillary thyroid microcarcinoma who have not undergone radioiodine therapy. J Clin Endocrinol Metab 2006;91(1):60–3.

5. Robbins RJ, Srivastava S, Shaha A, et al. Factors influencing the basal and recombinant human thyrotropin-stimulated serum thyroglobulin in patients with metastatic thyroid carcinoma. J Clin Endocrinol Metab 2004;89(12):6010–6.

6. Padovani RP, Robenshtok E, Brokhin M, et al. Even without additional therapy, serum thyroglobulin concentrations often decline for years after total thyroidectomy and radioactive remnant ablation in patients with differentiated thyroid cancer. Thyroid 2012;22(8):778–83.

7. Haugen BR, Alexander EK, Bible KC, et al. 2015 American Thyroid Association Management guidelines for adult patients with thyroid nodules and differentiated thyroid cancer: the American Thyroid Association guidelines task force on thyroid nodules and differentiated thyroid cancer. Thyroid 2016;26(1):1–133.

8. Chudgar AV, Shah JC. Pictorial review of false-positive results on radioiodine scintigrams of patients with differentiated thyroid cancer. Radiographics 2017; 37(1):298–315.

9. Yang SP, Bach AM, Tuttle RM, et al. Serial neck ultrasound is more likely to identify false-positive abnormalities than clinically significant disease in low-risk papillary thyroid cancer patients. Endocr Pract 2015;21(12):1372–9.

10. Refetoff S, Lever EG. The value of serum thyroglobulin measurement in clinical practice. JAMA 1983;250(17):2352–7.

11. Van Herle AJ, Uller RP, Matthews NI, et al. Radioimmunoassay for measurement of thyroglobulin in human serum. J Clin Invest 1973;52(6):1320–7.

12. Herle AJ, Uller RP. Elevated serum thyroglobulin. A marker of metastases in differentiated thyroid carcinomas. J Clin Invest 1975;56(2):272–7.

13. Spencer CA, LoPresti JS, Fatemi S, et al. Detection of residual and recurrent differentiated thyroid carcinoma by serum thyroglobulin measurement. Thyroid 1999;9(5):435–41.

14. Haugen BR, Pacini F, Reiners C, et al. A comparison of recombinant human thyrotropin and thyroid hormone withdrawal for the detection of thyroid remnant or cancer. J Clin Endocrinol Metab 1999;84(11):3877–85.

15. Torrens JI, Burch HB. Serum thyroglobulin measurement. Utility in clinical practice. Endocrinol Metab Clin North Am 2001;30(2):429–67.

16. Woodmansee WW, Haugen BR. Uses for recombinant human TSH in patients with thyroid cancer and nodular goiter. Clin Endocrinol 2004;61(2):163–73.

17. Giovanella L, Clark PM, Chiovato L, et al. Thyroglobulin measurement using highly sensitive assays in patients with differentiated thyroid cancer: a clinical position paper. Eur J Endocrinol 2014;171(2):R33–46.

18. Spencer CA, Takeuchi M, Kazarosyan M, et al. Serum thyroglobulin autoantibodies: prevalence, influence on serum thyroglobulin measurement, and prognostic significance in patients with differentiated thyroid carcinoma. J Clin Endocrinol Metab 1998;83(4):1121–7.

19. Kushnir MM, Rockwood AL, Straseski JA, et al. Comparison of LC-MS/MS to immunoassay for measurement of thyroglobulin in fine-needle aspiration samples. Clin Chem 2014;60(11):1452–3.

20. Netzel BC, Grebe SK, Algeciras-Schimnich A. Usefulness of a thyroglobulin liquid chromatography-tandem mass spectrometry assay for evaluation of suspected heterophile interference. Clin Chem 2014;60(7):1016–8.

21. Netzel BC, Grebe SK, Carranza Leon BG, et al. Thyroglobulin (Tg) testing revisited: Tg assays, TgAb assays, and correlation of results with clinical outcomes. J Clin Endocrinol Metab 2015;100(8):E1074–83.

22. Spencer CA. Clinical review: clinical utility of thyroglobulin antibody (TgAb) measurements for patients with differentiated thyroid cancers (DTC). J Clin Endocrinol Metab 2011;96(12):3615–27.
23. Gianoukakis AG. Thyroglobulin antibody status and differentiated thyroid cancer: what does it mean for prognosis and surveillance? Curr Opin Oncol 2015;27(1): 26–32.
24. Spencer C, Fatemi S. Thyroglobulin antibody (TgAb) methods—strengths, pitfalls and clinical utility for monitoring TgAb-positive patients with differentiated thyroid cancer. Best Pract Res Clin Endocrinol Metab 2013;27(5):701–12.
25. Piccardo A, Arecco F, Puntoni M, et al. Focus on high-risk DTC patients: high postoperative serum thyroglobulin level is a strong predictor of disease persistence and is associated to progression-free survival and overall survival. Clin Nucl Med 2013;38(1):18–24.
26. Giovanella L, Ceriani L, Ghelfo A, et al. Thyroglobulin assay 4 weeks after thyroidectomy predicts outcome in low-risk papillary thyroid carcinoma. Clin Chem Lab Med 2005;43(8):843–7.
27. Polachek A, Hirsch D, Tzvetov G, et al. Prognostic value of post-thyroidectomy thyroglobulin levels in patients with differentiated thyroid cancer. J Endocrinol Invest 2011;34(11):855–60.
28. Torres MR, Nobrega Neto SH, Rosas RJ, et al. Thyroglobulin in the washout fluid of lymph-node biopsy: what is its role in the follow-up of differentiated thyroid carcinoma? Thyroid 2014;24(1):7–18.
29. Matrone A, Gambale C, Piaggi P, et al. Postoperative thyroglobulin and neck ultrasound in the risk restratification and decision to perform 131I ablation. J Clin Endocrinol Metab 2017;102(3):893–902.
30. Frasoldati A, Pesenti M, Gallo M, et al. Diagnosis of neck recurrences in patients with differentiated thyroid carcinoma. Cancer 2003;97(1):90–6.
31. Leenhardt L, Erdogan MF, Hegedus L, et al. 2013 European Thyroid Association guidelines for cervical ultrasound scan and ultrasound-guided techniques in the postoperative management of patients with thyroid cancer. Eur Thyroid J 2013; 2(3):147–59.
32. Ying M, Ahuja A. Sonography of neck lymph nodes. Part I: normal lymph nodes. Clin Radiol 2003;58(5):351–8.
33. Peiling Yang S, Bach AM, Tuttle RM, et al. Frequent screening with serial neck ultrasound is more likely to identify false-positive abnormalities than clinically significant disease in the surveillance of intermediate risk papillary thyroid cancer patients without suspicious findings on follow-up ultrasound evaluation. J Clin Endocrinol Metab 2015;100(4):1561–7.
34. Shin JH, Han BK, Ko EY, et al. Sonographic findings in the surgical bed after thyroidectomy: comparison of recurrent tumors and nonrecurrent lesions. J Ultrasound Med 2007;26(10):1359–66.
35. Rondeau G, Fish S, Hann LE, et al. Ultrasonographically detected small thyroid bed nodules identified after total thyroidectomy for differentiated thyroid cancer seldom show clinically significant structural progression. Thyroid 2011;21(8): 845–53.
36. Chua WY, Langer JE, Jones LP. Surveillance neck sonography after thyroidectomy for papillary thyroid carcinoma: pitfalls in the diagnosis of locally recurrent and metastatic disease. J Ultrasound Med 2017;36(7):1511–30.
37. Leboulleux S, Girard E, Rose M, et al. Ultrasound criteria of malignancy for cervical lymph nodes in patients followed up for differentiated thyroid cancer. J Clin Endocrinol Metab 2007;92(9):3590–4.

38. Kuna SK, Bracic I, Tesic V, et al. Ultrasonographic differentiation of benign from malignant neck lymphadenopathy in thyroid cancer. J Ultrasound Med 2006; 25(12):1531–7 [quiz: 1538–40].

39. Steinkamp HJ, Cornehl M, Hosten N, et al. Cervical lymphadenopathy: ratio of long- to short-axis diameter as a predictor of malignancy. Br J Radiol 1995; 68(807):266–70.

40. Hoang JK, Branstetter BF, Gafton AR, et al. Imaging of thyroid carcinoma with CT and MRI: approaches to common scenarios. Cancer Imaging 2013;13:128–39.

41. Ahmed M, Saleem M, Al-Arifi A, et al. Obstructive endotracheal lesions of thyroid cancer. J Laryngol Otol 2002;116(8):613–21.

42. Moneke I, Kaifi JT, Kloeser R, et al. Pulmonary metastasectomy for thyroid cancer as salvage therapy for radioactive iodine-refractory metastases. Eur J Cardiothorac Surg 2018;53(3):625–30.

43. Wang R, Zhang Y, Tan J, et al. Analysis of radioiodine therapy and prognostic factors of differentiated thyroid cancer patients with pulmonary metastasis: an 8-year retrospective study. Medicine 2017;96(19):e6809.

44. Liu M, Shen Y, Ruan M, et al. Notable decrease of malignant pleural effusion after treatment with sorafenib in radioiodine-refractory follicular thyroid carcinoma. Thyroid 2014;24(7):1179–83.

45. Loevner LA, Kaplan SL, Cunnane ME, et al. Cross-sectional imaging of the thyroid gland. Neuroimaging Clin N Am 2008;18(3):445–61, vii.

46. Takashima S, Takayama F, Wang J, et al. Using MR imaging to predict invasion of the recurrent laryngeal nerve by thyroid carcinoma. AJR Am J Roentgenol 2003; 180(3):837–42.

47. Wang JC, Takashima S, Takayama F, et al. Tracheal invasion by thyroid carcinoma: prediction using MR imaging. AJR Am J Roentgenol 2001;177(4):929–36.

48. Wang J, Takashima S, Matsushita T, et al. Esophageal invasion by thyroid carcinomas: prediction using magnetic resonance imaging. J Comput Assist Tomogr 2003;27(1):18–25.

49. Mihailovic J, Prvulovic M, Ivkovic M, et al. MRI versus (1)(3)(1)I whole-body scintigraphy for the detection of lymph node recurrences in differentiated thyroid carcinoma. AJR Am J Roentgenol 2010;195(5):1197–203.

50. Lange MB, Nielsen ML, Andersen JD, et al. Diagnostic accuracy of imaging methods for the diagnosis of skeletal malignancies: a retrospective analysis against a pathology-proven reference. Eur J Radiol 2016;85(1):61–7.

51. Lu Y, Moreira AL, Hatzoglou V, et al. Using diffusion-weighted MRI to predict aggressive histological features in papillary thyroid carcinoma: a novel tool for pre-operative risk stratification in thyroid cancer. Thyroid 2015;25(6):672–80.

52. Kao CH, Yen TC. Stunning effects after a diagnostic dose of iodine-131. Nuklearmedizin 1998;37(1):30–2.

53. Urhan M, Dadparvar S, Mavi A, et al. Iodine-123 as a diagnostic imaging agent in differentiated thyroid carcinoma: a comparison with iodine-131 post-treatment scanning and serum thyroglobulin measurement. Eur J Nucl Med Mol Imaging 2007;34(7):1012–7.

54. Chong A, Song HC, Min JJ, et al. Improved detection of lung or bone metastases with an I-131 whole body scan on the 7th day after high-dose I-131 therapy in patients with thyroid cancer. Nucl Med Mol Imaging 2010;44(4):273–81.

55. Ladenson PW, Braverman LE, Mazzaferri EL, et al. Comparison of administration of recombinant human thyrotropin with withdrawal of thyroid hormone for radioactive iodine scanning in patients with thyroid carcinoma. N Engl J Med 1997; 337(13):888–96.

56. Ringel MD, Ladenson PW. Diagnostic accuracy of 131I scanning with recombinant human thyrotropin versus thyroid hormone withdrawal in a patient with metastatic thyroid carcinoma and hypopituitarism. J Clin Endocrinol Metab 1996; 81(5):1724–5.

57. Schroeder PR, Haugen BR, Pacini F, et al. A comparison of short-term changes in health-related quality of life in thyroid carcinoma patients undergoing diagnostic evaluation with recombinant human thyrotropin compared with thyroid hormone withdrawal. J Clin Endocrinol Metab 2006;91(3):878–84.

58. Lee M, Lee YK, Jeon TJ, et al. Low iodine diet for one week is sufficient for adequate preparation of high dose radioactive iodine ablation therapy of differentiated thyroid cancer patients in iodine-rich areas. Thyroid 2014;24(8):1289–96.

59. Iwano S, Kato K, Nihashi T, et al. Comparisons of I-123 diagnostic and I-131 post-treatment scans for detecting residual thyroid tissue and metastases of differentiated thyroid cancer. Ann Nucl Med 2009;23(9):777–82.

60. Triggiani V, Giagulli VA, Iovino M, et al. False positive diagnosis on (131)iodine whole-body scintigraphy of differentiated thyroid cancers. Endocrine 2016; 53(3):626–35.

61. Hannoush ZC, Palacios JD, Kuker RA, et al. False positive findings on I-131 WBS and SPECT/CT in patients with history of thyroid cancer: case series. Case Rep Endocrinol 2017;2017:8568347.

62. Campenni A, Giovinazzo S, Tuccari G, et al. Abnormal radioiodine uptake on post-therapy whole body scan and sodium/iodine symporter expression in a dermoid cyst of the ovary: report of a case and review of the literature. Arch Endocrinol Metab 2015;59(4):351–4.

63. Mi YX, Sui X, Huang JM, et al. Incidentally polycystic kidney disease identified by SPECT/CT with post-therapy radioiodine scintigraphy in a patient with differentiated thyroid carcinoma: a case report. Medicine 2017;96(43):e8348.

64. Zilioli V, Peli A, Panarotto MB, et al. Differentiated thyroid carcinoma: incremental diagnostic value of (131)I SPECT/CT over planar whole body scan after radioiodine therapy. Endocrine 2017;56(3):551–9.

65. Kohlfuerst S, Igerc I, Lobnig M, et al. Posttherapeutic (131)I SPECT-CT offers high diagnostic accuracy when the findings on conventional planar imaging are inconclusive and allows a tailored patient treatment regimen. Eur J Nucl Med Mol Imaging 2009;36(6):886–93.

66. Ciappuccini R, Heutte N, Trzepla G, et al. Postablation (131)I scintigraphy with neck and thorax SPECT-CT and stimulated serum thyroglobulin level predict the outcome of patients with differentiated thyroid cancer. Eur J Endocrinol 2011; 164(6):961–9.

67. Gonzalez Carvalho JM, Gorlich D, Schober O, et al. Evaluation of (131)I scintigraphy and stimulated thyroglobulin levels in the follow up of patients with DTC: a retrospective analysis of 1420 patients. Eur J Nucl Med Mol Imaging 2017;44(5): 744–56.

68. Farwell MD, Pryma DA, Mankoff DA. PET/CT imaging in cancer: current applications and future directions. Cancer 2014;120(22):3433–45.

69. Leboulleux S, Schroeder PR, Schlumberger M, et al. The role of PET in follow-up of patients treated for differentiated epithelial thyroid cancers. Nat Clin Pract Endocrinol Metab 2007;3(2):112–21.

70. Chin BB, Patel P, Cohade C, et al. Recombinant human thyrotropin stimulation of fluoro-D-glucose positron emission tomography uptake in well-differentiated thyroid carcinoma. J Clin Endocrinol Metab 2004;89(1):91–5.

71. Kim SJ, Lee SW, Pak K, et al. Diagnostic performance of PET in thyroid cancer with elevated anti-Tg Ab. Endocr Relat Cancer 2018;25(6):643–52.
72. Giovanella L, Ceriani L, De Palma D, et al. Relationship between serum thyroglobulin and 18FDG-PET/CT in 131I-negative differentiated thyroid carcinomas. Head Neck 2012;34(5):626–31.
73. Santhanam P, Solnes LB, Rowe SP. Molecular imaging of advanced thyroid cancer: iodinated radiotracers and beyond. Med Oncol 2017;34(12):189.
74. Lee JW, Lee SM, Lee DH, et al. Clinical utility of 18F-FDG PET/CT concurrent with 131I therapy in intermediate-to-high-risk patients with differentiated thyroid cancer: dual-center experience with 286 patients. J Nucl Med 2013;54(8):1230–6.
75. Kaneko K, Abe K, Baba S, et al. Detection of residual lymph node metastases in high-risk papillary thyroid cancer patients receiving adjuvant I-131 therapy: the usefulness of F-18 FDG PET/CT. Clin Nucl Med 2010;35(1):6–11.
76. Kunawudhi A, Pak-art R, Keelawat S, et al. Detection of subcentimeter metastatic cervical lymph node by 18F-FDG PET/CT in patients with well-differentiated thyroid carcinoma and high serum thyroglobulin but negative 131I whole-body scan. Clin Nucl Med 2012;37(6):561–7.
77. Santhanam P, Khthir R, Solnes LB, et al. The relationship of BRAF(V600E) mutation status to FDG PET/CT avidity in thyroid cancer: a review and meta-analysis. Endocr Pract 2018;24(1):21–6.
78. Gaertner FC, Okamoto S, Shiga T, et al. FDG PET performed at thyroid remnant ablation has a higher predictive value for long-term survival of high-risk patients with well-differentiated thyroid cancer than radioiodine uptake. Clin Nucl Med 2015;40(5):378–83.
79. Seiboth L, Van Nostrand D, Wartofsky L, et al. Utility of PET/neck MRI digital fusion images in the management of recurrent or persistent thyroid cancer. Thyroid 2008;18(2):103–11.
80. Sgouros G, Hobbs RF, Atkins FB, et al. Three-dimensional radiobiological dosimetry (3D-RD) with 124I PET for 131I therapy of thyroid cancer. Eur J Nucl Med Mol Imaging 2011;38(Suppl 1):S41–7.
81. Santhanam P, Taieb D, Solnes L, et al. Utility of I-124 PET/CT in identifying radioiodine avid lesions in differentiated thyroid cancer: a systematic review and meta-analysis. Clin Endocrinol 2017;86(5):645–51.
82. Rault E, Vandenberghe S, Van Holen R, et al. Comparison of image quality of different iodine isotopes (I-123, I-124, and I-131). Cancer Biother Radiopharm 2007;22(3):423–30.
83. Ziessman HA, O'Malley JP, Thrall JH, et al. Nuclear Medicine: The Requisites. Philadelphia: Elsevier Saunders; 2014.
84. Kuker R, Sztejnberg M, Gulec S. I-124 imaging and dosimetry. Mol Imaging Radionucl Ther 2017;26(Suppl 1):66–73.

Novel Drug Treatments of Progressive Radioiodine-Refractory Differentiated Thyroid Cancer

Steven P. Weitzman, MD, Steven I. Sherman, MD*

KEYWORDS

- Thyroid neoplasms • Mitogen-activated protein kinases • Angiogenesis
- MEK kinases • TOR serine-threonine kinases • Receptor tyrosine kinase RET
- Protooncogene protein TRK • Immunotherapy

KEY POINTS

- Patients with differentiated thyroid cancer (DTC) refractory to radioiodine have a worse prognosis compared with those with radioiodine-avid disease.
- Lenvatinib and sorafenib are aMKIs that are indicated for the treatment of rapidly progressive, radioiodine-refractory DTC.
- The currently available drugs are not curative and, therefore, the risks and benefits of treatment must be carefully assessed before starting therapy.
- There are many promising strategies that are novel in the treatment of thyroid cancer, such as immunotherapy or targeting BRAF, TRK, or RET.
- Testing for somatic genetic alterations is essential to assist in the selection of appropriate therapeutic agents and perhaps the identification of new potential targets.

INTRODUCTION

Most patients treated for differentiated thyroid cancer (DTC) fare quite well. Data from the Surveillance, Epidemiology, and End Results (SEER) program show that 98.1% of patients diagnosed with thyroid cancer are still alive 5 years after initial diagnosis.[1] However, the 5-year survival rates decline from 99.9% for those who present with localized disease to 55.5% for those presenting with distant spread. There is a standard of care for treatment of DTC as described in many of the earlier articles in this issue. Unfortunately, there are those for whom surgery, thyroid-stimulating hormone

Disclosure Statement: The authors have nothing to disclose.
Department of Endocrine Neoplasia and Hormonal Disorders, The University of Texas MD Anderson Cancer Center, 1400 Pressler Street, Unit 1461, Houston, TX 77030, USA
* Corresponding author.
E-mail address: sisherma@mdanderson.org

Endocrinol Metab Clin N Am 48 (2019) 253–268
https://doi.org/10.1016/j.ecl.2018.10.009
0889-8529/19/© 2018 Elsevier Inc. All rights reserved.

(TSH)-suppressive therapy, and radioiodine (RAI) are not sufficient to control disease progression. It is this subset of patients for whom novel treatment approaches are needed.

Because RAI has long been the primary tool in clinicians' armamentarium, DTC refractory to RAI presents a challenge. DTC is generally considered RAI-refractory when 1 of several conditions is present.[2–4] The first is known metastatic disease (1 or multiple lesions) that has either never demonstrated the capability to uptake RAI or has lost that ability, as determined by initial posttherapy or subsequent diagnostic scans. The second is when there is progression despite recent RAI therapy, typically within 1 year. The third condition is when a cumulative administered activity of greater than or equal to 600 mCi has already been administered. This is due to increasing risks with declining potential benefit. Higher cumulative administered activities of RAI have been associated with a significantly increased risk of secondary malignancies. The most frequent secondary malignancies are hematologic and those affecting the salivary glands and bone.[5]

The 10-year survival rate has been reported as 29% for those who had persistent disease despite RAI uptake and only 10% for those without any initial RAI uptake.[2] However, many patients with persistent disease may be asymptomatic with stable lesions, small volume of disease, or slow progression. For these patients, the toxicities of systemic treatments may outweigh the benefit. As a result, it is crucial to assess whether progression is sufficiently rapid to justify treatment of those patients most likely to benefit. Response evaluation criteria in solid tumors (RECIST) version 1.1 is widely used to assess whether rapid progression is present in clinical trials and can also be readily applied to routine clinical practice. Progressive disease is defined as a greater than or equal to 20% increase in the sum of diameters of target lesions or the appearance of a significant new lesion.[6]

When there is rapid progression that cannot be addressed with focal therapies such as surgery or radiotherapy, systemic therapies should be considered. Historically, treatment with cytotoxic chemotherapy has yielded disappointing results despite FDA approval of doxorubicin.[7,8] As a result, there has been much interest and investigation in the exploitation of targeting angiogenic pathways critical to tumor metastasis and progression as well as oncogenic alterations in signaling pathways. Further investigational approaches under evaluation include restoration of endogenous biologic processes to control the tumors, such as resensitization to RAI therapy, and use of immunotherapies.

ANTIANGIOGENIC MULTIKINASE INHIBITORS

The first class of agents to discuss is the antiangiogenic multikinase inhibitors (aMKIs). This is the only drug class that includes agents with US Food and Drug Administration (FDA) approval for the treatment of differentiated thyroid cancer. Although they all block multiple kinases with varied targets and potency, a shared mechanism of action is inhibition of the interaction between the vascular endothelial growth factor (VEGF) and its cognate VEGF receptor (VEGFR), thereby interfering with the angiogenesis necessary for tumor formation, metastasis, and growth.[9]

Lenvatinib

Lenvatinib is an aMKI that targets VEGFR 1 to 3, FGFRs 1 to 4, PDGFR, RET, and c-KIT kinases. During the initial phase I trial, responses were observed in subjects with thyroid cancer treated with lenvatinib. In a phase II trial, the objective response rate in 58 subjects with progressive, metastatic RAI-refractory DTC was 50% and the median progression-free survival (PFS) 12.6 months.[10] Median duration of response was 12.7 months. Lenvatinib was subsequently approved by the FDA in 2015 for patients with progressive, RAI-refractory DTC based on the findings of a phase III randomized, double-blind, placebo-controlled, multicenter trial.[11] This trial was known as the Study of (E7080) Lenvatinib in Differentiated Cancer of the Thyroid (SELECT). The SELECT trial enrolled subjects with RAI-refractory DTC with progression according to RECIST, and subjects were randomized in a 2:1 ratio to receive lenvatinib (starting dosage 24 mg daily) or placebo. The primary endpoint was improvement in PFS, defined as the time from randomization to progression or death. A total of 392 persons were randomized, and the primary endpoint was achieved; PFS significantly differed between the 2 groups (P<.001). The PFS was 18.3 months for those receiving lenvatinib versus 3.6 months for those on placebo (hazard ratio [HR] 0.21). The short PFS in the placebo arm suggests that this overall cohort of subjects had rapidly progressing disease. Improved PFS was seen in all histologic subgroups (papillary, follicular, poorly differentiated, and Hurthle cell) and regardless of whether subjects had previously been treated with another antiangiogenic therapy. Additionally, the objective response rate was 64.8% in the lenvatinib group, with a median time to response of only 2 months; 4 complete responses were observed that persisted through the last study assessment. Because crossover was permitted for subjects who progressed after randomization to placebo, the subsequent median PFS and objective response rate after crossover was 10.1 months and 52.3%, respectively. The efficacy of the drug was not affected by *BRAF* mutation status though, surprisingly, *BRAF* wild-type status may have itself been a negative prognostic indicator.[12] Although no improvement was seen in overall survival (OS) for the entire randomized cohort (potentially confounded by the crossover design), a further subanalysis showed a first of its kind OS benefit in subjects older than age 65 years with RAI-refractory, progressive DTC (HR 0.53, 95% CI 0.31–0.91, P = .020).[13]

Side effects were common in both treatment cohorts. Of all subjects on lenvatinib, 97.3% experienced a side effect versus 59.5% in the placebo group. The most common side effects of lenvatinib therapy included hypertension, diarrhea, fatigue, decreased appetite, and decreased weight. Of note, 2.3% of subjects on lenvatinib suffered a fatal side effect that was believed to be treatment-related. This highlights the need for thoughtful patient selection and vigilant surveillance while receiving lenvatinib. Unless the risks associated with this drug are unusually great for a specific individual, lenvatinib is generally considered first-line treatment of patients with progressive, metastatic, RAI-refractory DTC owing to the impressive improvement in PFS in all patients, prolongation of OS seen in those older than age 65 years, and considerable cost-effectiveness compared with placebo.[14,15]

Sorafenib

Sorafenib is another aMKI that targets VEGFRs 1 to 3, RET, RET/PTC, and BRAF kinases. Two single-institution phase II trials initially suggested efficacy in patients with metastatic RAI-refractory DTC, reporting objective response rates of 23% and 15%, respectively.[10,17] Sorafenib was approved by the FDA in 2013 as first-line therapy for patients with locally recurrent or metastatic, progressive, DTC refractory to RAI based on the findings of a phase III randomized, double-blind, placebo-controlled, multicenter trial.[18] This was the stuDy of sorafEnib in loCally advanced or metastatic patientS with radioactive Iodine-refractory thyrOid caNcer (DECISION) trial. This study enrolled previously untreated subjects with RAI-refractory DTC that was progressive according to RECIST, randomized in a 1:1 ratio to receive sorafenib, starting at

400 mg twice daily, or placebo. The primary endpoint was improvement in PFS. A total of 417 subjects were randomized and a significant difference in PFS was found between the 2 groups (P<.0001). The PFS was 10.8 months for those receiving sorafenib versus 5.8 months for those on placebo (HR 0.59), and objective response rate was 12.2% on sorafenib. No significant difference was seen in OS, however. Similar to the SELECT trial, the efficacy of sorafenib was not affected by BRAF mutation status, and BRAF wild-type status was associated with worse PFS in both study arms. Of all subjects on sorafenib, 98.6% experienced a side effect versus 87.6% in the placebo group. The most common side effects of therapy included hand–foot skin reactions, diarrhea, alopecia, rash, and fatigue. There were 2 deaths, 1 in each arm, that were believed to be related to treatment.

Although the SELECT and DECISION trials cannot be directly compared, lenvatinib showed a greater improvement in PFS despite a shorter PFS in the placebo group and was assessed to be considerably more cost-effective than sorafenib, suggesting to the authors that this should be the initial antiangiogenic drug of choice.[14,15] Nonetheless, for patients in whom a more potent antiangiogenic might be contraindicated, such as those at higher risk for tracheoesophageal fistula or bowel perforation, sorafenib might be a more reasonable initial therapy.

Vandetanib

Vandetanib is an aMKI that targets RET, RET/PTC, VEGFR2, VEGFR3 and epithelial growth factor (EGFR) kinases. It was approved by the FDA in 2011 for the treatment of symptomatic or progressive medullary thyroid cancer (MTC) in patients with unresectable locally advanced or metastatic disease. Due to the array of kinases inhibited, a phase II randomized, double-blind, placebo-controlled multicenter trial was performed that enrolled subjects with locally advanced or metastatic DTC deemed unsuitable for RAI.[19] A total of 145 subjects were randomized in a 1:1 ratio to receive vandetanib, starting at 300 mg daily, or placebo, with the primary endpoint of improvement in PFS. The primary endpoint was achieved because the PFS was 11.1 months for those receiving vandetanib versus 5.9 months for those on placebo (HR 0.63); the overall response rate was only 8% in the vandetanib-treated subjects and 5% in the placebo group, which did not differ significantly.

The most common side effects reported were diarrhea, hypertension, acne, asthenia, decreased appetite, rash, fatigue, and QT_c prolongation. In fact, grade 3 or greater QT_c prolongation was seen in 14% of those in the safety population.[19] It is for this reason prescribers must be enrolled in the Risk Evaluation and Mitigation Strategies program before prescribing vandetanib. Given the plethora of nononcologic drugs that prolong the QT interval, it can be challenging to treat patients who have a slightly prolonged QT before vandetanib treatment.

Cabozantinib

Cabozantinib is an aMKI that targets VEGFR2, cMET, and RET kinases. It is FDA approved for the treatment of progressive metastatic MTC. However, an open-label phase I trial, which was performed primarily to evaluate potential drug–drug interactions, enrolled 15 subjects from 2 centers with RAI-refractory metastatic or unresectable DTC.[20] Secondary endpoints included overall response and OS rates. A partial response was seen in 8 subjects (53%) and stable disease was seen in another 6 subjects (40%). Unfortunately, there was 1 death in this trial due to fistula formation.[20,21] Subsequently, a multicenter phase II trial enrolled 25 subjects with RAI-refractory DTC who developed progression on at least 1 prior VEGFR-targeted therapy.[22] The starting dosage was 60 mg daily, and the primary endpoint was overall response rate. Of these subjects, 40% had a partial response, 52% had stable disease, and 8% were not evaluable (due to clinical progression or intolerable side effects). Median PFS was 12.7 months and the median OS was 34.7 months. This trial was the first prospective trial to show efficacy in subjects who were previously treated with an aMKI. Another phase II study has also been preliminarily reported, examining cabozantinib in the first-line setting at a starting dosage of 60 mg daily.[23] Overall response was 54%, with a median duration of response of 40 weeks and median PFS had not yet been reached. A phase III trial is anticipated, evaluating cabozantinib therapy in DTC subjects who have progressed on previous antiangiogenic therapy.

Pazopanib

Pazopanib is another aMKI that targets VEGFRs 1 to 3, FGFRs 1 to 3, PDGFR, and c-Kit kinases. A phase II trial enrolled subjects with metastatic, rapidly progressive, RAI-refractory DTC to be treated with pazopanib, starting at 800 mg daily.[24] The primary endpoint was objective response rate. Of 37 evaluable subjects, the objective response rate was 49%, PFS at 1 year was 47%, and 1 year OS was 81%. The drug was well-tolerated overall, with the most common adverse events reported as fatigue, skin and hair hypopigmentation, diarrhea, and nausea. Although pazopanib shows promise in the treatment of thyroid cancer, further trials confirming its efficacy are lacking.

Sunitinib

Sunitinib is an aMKI that targets VEGFR, PDGFR, and RET kinases. There have been 2 phase II trials assessing the utility of sunitinib in subjects with DTC. The first trial was a single-institution study that evaluated its potential utility in subjects with fluorodeoxyglucose PET-avid metastatic or RAI-refractory metastatic DTC or MTC. In the 28 subjects with DTC, the disease control rate (defined as subjects with objective response or prolonged stable disease at 3 months) was 78%.[25] The more recent study was a single-center, open-label, nonrandomized trial that enrolled 23 subjects with DTC and either metastatic, residual, recurrent, or progressive disease. There were 6 subjects (26%) who had a partial response.[26]

Axitinib

Axitinib is an aMKI that inhibits VEGFR and PDGFR kinases. There was a multicenter, open-label, single arm, phase II study using axitinib in subjects with RAI-refractory, metastatic, or unresectable locally advanced thyroid cancer.[27] Included in this study were 45 subjects with DTC. Of these subjects, 38% had a partial response and 29% had stable disease. Unfortunately, the subjects with DTC were not further evaluated as a subgroup but this trial shows some likely degree of efficacy.

Using Antiangiogenic Multikinase Inhibitors Safely

Given the high incidence of adverse events related to the use of aMKIs, careful monitoring and aggressive management of adverse events are of the utmost importance. The side effects that are either most frequently seen or most serious (but uncommon) include hypertension, fatigue, chronic weight loss, diarrhea, QT prolongation, congestive heart failure, proteinuria, hepatic injury, myelosuppression, hemorrhage, thrombosis, hand–foot skin reaction, and other rash. Guidance regarding the safe use of these drugs and the management of drug-related adverse effects are outlined elsewhere.[28–30]

PRECISION ONCOLOGY–DIRECTED THERAPIES

Given the importance of activated signaling through the mitogen-activated protein kinase (MAPK) and phosphatidylinositol 3-kinase/AKT pathways in both the oncogenesis and biologic behavior of DFCs, there has been considerable interest in the use of more selective kinase inhibitors that precisely target these pathways. (See Veronica Valvo and Carmelo Nucera's article, "Coding Molecular Determinants of Thyroid Cancer Development and Progression," in this issue.) In particular, tumors with activating mutations of BRAF have been found to be typically more aggressive and associated with the loss of differentiated functioning such as radioactive iodine responsiveness. Multiple clinical trials have focused on evaluating the outcomes of using BRAF kinase inhibitors either to reduce tumor growth or to reinduce sensitivity to radioactive iodine therapy. Inhibitors targeting other kinases in these pathways have been less intensively studied but they remain of interest either for monotherapy or in combination with other agents, including as possible adjuncts to enhance or restore responsiveness to RAI therapy. Newer therapies currently in early clinical trials are focused on targeting uncommon fusion mutations associated with development of DTC and are yielding promising early results.

BRAF-Directed Therapies

Two BRAF kinase inhibitors currently approved for treating mutated melanoma have been studied and found to be effective in BRAF-mutated DTC: vemurafenib and dabrafenib.[31] Both of these agents are type I inhibitors, which function as ATP-competitive inhibitors that preferentially bind to the V600E-mutated kinase.[32] However, they also enhance heterodimerization of wild-type BRAF with and transactivation of CRAF, which can paradoxically increase MAPK signaling especially in the setting of RAS mutation. Thus, their use is limited to patients with documented BRAF mutations and specifically contraindicated with RAS mutations.

Vemurafenib was initially considered for BRAF-mutated papillary thyroid carcinoma in the phase I trial based on its 3-fold greater selectivity for the V600E mutant kinase (IC_{50} 31 nM) compared with wild-type.[33,34] One of 3 treated subjects with BRAF-mutated, RAI-refractory metastatic disease experienced a confirmed partial response to therapy with shrinkage of pulmonary metastases.[33] In a subsequent multicenter phase II trial, 2 cohorts of subjects with progressive, RAI-refractory metastatic BRAF V600E-mutated papillary carcinoma were treated with vemurafenib, starting at 960 mg twice daily.[35] Of 26 subjects who had never been treated with antiangiogenic multitargeted kinase inhibitors, 38.5% experienced partial response, with a median duration of response of 16.5 months, and median PFS of 18.2 months. In the second cohort of 25 subjects previously treated with antiangiogenic multitargeted kinase inhibitors, including sorafenib, 27.3% experienced partial response, with a median duration of response 7.4 months and a median PFS 8.9 months. Thus, as second-line therapy after antiangiogenic kinase inhibitor, vemurafenib may have been somewhat less effective than in kinase-inhibitor naïve subjects. The profile of adverse events reported in the trial were similar to those seen in other studies, including rash (69%), fatigue (67%), weight loss (51%), decreased appetite (45%), alopecia (41%), and arthralgia (41%). Elevations in serum creatinine were also seen in about one-third of subjects, which can occasionally be marked and dose-limiting. One-fifth of subjects developed cutaneous squamous cell carcinomas, and 2 subjects developed noncutaneous squamous cell carcinoma of the head or neck, perhaps as a result of dedifferentiation of their thyroid primary. In a report of real-world use of vemurafenib in 15 subjects (12 of whom were kinase inhibitor naïve), the partial response rate was 47% and median time to treatment failure 13 months.[36] These studies suggest that vemurafenib may be effective for treatment of RAI-refractory *BRAF* V600E-mutated papillary carcinoma, especially in the first-line setting.

Given the efficacy of vemurafenib for treating progressive metastatic disease, a single-institution trial was recently completed that studied neoadjuvant use of the drug to shrink bulky cervical tumors before attempted resection.[37] Although the primary translational endpoints have not yet been reported, secondary clinical endpoints indicated that 8 weeks of preoperative vemurafenib therapy for patients with locally advanced *BRAF*-mutated papillary carcinoma could lead to clinically significant tumor reduction in more than two-thirds, probably increasing the likelihood that surgery would result in minimally residual or no residual disease.

Dabrafenib is a highly potent inhibitor of activating mutations of *BRAF* at codon 600 (IC50 0.5 nM for V600E). Three of 9 treated subjects with *BRAF*-mutated, radioactive iodine-refractory metastatic papillary thyroid carcinoma experienced partial response to therapy in the initial report of a phase I clinical trial.[38] Subsequently, a full report of the expansion cohort of *BRAF*-mutated thyroid subjects with cancer from that trial described a partial response rate of 29% in 14 subjects with progressive radioactive iodine refractory disease, treated with dabrafenib 150 mg twice daily.[39] The median PFS was 11.3 months. Among subjects with thyroid cancer, the most commonly reported adverse events included cutaneous papilloma, hyperkeratosis, alopecia, arthralgia, and pyrexia.

Given the efficacy and tolerability of dabrafenib combined with the MEK inhibitor trametinib reported in melanoma, a randomized phase II clinical trial was performed comparing monotherapy with dabrafenib with the combination of dabrafenib and trametinib.[40] Of subjects with radioactive iodine refractory *BRAF*-mutated papillary thyroid carcinoma, 53 were randomized to dabrafenib (150 mg twice daily) or dabrafenib (150 mg twice daily) and trametinib (2 mg daily). No significant difference was seen in objective response rates between the 2 arms of the study, with objective response (defined as partial plus minor responses) of 50% in the monotherapy arm (median duration of response 15.6 months) and 54% in the combination arm (median duration of response 13.3 months). Toxicities were also similar in the 2 arms of the study. In an effort to improve the tolerability of the combination regimen, dosing modifications are being described that may prolong the ability of patients to remain stable on treatment.[41]

Further, the combination of dabrafenib and trametinib seems to be particularly effective in *BRAF*-mutated anaplastic thyroid cancer and thus BRAF kinase–targeted therapy may have a more significant role in more aggressive forms of differentiated carcinoma.[42] As an example, the authors have recently treated a patient with rapidly progressing neck metastases from *BRAF*-mutated poorly differentiated carcinoma with cutaneous involvement, anticipating therapy with dabrafenib and trametinib as a neoadjuvant approach to try to facilitate subsequent surgery. The patient experienced radiographic complete response after 2 months of therapy with the combination, and surgical consideration was subsequently deferred in the absence of demonstrable disease (**Fig. 1**).

MEK-Directed Therapies

Use of inhibitors targeting MEK has not been extensively studied in this disease other than in combination with BRAF kinase inhibitors, despite this kinase being a common downstream effector of activated signaling from either RAS or BRAF. A single phase II clinical trial has been published of the MEK inhibitor selumetinib.[43] Of 39 subjects with progressive radioactive iodine refractory papillary carcinoma, confirmed partial

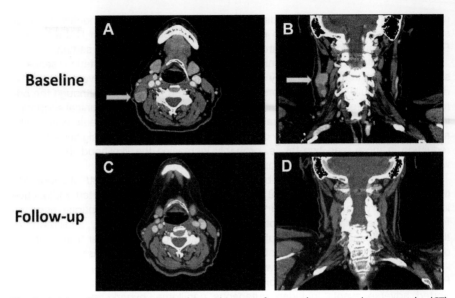

Fig. 1. Axial and coronal contrast-enhanced images from neck computed tomography (CT) scans in a patient treated for *BRAF* V600E-mutated poorly differentiated thyroid carcinoma. The baseline images (*A, B*), obtained before therapy, demonstrate enhancing metastases (*arrows*) in the right lateral neck with subcutaneous involvement. The follow-up images (*C, D*), obtained 2 months later, demonstrate that these lesions have completely resolved and are undetectable.

response was reported in only 1 subject and the median PFS was 32 weeks. Significant adverse events were reported that were thought to limit the long-term tolerability of the drug and subsequent trials have not been performed in this population. Although commercially available in the United States for treatment of melanoma, no studies have been reported of the MEK inhibitor cobimetinib.

PI3K Pathway–Directed Therapies

Three recent phase II studies have evaluated the PI3K inhibitor everolimus in subjects with RAI-refractory metastatic DTC. In the first study, 28 subjects with progressive disease were treated with everolimus, starting at 10 mg daily.[44] No objective responses were observed, and median PFS and OS were 9 months and 18 months, respectively. In the second study, 33 subjects with progressive RAI-refractory DTC received everolimus, also starting at 10 mg daily.[45] As the primary endpoint, the median PFS was 12.9 months, with 2-year estimates of PFS and OS of 23.6% and 73.5%, respectively. Only 1 partial response was observed. Although the numbers of subjects in each genomic characterized subgroup were quite small, subjects with *BRAF* V600E mutations experienced the longest PFS. In the third trial, 24 subjects with RAI-refractory metastatic DTC were treated with everolimus, starting at 10 mg daily.[46] Partial response was reported in 2 subjects, and median PFS was 43 weeks. In these 3 studies, commonly recorded adverse effects included mucositis or stomatitis, anemia, cough, and hyperglycemia.

Both everolimus and temsirolimus have been studied in combination with sorafenib in 3 separate phase II studies. In a trial of 36 subjects with progressive RAI-refractory carcinoma (including 2 cases of anaplastic carcinoma), temsirolimus and sorafenib (starting dosages 25 mg weekly and 200 mg twice daily, respectively) yielded a

22% partial response rate.[47] The PFS rate was 31% after one year, and median OS was 24.6 months. The most common grade 3 to 5 adverse events were hyperglycemia, fatigue, anemia, and oral mucositis, though no detail was provided about lower grade events. The combination of everolimus and sorafenib was studied in 28 subjects with RAI-refractory DTC, starting at 5 mg daily and 400 mg twice daily, respectively.[48] In a preliminary report, the partial response rate was 61%, including 7 of 9 subjects with the Hürthle cell variant. In the third trial, everolimus, 10 mg daily, was added to sorafenib in 33 DTC subjects already treated and progressing while taking sorafenib alone.[49] Sorafenib was also dosage-escalated at the time of adding everolimus. The median PFS following addition of everolimus and higher dosage sorafenib was 13.7 months but only 1 partial response was reported.

Resensitization with MAPK-Directed Therapies

Recognition that DTCs with highly activated signaling along the MAPK pathway are less likely to be radioactive iodine–avid led to the suggestion that inhibition of this signaling might allow restoration of RAI uptake. This hypothesis was elegantly tested in a transgenic mouse model with a doxycycline inducible *BRAF* V600E mutation, in which radioactive iodine uptake was restored by use of either a BRAF or MEK inhibitor.[50] In a subsequent pilot trial, the MEK inhibitor selumetinib was administered for 4 weeks to 20 subjects with radioactive iodine refractory DTC, though entry was not limited to subjects with *BRAF* or *RAS* mutations.[51] Using [124]I-PET imaging and dosimetry, 60% of subjects experienced significant restoration of radioactive iodine uptake, which allowed 7 subjects to proceed to receive therapeutic radioactive iodine treatment. Of the 20 subjects initially treated, 5 subjects experienced partial response with significant tumor reduction, yielding an objective response rate of 25%. Short-term toxicities were insignificant, although 1 subject who had previously received nearly 1000 mCi of radioactive iodine, as well as pelvic irradiation for prostate cancer, subsequently developed myelodysplastic syndrome about 1 year after treatment. The BRAF inhibitor dabrafenib was also tested in a 10-subject protocol, examining the ability to restore radioactive iodine uptake after 25 days of therapy.[52] Radioactive iodine scanning demonstrated uptake in 6 subjects who went on to receive therapeutic radioactive iodine, and an overall response rate of 20% was observed because 2 subjects experienced partial response.

A recent report from our institution reviewed 13 subjects who underwent radioactive iodine scanning as part of routine clinical follow-up while being treated with BRAF-directed or MEK-directed therapy for progressive metastatic radioactive iodine refractory thyroid carcinoma.[53] Nine of the subjects were treated with a BRAF inhibitor because of the presence of *BRAF* mutation and 4 were treated with a MEK inhibitor. Nine subjects, treated for a median of 14 months with kinase inhibitor, experienced significant restoration of radioactive iodine uptake leading to subsequent therapy with approximately 200 mCi. Kinase inhibitor therapy was then discontinued, and 7 subjects remained progression-free after a median follow-up of about 8 months. Despite use of radioactive iodine dosimetry, transient radiation pneumonitis was experienced by 2 subjects, further evidence of the marked restoration of uptake and retention facilitated by the kinase inhibitor therapy.

Further studies are ongoing investigating possible clinical roles for RAI resensitization therapy, reflecting the great excitement in the field for this approach. Two currently recruiting multicenter studies are attempting to expand on the initial observations in subjects with metastatic disease previously responsive to RAI therapy, including 1 placebo-controlled trial.[54,55] In a different treatment paradigm, the ASTRA trial is evaluating the hypothesis that 5 weeks of selumetinib would improve the 18-month complete remission rate compared with placebo, administered before RAI therapy in subjects at intermediate to high risk for recurrence after initial surgery.[56] Unfortunately, it was recently announced that the study failed to achieve the primary endpoint.[57]

Rearranged Gene-Directed Therapies

In addition to activating point mutations, gene rearrangements leading to novel chimeric kinases with altered expression or function are oncogenic in thyroid cancer and of therapeutic interest.[58] RET kinase fusion rearrangements, first identified in papillary thyroid carcinoma, have recently been identified as actionable mutations in nearly 2% of solid malignancies, including non-small cell lung carcinoma.[59] With a broad array of tumor types potentially susceptible to RET-targeted therapy, interest has focused on developing RET inhibitors that are more selective than the existing agents, such as lenvatinib or sorafenib, whose toxicities are thought to be in part due to their antiangiogenic properties. Currently, preliminary efficacy and safety data exist for 3 such agents in phase I trials: RXDX-105, BLU-667, and LOXO-292. Each of these drugs has an IC_{50} for wild-type RET kinase that is markedly lower than for VEGFR, and clinical responses seem to be broad regardless of actual tumor type.[60–62] Using LOXO-292, the partial response rate in metastatic *RET* fusion papillary carcinoma was 83% (5 of 6 evaluable subjects) compared with 65% in non-small cell lung carcinoma.[63] With BLU-667, a nearly 80% tumor reduction was noted in 1 evaluable PTC with a *RET/PTC1 (CCDC6)* fusion rearrangement and a 50% response rate in non-small cell lung carcinoma.[64]

Rearrangements of *NTRK* genes causing kinase activation are also seen in some papillary carcinomas, as well as a variety of other solid tumors, leading to development of selective TRK inhibitors. Larotrectinib is an inhibitor of all 3 TRK proteins at nanomolar concentrations.[65] In a report summarizing subjects treated in several phase I trials, the overall response rate was 100% for DTCs with *TRK* gene rearrangements (4 partial responses, 1 complete response) compared with about 75% in the overall larger set of subjects with solid tumors.[66,67] Abnormal liver function tests, fatigue, vomiting, dizziness, and nausea are the most common side effects noted in these studies. Ongoing basket trials of larotrectinib, as well as entrectinib (which also inhibits ROS1 and ALK-rearranged kinases) are actively enrolling subjects with thyroid cancer, among others with NTRK abnormalities. Larotrectinib has recently been approved by the Food and Drug Administration for any solid tumor bearing an NTRK mutation requiring systemic therapy. Rearrangements have also been reported in other kinases, including BRAF, ALK, and ROS1 as potentially oncogenic in DTC, though studies of therapeutic targeting have yet to be reported.

The product of fusion between the genes for the transcription factor paired box 8 (*PAX8*) and peroxisome proliferator-activated receptor gamma (*PPARG*) is an uncommon driver in DTC, especially with follicular-patterned histologies. Based on preclinical data showing that a PPARγ agonist, pioglitazone, could markedly shrink metastatic thyroid carcinoma bearing this gene fusion, there was a report of 1 subject who experienced a remarkable tumor shrinkage and symptomatic relief from pioglitazone therapy for skeletal spread from follicular carcinoma.[68] A multicenter trial was initiated to assess efficacy in a similar population but additional subjects with documented gene rearrangement could not be identified for participation. The challenging experience in this study, along with lessons learned from phase I trials of other therapies targeting rearranged genes, points out the need to incorporate massive parallel sequencing methods such as whole transcriptome sequencing (RNA-Seq) in the evaluation of patients with metastatic disease who might be eligible for such therapies.[58]

IMMUNOTHERAPY

Given the success of novel therapies directed against T cell–associated immune checkpoints that are suppressing anticancer immunologic responses, interest has emerged in applying new immunotherapies to metastatic DTC.[69] The low rate of non-synonymous mutations and, therefore, neoantigens seen in DTC might suggest that this would be a poor target for monotherapy with inhibitors of CTLA-4, PD-1, or PD-L1.[70] In fact, a preliminary report from a large basket trial of the PD-1 inhibitor pembro-lizumab confirmed that suggestion.[71] Of 22 subjects with RAI-refractory DTC treated with pembrolizumab, starting at 10 mg/kg every 2 weeks, the partial response rate was only 9.1%, despite the presence of PD-L1 expression on at least 1% of tumor cells in each subject. Typical of other trials with this PD-1 inhibitor, common side effects included diarrhea and fatigue, with 1 case of colitis.

Despite a cold immunogenic environment, some cancers have been shown to develop responsiveness to checkpoint inhibitors when combined with other treatments that increase the expression of the checkpoint proteins themselves, and this may well apply to DTC.[69] Pursuing this approach, a multicenter trial is currently under-way evaluating the response to combining lenvatinib with pembrolizumab, either following progression on lenvatinib alone or as first-line combination therapy (NCT02973997). An expansion cohort of subjects with metastatic thyroid carcinoma, including RAI-refractory DTC, is included in a study of the CTLA-4 inhibitor ipilimumab administered with stereotactic ablative radiotherapy for a lung, liver, or adrenal metas-tasis (NCT02239900), attempting to build on the abscopal effect from radiotherapy alone.[72]

CHOICE OF INITIAL THERAPY

Currently, there are only 2 effective FDA-approved therapies available to treat patients with progressive, metastatic, RAI-refractory DTC: lenvatinib and sorafenib. There have been no randomized trials comparing these 2 approved agents. In fact, other than the study of dabrafenib versus dabrafenib plus trametinib, there have been no randomized trials comparing any 2 drugs or regimens that might inform the choice of initial therapy for a patient with RAI-refractory DTC. Thus, any decision about selection of these treatments is based primarily on judgment rather than definitive data.[14] Further, selec-tion of patients appropriate for treatment with precision oncology therapies that target specific oncogenic alterations, such as BRAF mutations or TRK rearrangements,

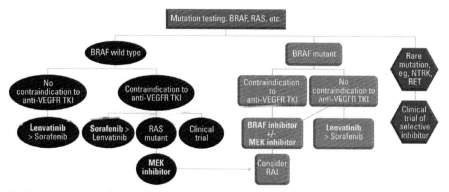

Fig. 2. An algorithm for determining selection of initial therapy for progressive metastatic RAI-refractory DTC. TKI, tyrosine kinase inhibitor.

require demonstration of the specific somatic gene abnormality, which is not necessarily routine practice.

At the authors' institution, the selection of initial systemic therapy involves assessment of a patient's risk from potent antiangiogenic therapy because lenvatinib is considered the drug of choice based on its demonstrated efficacy to markedly improve PFS, to yield significant tumor shrinkage, and to improve OS (at least in older patients). Tumor somatic mutation profiling is generally performed to assess suitability for precision oncology treatments, such as commercially available BRAF inhibitors or investigational agents. If appropriate, consideration is given to eventual assessment of possible resensitization to allow further RAI therapy. These various factors are then considered in aggregate, as outlined in **Fig. 2**.

REFERENCES

1. Noone A, Howlader N, Krapcho M, et al. SEER cancer statistics review, 1975-2015. Bethesda (MD): National Cancer Institute; 2018. Available at: https://seer.cancer.gov/csr/1975_2015/. Based on November 2017 SEER data submission. Accessed September 1, 2018.
2. Durante C, Haddy N, Baudin E, et al. Long-term outcome of 444 patients with distant metastases from papillary and follicular thyroid carcinoma: benefits and limits of radioiodine therapy. J Clin Endocrinol Metab 2006;91(8):2892–9.
3. Schlumberger M, Brose M, Elisei R, et al. Definition and management of radioactive iodine-refractory differentiated thyroid cancer. Lancet Diabetes Endocrinol 2014;2(5):356–8.
4. Haugen BR, Alexander EK, Bible KC, et al. 2015 American Thyroid Association Management Guidelines for Adult Patients with Thyroid Nodules and Differentiated Thyroid Cancer: the American Thyroid Association Guidelines Task Force on Thyroid Nodules and Differentiated Thyroid Cancer. Thyroid 2016;26(1):1–133.
5. Endo M, Liu JB, Dougan M, et al. Incidence of second malignancy in patients with papillary thyroid cancer from surveillance, epidemiology, and end results 13 dataset. J Thyroid Res 2018;2018:8765369.
6. Eisenhauer EA, Therasse P, Bogaerts J, et al. New response evaluation criteria in solid tumours: revised RECIST guideline (version 1.1). Eur J Cancer 2009;45(2):228–47.
7. Shimaoka K, Schoenfeld DA, DeWys WD, et al. A randomized trial of doxorubicin versus doxorubicin plus cisplatin in patients with advanced thyroid carcinoma. Cancer 1985;56(9):2155–60.
8. Sherman SI. Cytotoxic chemotherapy for differentiated thyroid carcinoma. Clin Oncol (R Coll Radiol) 2010;22:464–8.
9. Lin JD, Chao TC. Vascular endothelial growth factor in thyroid cancers. Cancer Biother Radiopharm 2005;20(6):648–61.
10. Cabanillas ME, Schlumberger M, Jarzab B, et al. A phase 2 trial of lenvatinib (E7080) in advanced, progressive, radioiodine-refractory, differentiated thyroid cancer: a clinical outcomes and biomarker assessment. Cancer 2015;121(16):2749–56.
11. Schlumberger M, Tahara M, Wirth LJ, et al. Lenvatinib versus placebo in radioiodine-refractory thyroid cancer. N Engl J Med 2015;372(7):621–30.
12. Tahara M, Schlumberger M, Elisei R, et al. Exploratory analysis of biomarkers associated with clinical outcomes from the study of lenvatinib in differentiated cancer of the thyroid. Eur J Cancer 2017;75:213–21.

13. Brose MS, Worden FP, Newbold KL, et al. Effect of age on the efficacy and safety of lenvatinib in radioiodine-refractory differentiated thyroid cancer in the phase III select trial. J Clin Oncol 2017;35(23):2692–9.
14. Rao SN, Cabanillas ME. Navigating systemic therapy in advanced thyroid carcinoma: from standard of care to personalized therapy and beyond. J Endocr Soc 2018;2(10):1109–30.
15. Wilson L, Huang W, Chen L, et al. Cost effectiveness of lenvatinib, sorafenib and placebo in treatment of radioiodine-refractory differentiated thyroid cancer. Thyroid 2017;27(8):1043–52.
16. Kloos RT, Ringel MD, Knopp MV, et al. Phase II trial of sorafenib in metastatic thyroid cancer. J Clin Oncol 2009;27(10):1675–84.
17. Gupta-Abramson V, Troxel AB, Nellore A, et al. Phase II trial of sorafenib in advanced thyroid cancer. J Clin Oncol 2008;26(29):4714–9.
18. Brose MS, Nutting CM, Jarzab B, et al. Sorafenib in radioactive iodine-refractory, locally advanced or metastatic differentiated thyroid cancer: a randomised, double-blind, phase 3 trial. Lancet 2014;384(9940):319–28.
19. Leboulleux S, Bastholt L, Krause T, et al. Vandetanib in locally advanced or metastatic differentiated thyroid cancer: a randomised, double-blind, phase 2 trial. Lancet Oncol 2012;13(9):897–905.
20. Cabanillas ME, Brose MS, Holland J, et al. A phase I study of cabozantinib (XL184) in patients with differentiated thyroid cancer. Thyroid 2014;24(10):1508–14.
21. Blevins DP, Dadu R, Hu M, et al. Aerodigestive fistula formation as a rare side effect of antiangiogenic tyrosine kinase inhibitor therapy for thyroid cancer. Thyroid 2014;24(5):918–22.
22. Cabanillas ME, de Souza JA, Geyer S, et al. Cabozantinib as salvage therapy for patients with tyrosine kinase inhibitor-refractory differentiated thyroid cancer: results of a multicenter phase II international thyroid oncology group trial. J Clin Oncol 2017;35(29):3315–21.
23. Brose MS, Shenoy S, Bhat N, et al. A phase II trial of cabozantinib (CABO) for the treatment of radioiodine (RAI)-refractory differentiated thyroid carcinoma (DTC) in the first-line setting. J Clin Oncol 2018;36(15_suppl):6088.
24. Bible KC, Suman VJ, Molina JR, et al. Efficacy of pazopanib in progressive, radioiodine-refractory, metastatic differentiated thyroid cancers: results of a phase 2 consortium study. Lancet Oncol 2010;11(10):962–72.
25. Carr LL, Mankoff DA, Goulart BH, et al. Phase II study of daily sunitinib in FDG-PET-positive, iodine-refractory differentiated thyroid cancer and metastatic medullary carcinoma of the thyroid with functional imaging correlation. Clin Cancer Res 2010;16(21):5260–8.
26. Bikas A, Kundra P, Desale S, et al. Phase 2 clinical trial of sunitinib as adjunctive treatment in patients with advanced differentiated thyroid cancer. Eur J Endocrinol 2016;174(3):373–80.
27. Locati LD, Licitra L, Agate L, et al. Treatment of advanced thyroid cancer with axitinib: phase 2 study with pharmacokinetic/pharmacodynamic and quality-of-life assessments. Cancer 2014;120(17):2694–703.
28. Carhill AA, Cabanillas ME, Jimenez C, et al. The noninvestigational use of tyrosine kinase inhibitors in thyroid cancer: establishing a standard for patient safety and monitoring. J Clin Endocrinol Metab 2013;98(1):31–42.
29. Resteghini C, Cavalieri S, Galbiati D, et al. Management of tyrosine kinase inhibitors (TKI) side effects in differentiated and medullary thyroid cancer patients. Best Pract Res Clin Endocrinol Metab 2017;31(3):349–61.

30. Lacouture ME. Management of dermatologic toxicities. J Natl Compr Canc Netw 2015;13(5 Suppl):686–9.
31. Cabanillas ME, Patel A, Danysh BP, et al. BRAF inhibitors: experience in thyroid cancer and general review of toxicity. Horm Cancer 2015;6(1):21–36.
32. Holderfield M, Deuker MM, McCormick F, et al. Targeting RAF kinases for cancer therapy: BRAF-mutated melanoma and beyond. Nat Rev Cancer 2014;14(7): 455–67.
33. Kim KB, Cabanillas ME, Lazar AJ, et al. Clinical responses to vemurafenib in patients with metastatic papillary thyroid cancer harboring BRAF(V600E) mutation. Thyroid 2013;23(10):1277–83.
34. Sala E, Mologni L, Truffa S, et al. BRAF silencing by short hairpin RNA or chemical blockade by PLX4032 leads to different responses in melanoma and thyroid carcinoma cells. Mol Cancer Res 2008;6(5):751–9.
35. Brose MS, Cabanillas ME, Cohen EE, et al. Vemurafenib in patients with BRAF(V600E)-positive metastatic or unresectable papillary thyroid cancer refractory to radioactive iodine: a non-randomised, multicentre, open-label, phase 2 trial. Lancet Oncol 2016;17(9):1272–82.
36. Dadu R, Shah K, Busaidy NL, et al. Efficacy and tolerability of vemurafenib in patients with BRAF(V600E) -positive papillary thyroid cancer: M.D. Anderson Cancer Center off label experience. J Clin Endocrinol Metab 2015;100(1):E77–81.
37. Cabanillas ME, Busaidy NL, Zafereo M, et al. Neoadjuvant vemurafenib in patients with locally advanced papillary thyroid cancer (PTC). Eur Thyroid J 2017; 6(Suppl 1):38.
38. Falchook GS, Long GV, Kurzrock R, et al. Dabrafenib in patients with melanoma, untreated brain metastases, and other solid tumours: a phase 1 dose-escalation trial. Lancet 2012;379(9829):1893–901.
39. Falchook GS, Millward M, Hong D, et al. BRAF inhibitor dabrafenib in patients with metastatic BRAF-mutant thyroid cancer. Thyroid 2015;25(1):71–7.
40. Shah MH, Wei L, Wirth LJ, et al. Results of randomized phase II trial of dabrafenib versus dabrafenib plus trametinib in BRAF-mutated papillary thyroid carcinoma. J Clin Oncol 2017;35(15_suppl):6022.
41. White PS, Pudusseri A, Lee SL, et al. Intermittent dosing of dabrafenib and trametinib in metastatic BRAFV600E mutated papillary thyroid cancer: two case reports. Thyroid 2017;27(9):1201–5.
42. Subbiah V, Kreitman RJ, Wainberg ZA, et al. Dabrafenib and trametinib treatment in patients with locally advanced or metastatic BRAF V600-mutant anaplastic thyroid cancer. J Clin Oncol 2018;36(1):7–13.
43. Hayes DN, Lucas AS, Tanvetyanon T, et al. Phase II efficacy and pharmacogenomic study of selumetinib (AZD6244; ARRY-142886) in iodine-131 refractory papillary thyroid carcinoma (IRPTC) with or without follicular elements. Clin Cancer Res 2012;18(7):2056–65.
44. Schneider TC, de Wit D, Links TP, et al. Everolimus in patients with advanced follicular-derived thyroid cancer: results of a phase II clinical trial. J Clin Endocrinol Metab 2017;102(2):698–707.
45. Hanna GJ, Busaidy NL, Chau NG, et al. Genomic correlates of response to everolimus in aggressive radioiodine-refractory thyroid cancer: a phase II study. Clin Cancer Res 2018;24(7):1546–53.
46. Lim SM, Chang H, Yoon MJ, et al. A multicenter, phase II trial of everolimus in locally advanced or metastatic thyroid cancer of all histologic subtypes. Ann Oncol 2013;24(12):3089–94.

47. Sherman FJ, Dunn LA, Ho AL, et al. Phase 2 study evaluating the combination of sorafenib and temsirolimus in the treatment of radioactive iodine-refractory thyroid cancer. Cancer 2017;123(21):4114–21.

48. Sherman EJ, Ho AL, Fury MG, et al. Combination of everolimus and sorafenib in the treatment of thyroid cancer: update on phase II study. J Clin Oncol 2015; 33(15suppl):6069.

49. Brose MS, Troxel AB, Yarchoan M, et al. A phase II study of everolimus (E) and sorafenib (S) in patients (PTS) with metastatic differentiated thyroid cancer who have progressed on sorafenib alone. J Clin Oncol 2015;33(15suppl):6072.

50. Chakravarty D, Santos E, Ryder M, et al. Small-molecule MAPK inhibitors restore radioiodine incorporation in mouse thyroid cancers with conditional BRAF activation. J Clin Invest 2011;121(12):4700–11.

51. Ho AL, Grewal RK, Leboeuf R, et al. Selumetinib-enhanced radioiodine uptake in advanced thyroid cancer. N Engl J Med 2013;368(7):623–32.

52. Rothenberg SM, McFadden DG, Palmer EL, et al. Redifferentiation of iodine-refractory BRAF V600E-mutant metastatic papillary thyroid cancer with dabrafenib. Clin Cancer Res 2015;21(5):1028–35.

53. Jaber T, Waguespack SG, Cabanillas ME, et al. Targeted therapy in advanced thyroid cancer to resensitize tumors to radioactive iodine. J Clin Endocrinol Metab 2018;103(10):3698–705.

54. Iodine I-131 with or without selumetinib in treating patients with recurrent or metastatic thyroid cancer. 2018. Available at: https://clinicaltrials.gov/ct2/show/NCT02393690?term=selumetinib&cond=Thyroid+Cancer&rank=3. Accessed September 3, 2018.

55. Wadsley J, Gregory R, Flux G, et al. SELIMETRY-a multicentre I-131 dosimetry trial: a clinical perspective. Br J Radiol 2017;90(1073):20160637.

56. Ho A, Keating K, Skolnik J, et al. The ASTRA study: adjuvant selumetinib for differentiated thyroid cancer (DTC); remission after radioiodine. Paper presented at: World Congress on Thyroid Cancer. Boston, MA, July 2013.

57. Soriot P, Frederickson D, Mallon M, et al. H1 2018 results. 2018. Available at: https://www.astrazeneca.com/content/dam/az/PDF/2018/h1-2018/H1%202018%20Results%20Presentation.pdf. Accessed September 3, 2018.

58. Yakushina VD, Lerner LV, Lavrov AV. Gene fusions in thyroid cancer. Thyroid 2018; 28(2):158–67.

59. Kato S, Subbiah V, Marchlik E, et al. RET aberrations in diverse cancers: next-generation sequencing of 4,871 patients. Clin Cancer Res 2017;23(8):1988–97.

60. Subbiah V, Velcheti V, Tuch BB, et al. Selective RET kinase inhibition for patients with RET-altered cancers. Ann Oncol 2018;29(8):1869–76.

61. Li GG, Somwar R, Joseph J, et al. Antitumor activity of RXDX-105 in multiple cancer types with RET rearrangements or mutations. Clin Cancer Res 2017;23(12): 2981–90.

62. Rahal R, Evans EK, Hu W, et al. The development of potent, selective RET inhibitors that target both wild-type RET and prospectively identified resistance mutations to multi-kinase inhibitors. Cancer Res 2016;76(14 Supplement):2641.

63. Drilon AE, Subbiah V, Oxnard GR, et al. A phase 1 study of LOXO-292, a potent and highly selective RET inhibitor, in patients with RET-altered cancers. J Clin Oncol 2018;36(15_suppl):102.

64. Subbiah V, Taylor M, Lin J, et al. Highly potent and selective RET inhibitor, BLU-667, achieves proof of concept in a phase I study of advanced, RET-altered solid tumors. Cancer Res 2018;78(13 Supplement):CT043.

65. Khotskaya YB, Holla VR, Farago AF, et al. Targeting TRK family proteins in cancer. Pharmacol Ther 2017;173:58–66.
66. Wirth L, Drilon A, Albert C, et al. Larotrectinib is highly active in patients with advanced recurrent TRK fusion thyroid (TC) and salivary gland cancers (SGC). Int J Radiat Oncol Biol Phys 2018;100(5):1318.
67. Drilon A, Laetsch TW, Kummar S, et al. Efficacy of larotrectinib in TRK fusion-positive cancers in adults and children. N Engl J Med 2018;378(8):731–9.
68. Giordano TJ, Haugen BR, Sherman SI, et al. Pioglitazone therapy of PAX8-PPARgamma fusion protein thyroid carcinoma. J Clin Endocrinol Metab 2018; 103(4):1277–81.
69. French JD, Bible K, Spitzweg C, et al. Leveraging the immune system to treat advanced thyroid cancers. Lancet Diabetes Endocrinol 2017;5(6):469–81.
70. Colli LM, Machiela MJ, Myers TA, et al. Burden of nonsynonymous mutations among TCGA cancers and candidate immune checkpoint inhibitor responses. Cancer Res 2016;76(13):3767–72.
71. Mehnert JM, Varga A, Brose M, et al. Pembrolizumab for advanced papillary or follicular thyroid cancer: preliminary results from the phase 1b KEYNOTE-028 study. J Clin Oncol 2016;34(15_suppl):6091.
72. Welsh JW, Tang C, de Groot P, et al. Phase 2 5-arm trial of ipilimumab plus lung or liver stereotactic radiation for patients with advanced malignancies. Int J Radiat Oncol Biol Phys 2017;99(5):1315–U1337.

Diagnosis and Management of Anaplastic Thyroid Cancer

Ashish V. Chintakuntlawar, MBBS, PhD[a], Robert L. Foote, MD[b],
Jan L. Kasperbauer, MD[c], Keith C. Bible, MD, PhD[a],*

KEYWORDS

- Anaplastic thyroid cancer • Chemoradiotherapy • Multimodality therapy
- Systemic therapy

KEY POINTS

- Anaplastic thyroid cancer (ATC) remains a devastating diagnosis with near universal mortality.
- Chemoradiotherapy, with or without surgery, is the preferred therapy with locally advanced ATC.
- New data with targeted therapies, including BRAF and MEK inhibitors, are paving the way for more effective therapeutic options in metastatic settings.

INTRODUCTION

Anaplastic thyroid cancer (ATC) is an extremely aggressive but rare form of thyroid malignancy, making up only 1% to 2% of all thyroid cancers.[1] Although the incidence of differentiated thyroid cancer (DTC) is increasing, principally due to increased diagnoses of micropapillary thyroid cancer, the incidence of ATC seems most likely stable over the last few decades. On the contrary, mortality from this cancer is almost universal and, therefore, disproportionately accounts for 20% to 50% of all deaths from thyroid cancer.[2] Median survival in many population-based studies has been noted to be anywhere from 3 to 6 months and population-based studies indicate that survival does not seem to be improving over the decades.[3,4] Therefore, ATC remains a devastating diagnosis even in 2018. However, there is a ray of hope consequent to greater understanding of pathophysiology, new advances in treatment technologies, and the formulation and development of multiple innovative therapeutic clinical trials. This article

Disclosure: The authors have nothing to disclose.
[a] Division of Medical Oncology, Mayo Clinic, 200 First Street Southwest, Rochester, MN 55905, USA; [b] Department of Radiation Oncology, Mayo Clinic, 200 First Street Southwest, Rochester, MN 55905, USA; [c] Division of Head and Neck Surgery, Mayo Clinic, 200 First Street Southwest, Rochester, MN 55905, USA
* Corresponding author.
E-mail address: Bible.Keith@mayo.edu

Endocrinol Metab Clin N Am 48 (2019) 269–284
https://doi.org/10.1016/j.ecl.2018.10.010
0889-8529/19/© 2018 Elsevier Inc. All rights reserved.

elaborates on these issues and outlines current stage-based approaches to the management of ATC.

PRESENTATION

Patients with ATC usually present with a rapidly enlarging neck mass, possibly associated with erythema and edema of the overlying skin, and symptoms associated with compression of local structures, such as neck vessels, esophagus, or trachea. It is also commonly associated with unilateral vocal cord palsy due to invasion of the adjacent recurrent laryngeal nerve,[5] leading to hoarseness of the voice, dysphonia, and sometimes frank stridor from local invasion and compression of the trachea causing impending airway distress. Patients can also present with dysphagia, dyspnea, cough, pain, or symptoms from distant or brain metastases.[6] Rarely, hemoptysis is present. Sometimes, ATC is found incidentally in a surgical pathologic specimen from a known DTC patient[7,8] or, rarely, develops in a deposit of dedifferentiated distantly metastatic DTC.[9]

ATC usually occurs in patients in their fifth to seventh decades of life but can occasionally also be seen in younger patients. Unlike DTC, ATC almost never occurs before the second or third decade of life; women are more commonly affected by ATC.[10] A past history of DTC could be present in up to about half of all ATC patients. Unlike primary thyroid lymphoma, history of Hashimoto disease is not associated with ATC.[5]

DIFFERENTIAL AND PATHOLOGIC DIAGNOSIS

Differential diagnosis of a rapidly enlarging neck mass includes aggressive thyroid cancers, such as poorly differentiated thyroid cancer (PDTC), and ATC, primary thyroid lymphoma, and sarcoma. Very rarely, primary squamous cell carcinoma of the thyroid could also be encountered. Metastatic adenopathy from poorly differentiated upper aerodigestive tract malignancies may also present with rapidly enlarging neck masses. It is paramount to quickly differentiate these possibilities because management differs substantially. Thus, an adequate biopsy is key to diagnosis. The role of the pathologist to differentiate between these tumors quickly becomes extremely important during initial presentation.

Thyroid cancer has a broad histologic spectrum ranging from indolent tumor, such as papillary microcarcinoma, to aggressive tumors, such as undifferentiated carcinoma or ATC. It is extremely important to separate ATC from thyroid cancer that is poorly differentiated; however, the features that segregate these malignancies can be subtle at times and should rely on experienced pathologist review of the histology. Fine-needle aspirates are usually cellular, with cells exhibiting a variety of shapes and mixed with acute inflammatory cells, such as neutrophils. Approximately 20% to 50% of ATC cases are associated with coexisting DTC; therefore, cells demonstrating features of DTC could also be admixed within the smear.[5] ATC has various histologic subtypes, including sarcomatoid, squamoid, osteoclastic, paucicellular, rhabdoid, and carcinosarcoma variant. Even though these histologic variants have been described, they do not ultimately affect clinical management. Specific subtyping is usually not possible on a fine-needle aspirate and may require a larger biopsy sample or at least a core needle biopsy. Pathologic samples often show necrosis and cellular debris with frequent mitotic figures, raising suspicion of ATC. They are usually focally immunohistochemically positive for keratin. Vimentin could also be expressed, especially in spindle cells; however, ATCs are negative for thyroid transcription factor-1, thyroglobulin, and calcitonin, and usually show diffuse expression of PAX-8 and P53.[11] Except for the paucicellular variant, most ATCs are heavily infiltrated with inflammatory cells that include tumor-associated macrophages and T cells.[12,13] ATC cells also show high expression of PD-L1.[14] Core needle biopsy has a very high sensitivity and positive predictive value, and usually obviates surgery for diagnostic purposes.[15]

Critically, ATC is almost indistinguishable from any other poorly differentiated carcinoma; however, positive PAX8 immunohistochemical staining, and association with adjacent thyroid cancer that is more differentiated are often distinguishing characteristics that allow for more expeditious diagnosis.

PATHOPHYSIOLOGY

About half of all ATCs arise in the setting of previous or concurrent DTC, suggesting that a large proportion of ATCs reflect dedifferentiation of preexistent DTC into the more aggressive phenotype. Moreover, genomic interrogations of DTCs versus ATCs indicate many overlapping but some additional alterations that are seen more commonly but not exclusively in conjunction with the DTC to PDTC to ATC transition, also suggesting a continuum of acquired alterations ultimately leading to ATC. In particular, *TP53* alterations, and combined *BRAF* and *TERT* mutations, are more frequent in in ATC than in DTC. ATCs also carry a larger mutational load than DTC. Landa and colleagues[16] and Kunstman and colleagues[17] published the first experience with a large cohort of ATCs and showed that they frequently carry BRAF, P53, and RAS mutations. Landa and colleagues[16] also demonstrated a high rate of mutation in TERT promoter. ATCs harbor higher somatic mutational burden, including mutations that are implicated in DTC such as BRAF and RAS but likely accumulate further mutations such as P53 and TERT promoter that lead to their virulence. These findings were confirmed in later studies with more patients.[18–20] In a cohort of Chinese and American patients, TERT promoter mutations were shown to be associated with BRAF mutation, older age, and distant metastases.[21] Indeed, the noted genetic alterations lead to activation of proliferative and antiapoptotic pathways.[22] Mutational frequencies of some major genes are noted in **Table 1**; differences are likely due to investigational techniques and population variance. These studies support a model in which DTC harboring a driver mutation further mutates into virulent pathogenic varieties such as thyroid cancer that is poorly differentiated or a frankly undifferentiated variety such as ATC.[19,23]

However, there is more to the underlying complexity that leads to the aggressiveness of these tumors. There are alterations in many other genes, including PI3-kinase pathway (PTEN, PIK3CA, mTOR), transcription factors (EIF1AX, NF1), cell cycle regulators (CDKN1B), receptor tyrosine kinases (FLT1), and histone methyltransferases (KMT). Other genetic aberrations such as copy number alterations and fusions (ALK) may also contribute.[16]

Major, and potentially therapeutically targetable, signaling pathways that are also implicated in ATC pathogenesis are depicted in **Fig. 1**. Exactly how these alterations

Table 1
Mutational frequencies of major genes

Study	N	P53 (%)	TERT (%)	BRAF (%)	RAS(N-,H-,K) (%)
Kunstman et al,[17] 2015	22	29	NR	20	32
Landa,[16] 2016	33	73	73	45	24
Bonhomme et al,[18] 2017	144	54	54	14	42
Tiedje et al,[20] 2017	118	55	73	11	19
Pozdeyev et al,[19] 2018	196	65	65	41	27

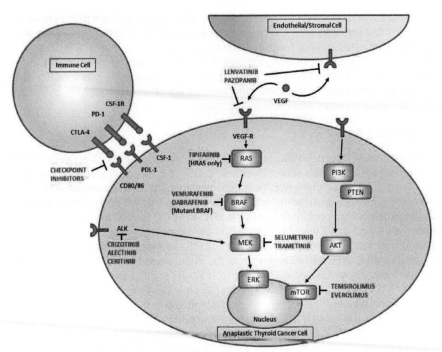

Fig. 1. Simplified schematic of active immune and signaling pathways in anaplastic thyroid carcinoma.

lead to tumorigenesis in ATC is gradually being elucidated. It seems that downstream effects of altered kinase activities lead to not only canonical pathway activation but also to effects such as activation of TERT[24] or dysregulation of the cell cycle checkpoint kinases.[25,26] Although genetic studies have not implicated the sonic hedgehog pathway in ATC, it interacts with commonly altered pathways in ATC,[27] maintains stem cell like properties,[28] and contributes to resistance. Epigenetic mechanisms such as methylation[29] are also being revealed and could be explored as clinical treatments.[30] In contrast, the role of micro-RNA is just being explored, adding to the complexity of understanding but likely will not see clinical use in the near future.[31,32]

That the canonical signaling pathways do not operate in isolation and interact with each other is also an important consideration in ATC pathogenesis. Also, pharmacologic inhibition of one pathway can trigger activation of others, leading to drug resistance[33] and sometimes, surprisingly, to immunologic resistance in the ATC tumor microenvironment.[34,35] ATC is a tumor wherein many mechanisms of immune evasion appear operative, making immunotherapeutics attractive candidate therapeutics in ATC.[36,37] It has been shown that ATCs are enriched in neutrophils, T cells, and tumor-associated macrophages,[13] and have high expression of PD-L1.[12,14] These features are also associated with poor survival, suggesting an immune rich but exhausted environment.[14] Immunotherapies targeting these pathways (CSF-1/CSF-1R, CTLA4, PD-1/PD-L1) and other immunoregulatory molecules, such as OX-40, 4-1BB, GITR, and NK-cells, are already US Food and Drug Administration (FDA)-approved or in clinical development. Antibodies targeting CTLA4 and PD-1 are currently being tested in subjects with ATC, alone or in combination, with kinase inhibitors paving pathways for future treatments.

DIAGNOSTIC TESTS AND IMAGING

Unlike DTC, wherein thyroglobulin is a valuable tumor marker, there are no specific tumor markers associated with ATC. Usually, thyroglobulin staining is negative in ATC if there are no intermixed DTC tumor components. Nevertheless, ATC patients require evaluation of bone marrow and organ function with basic laboratory tests.

Ultrasound examination of the primary lesion in the neck will usually show a hypoechoic irregular structure with local invasion suggestive of a malignant lesion and help characterize neck node metastases. For surgical planning, however, additional imaging, such as contrast-enhanced neck computed tomography (CT) is required. For evaluation of distant metastases, the authors usually prefer fluorodeoxyglucose (FDG) PET-CT.[38] CT scan of the neck, chest, abdomen, and pelvis is also acceptable for staging if PET scan is not available. ATC has significant risk of brain metastases and hence MRI of the brain to rule out intracranial metastases is recommended at initial staging.[39]

Although there are no prospective data, analysis from retrospective studies show that PET imaging is more sensitive and more efficient in detecting therapeutic response in ATC.[40] In the postchemoradiotherapy setting, a persistent mass is often seen in the neck and takes a few months to demonstrate maximal response. Retrospective analysis has shown that patients with persistent uptake might fare poorly but this has not been confirmed in a prospective analysis.[40]

In the new (8th edition) American Joint Committee on Cancer (AJCC) staging manual[41] the tumor (T) and the nodal (N) categories have changed slightly; however, the prognostic grouping with stage IVA, IVB, and IVC remains largely unchanged. ATCs confined to the thyroid gland are staged as IVA, those with gross extrathyroidal extension or lymph node involvement in the neck are staged as IVB, and those with distant metastases are staged as IVC. However, in many cases, the presence of subcentimeter lung nodules or the presence of distant disease that could potentially be related to DTC can lead to confusion in staging and should be interpreted cautiously within the clinical context and patient goals of care.

MANAGEMENT

ATC is best considered an oncology emergency, given the potential for rapid threat to airway and esophageal patency that can end life within days if not rapidly palliated. Rapid diagnosis is critical to expedite care, with comprehensive and expeditious evaluation by a coordinated and experienced multidisciplinary team, including an expert endocrine pathologist, head and neck surgeon, medical oncologist, radiation oncologist, and an endocrinologist. Ideally, a palliative care physician is also part of the team. Because ATC still has an extremely poor prognosis overall, ATC patients and families deserve an in-depth discussion about the natural history of the disease, goals of treatment, treatment toxicities, and expected outcomes in response to various care options.[42]

Because of the historically terrible prognosis, ATCs have been treated nihilistically and potentially neglected. Most ATC patients, if not all, will die of asphyxiation if the neck tumor is left untreated, and disease in the neck is most commonly the first threat to life even in stage IVC or metastatic ATC. Therefore, approaches to care must prioritize palliation of the primary neck disease (thyroid and nodal) as a first order of business.

Reports before initiation of multimodality treatment of ATC show that two-thirds of the patients died of asphyxiation.[43] A Canadian population-based registry study reported that 11 of 13 nonreferred patients died within 1 month, with a median survival of 6 days. Similar results were seen with no treatment indicating extremely poor survival in a cohort of patients from Europe.[44]

Initial evaluation should include careful history and symptom assessment, physical examination, including endoscopic examination for evaluation of the larynx, subglottis, and trachea, and anatomic staging via imaging. Critically, a thorough discussion among the multidisciplinary team with regard to the patient's clinical status and appropriate treatment pathways that are available must be completed. A mindful discussion with the patient and family regarding the dire natural history, prognosis, and treatment goals of each individual patient must be incorporated throughout the process. Establishing personalized goals of care is essential to therapeutic decision-making and planning because all therapeutic decisions in ATC involve serious trade-offs between risks of disease and risks of therapies. A framework for considering approaches to the initial care of ATC patients is shown in **Fig. 2**.

Best Supportive Care or Hospice

First, it is critical to distinguish palliative care, which is an approach focused on symptom palliation that is required in all ATC patients regardless of elected aggressiveness of care, from best supportive care or hospice, wherein the only goal of care is symptom management and no anticancer therapy is pursued. The election of best supportive care or hospice is optimal for patients who do not wish to pursue aggressive

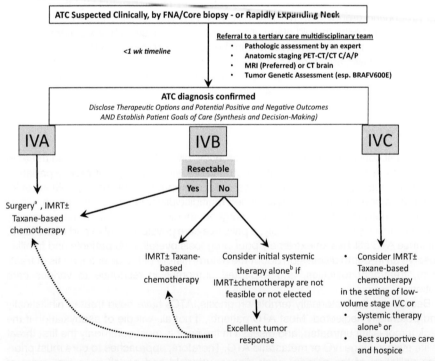

Fig. 2. Algorithm of the evaluation and management of anaplastic thyroid cancer. C/A/P; chest, abdomen and pelvis. [a] Goal is R0 or R1 resection, not debulking. Avoid procedures that delay prompt onset of chemoradiation (partial pharyngectomy, partial esophagectomy, tracheal resection, laryngectomy). [b] Dabrafenib or trametinib if BRAFV600E-mutated (FDA-approved), clinical trial, or cytotoxic chemotherapy. FNA, fine-needle aspirate.

multimodality therapy or for those who have poor performance status precluding safe pursuit of cancer-directed treatments. However, best supportive care should be applied with caution because most patients will experience a miserable death in this context.[43] Tracheostomy to relieve airway obstruction as a part of best supportive care is controversial but could be used in selected cases in which there is impending airway compromise that can be relieved by tracheostomy to attain patient respiratory comfort. In addition, a tracheostomy can relieve acute symptoms while the diagnosis and staging steps are completed and provide a less overwhelming environment in which to make treatment decisions. However, tracheostomy itself has significant negative effects on quality of life and function, and requires incremented care to manage the appliance, wound, and secretions. Other supportive measures, such as analgesics, opiates for air hunger, oxygenation for relief of dyspnea, and corticosteroids, can represent alternative approaches to tracheostomy. ATC patients electing best supportive care alone have an almost uniformly short life span, generally measured in days.[44]

Multimodality Therapy

Table 2 summarizes better-established prognostic factors in ATC, including age, extent of the disease (including absence of distant metastases), primary tumor and regional node radiotherapy dose, and combined modality treatment.[3,4,6,8,10] Based on these studies and some single-institution consecutive experiences, the authors think that patients with neck and, especially, thyroid-limited disease (stage IVA and IVB) should be treated with initial surgery followed by chemoradiotherapy (intensity-modulated radiotherapy [IMRT] plus taxane-based chemotherapy) as a standard of care when feasible, unless hospice is alternatively elected. However, such multimodality therapy is very toxic and morbid, and trade-offs in electing such an approach must be fully disclosed because most stage IVB (and IVC) patients will still succumb to their disease within 1 year of diagnosis regardless of approach.

One of the first reports of outcomes resulting from combining chemotherapy with radiotherapy was published by Wallgren and Norin.[45] Subsequent studies demonstrated that multimodality treatment that included surgery, chemotherapy, and radiotherapy resulted in improved local tumor control compared with less aggressive historical approaches.[43] Earlier studies from Sweden and France experimented with various chemotherapy regimens, fractionation of radiotherapy, and sequencing of various modalities of treatment, indicating better local tumor control but poor overall survival primarily due to inadequate control of distant disease (**Table 3**).[46–48]

Treatment with multimodality therapy has continued to evolve to become a cornerstone of initial ATC therapy, with better results attained when cytotoxic chemotherapy is used alongside external beam radiotherapy, especially IMRT. **Table 3** shows median overall survival, local tumor control, and distant disease control rates of selected single-institution reports. Data from the authors' center has consistently shown excellent local tumor control also associated with improvement in overall survival when compared with historical studies or population-based studies.[49,50] What has been striking is the improvement in the survival of stage IVB and, especially, IVA, patients. In stage IVB patients, treatment with palliative intent resulted in a poor survival when compared with a more aggressive treatment with multimodality therapy (4 months vs 22.4 months; hazard ratio 0.12, $P = .0001$).[50] However, all such studies continue to show poor control of distant disease. A more effective approach to control the seemingly universally present occult distant disease present at initial diagnosis is greatly needed.

Table 2
Prognostic factors in anaplastic thyroid cancer

Author, Year	Study Setting	N	Female Subjects/ Male Subjects (n)	Age (y)	Med OS (mo)	Favorable Factors
Goutsouliak et al,[3] 2005	Registry	75	51/24	74	5.1	Radical treatment
Kebebew et al,[10] 2005	Registry	516	345/171	71	3	Age, localized, absence of distant metastasis, surgery combined with radiotherapy
Sugitani et al,[8] 2012	Multiinstitution	547	339/208	~70		Age, acute symptoms, leukocytosis, tumor size, absence of metastasis, surgical resection, and chemoradiotherapy
Wendler et al,[6] 2016	Multiinstitution	100	52/48	70	5.7	Age, absence of metastasis, surgical resection, XRT >40 Gy, and chemotherapy
Pezzi et al,[4] 2017	Registry	1288	769/519	70	2.2	Age, no comorbidity, absence of distant metastasis, surgery, chemotherapy, XRT >45 Gy

Abbreviations: Med OS, median overall survival; XRT, external beam radiotherapy.

There is no established clear standard radiosensitizing agent that has emerged as superior in the treatment ATC. Initial studies from Europe involved mostly combined cytotoxic chemotherapy.[46,51] Later, Kim and Leeper[52] and others developed protocols using doxorubicin.[53,54] However, in the last few decades, taxane-based therapy has been shown to be effective in ATC.[50,55,56] Although there are no randomized data yet, combination systematic therapy might be more effective[25] and results from Radiation Therapy Oncology Group 0912 should help answer that question. Currently, the authors aim to use combination cytotoxic chemotherapy concurrently with radiotherapy in our practice, either docetaxel and doxorubicin, or carboplatin and paclitaxel, generally administered weekly concurrently with IMRT.[50]

Radiotherapy modalities and planning techniques have changed considerably over the years. Hyperfractionated or accelerated radiotherapy was attempted in the treatment of ATC but has been reported to be associated with increased toxicities.[57,58] However, they have also been apparently associated with improved local tumor control.[47] Over the years it has been very clear from both population-based and single-institution studies that a radiotherapy dose of greater than 40 to 45 Gy is optimal in the treatment of ATC.[4,8,59,60] With the advent of IMRT and other more conformal radiotherapeutic approaches, it has been possible to achieve complete tumor volume coverage with higher localized doses with less toxicity.[61] The authors' institution routinely aims to achieve a dose of 66 to 70 Gy in 33 to 35 fractions over 6.5 to 7 weeks with IMRT, especially in stage IVA and IVB ATC patients (R1 resection, R2 resection, or unresectable disease) wherein we are treating unresectable disease with curative

Table 3
Key multimodality studies in anaplastic thyroid cancer

Study	Years	N	Female Subjects/ Male Subjects (n)	Age (y)	Surgery (%)	RT Dose (Gy)	Chemotherapy Regimen	Median OS (mo)	Local Control (%)	Distant Control (%)
Werner	1975–80	19	14/5	68–72	63	30–40	BCF	7–12	NR	16
Kim	1979–87	19	13/6	60	53	56	Doxorubicin	12	68	21
Schlumberger	1981–90	20	11/9	NR	60	52	Mitoxantrone or doxorubicin plus cisplatin	2–6	75	35
Tennvall	1984–99	55	38/17	76	73	46	Doxorubicin	2–4.5	60	22
Crevoisier	1999–00	30	18/12	59	24	40	Doxorubicin and cisplatin	10	47	37
Sherman	1984–07	37	20/17	63	51	58	Doxorubicin	6	50	NR
Prasongsook	2003–15	30	8/22	60	90	66	Doxorubicin and docetaxel	21	93	22

Abbreviation: BCF, bleomycin, cyclophosphamide, 5-fluorouracil.

intention.[62] Sixty-six Gy in 30 fractions can be considered for small volume disease. In cases with R0 resection, we use an adjuvant dose of 60 Gy in 30 fractions over 6 weeks.

The utility of surgical resection is harder to answer considering the lack of any studies looking at this particular question, definition of resectability, and how resection was defined in these studies in any prospective way. However, it is evident from multiple population-based studies that surgery is an independent variable implicated in improved survival of ATC subjects,[4,10,63] which was also confirmed by a recent systematic review of more than 40 studies.[64] Of note is that overall survival seems especially improved with surgery in stage IVA and IVB ATC.[8,65] An operation with a goal of debulking is likely not very helpful and should be avoided in deference to a goal of R0 or R1 resection.[57] Tracheostomy alone should be avoided if possible[39] and may be difficult to perform because of overlying tumor mass in most patients.[66] We also advise surgical restraint in patients with metastatic or clearly locally unresectable tumors. Procedures that delay the prompt postoperative onset of chemotherapy and radiation therapy are difficult to justify given the high likelihood of distant metastasis; for example, partial pharyngectomy, tracheal resection, esophageal resection, and laryngectomy.

Based on the multiple studies previously detailed, the authors propose a clinical stage-based treatment algorithm as depicted in **Fig. 2**. After expedited initial evaluation is complete, we believe that most stage IVA and IVB patients should undergo surgical resection (if feasible) followed by adjuvant chemoradiotherapy. This approach, however, is only relevant in patients fit to undertake, and commit to, an aggressive and toxic multimodality approach. Because our experience using this approach in stage IVA disease has resulted in consistently favorable long-term survival, IVA patients should in particular strongly consider this approach; however, we believe that stage IVB patients should also consider this regimen because we have found it associated with improved overall survival, albeit not as dramatically as among stage IVA patients.

Alternatively, it is our recommendation that stage IVB patients who have unresectable disease should undergo combination cytotoxic chemotherapy concurrently with conventional radiotherapy, preferably IMRT. Unresectable stage IVB patients could also be eligible for neoadjuvant treatment followed by surgical resection.[67] However, this approach has not been rigorously tested and also poses a risk of asphyxiation if there is no response to the systemic therapeutic approach, making our group very reluctant to forgo definitive intention therapy to the primary tumor in the neck in favor of initial systemic therapy alone.

Patients who clearly have widely metastatic or stage IVC disease should instead be treated with palliative systemic therapy or best supportive care tailored to their individual goals of care. In the very limited number of ATC patients who present with or subsequently develop oligometastatic distant disease, multimodality therapy could be considered, enhanced by focal therapy for the few distant macrometastases (eg, stereotactic body radiotherapy, stereotactic radiosurgery, radiofrequency ablation, cryoablation). However, the benefit in this setting seems to be restricted to local control and does not clearly result in improved overall survival.[50]

Systemic Therapies, Including Targeted and Immunotherapies

Systemic therapy for ATC has seen significant change in the last few years. Taxane-based or doxorubicin-based chemotherapy has mostly been used in the context of chemoradiotherapy; however, is plagued by poor efficacy and short duration of response when used alone for metastatic disease.[55,56,68] However, about 40% to

50% of ATCs carry a BRAFV600E somatic mutation (those apparently derived from an underlying previously more differentiated papillary neoplasm wherein this mutation is a common oncologic driver).[16] Acting on these data, a recent study by Subbiah and colleagues[69] demonstrated multiple exceptional responses in a study of 16 ATC subjects who received the BRAF inhibitor dabrafenib and the MEK-inhibitor trametinib; the median overall survival was not reached and 1-year survival was reported to be 80%. Based on this study, and prior approval of the combination in melanoma, the FDA has approved this combination for treatment of ATC patients who have no satisfactory locoregional treatment options. We also have seen exceptional responses to BRAFV600E-targeted approaches; however, in our experience, observed responses have been only a few months duration. Other kinase inhibitors, such as lenvatinib[70] and pazopanib,[71] have also shown some activity in ATC patients and could be considered as salvage therapies in the absence of BRAF mutation or after failure of these agents but also suffer from short periods of benefit, if attained. Although any therapy that benefits ATC patients with metastatic disease represents progress, additional progress is still sorely needed in metastatic ATC.

Immunotherapy has been shown to be effective in preclinical ATC models[35,72] but has only recently become more attractive with the emergence of more effective and tolerable immunotherapeutics. Results from immune studies in ATC are provocative but currently limited.[67] Therefore, these agents are yet to be incorporated in the treatment of ATC outside of the context of clinical trials. Based on preclinical studies,[12,14] case reports,[73] and early results from a prospective study of Wirth and colleagues[74] (phase I-II study of spartalizumab, an anti-PD1 monoclonal antibody), it is reasonable to consider PD-1 inhibitors if there are no clinical trials and providing that immunotherapy is available with no financial burden or medical contraindications.

Multiple clinical studies with newer agents such as the PPAR-γ agonist efatutazone (NCT02152137),[75] immunotherapy combinations (NCT03122496, NCT03181100), and mTOR inhibitors (NCT02244463) are currently recruiting ATC subjects, with some responses noted. The authors eagerly await the results of these and other trials developed in pursuit of improved systemic therapy for advanced ATC.

SUMMARY

ATC is a rare and historically highly fatal cancer. Nonetheless, recent studies have indicated improvements in overall survival in response to early aggressive multimodality therapy, especially in stage IVA and IVB but at the cost of considerable toxicities and with no guarantee of benefit in any individual patient. Hence, in electing such an initial aggressive multimodality approach, patients and providers must be very thoughtful in counterbalancing potential benefits with associated morbidity and risks of therapy within the context of individual goals of care. The recent FDA approval of the combination of dabrafenib and trametinib adds to the previous FDA approval of doxorubicin for treatment of ATC, and represents another therapeutic option in advanced BRAFV600E mutated ATC. Metastatic, stage IVC ATC nevertheless still engenders a dire prognosis regardless of approach used despite a modicum of recent progress. Although ATC has been previously considered universally fatal and hard to treat, there is glimmer of hope with new approaches and clinical trials being designed with the incorporation of biologically targeted agents and immunotherapeutics in multimodality therapy protocols. The authors look forward to further progress, optimized via highly coordinated collaborative efforts across institutions of many nations.

ACKNOWLEDGMENTS

The authors stand in admiration of the dedicated commitment of patients with anaplastic thyroid cancer who have generously participated in many of the cited studies in pursuit of improved outcomes for future patients. We also apologize to numerous esteemed colleagues whose work could not be cited simply due to space constraints.

REFERENCES

1. Mao Y, Xing M. Recent incidences and differential trends of thyroid cancer in the USA. Endocr Relat Cancer 2016;23(4):313–22.
2. Lim H, Devesa SS, Sosa JA, et al. Trends in thyroid cancer incidence and mortality in the United States, 1974-2013. JAMA 2017;317(13):1338–48.
3. Goutsouliak V, Hay JH. Anaplastic thyroid cancer in British Columbia 1985-1999: a population-based study. Clin Oncol 2005;17(2):75–8.
4. Pezzi TA, Mohamed ASR, Sheu T, et al. Radiation therapy dose is associated with improved survival for unresected anaplastic thyroid carcinoma: outcomes from the National Cancer Data Base. Cancer 2017;123(9):1653–61.
5. Nel CJ, van Heerden JA, Goellner JR, et al. Anaplastic carcinoma of the thyroid: a clinicopathologic study of 82 cases. Mayo Clin Proc 1985;60(1):51–8.
6. Wendler J, Kroiss M, Gast K, et al. Clinical presentation, treatment and outcome of anaplastic thyroid carcinoma: results of a multicenter study in Germany. Eur J Endocrinol 2016;175(6):521–9.
7. Yoshida A, Sugino K, Sugitani I, et al. Anaplastic thyroid carcinomas incidentally found on postoperative pathological examination. World J Surg 2014;38(9): 2311–6.
8. Sugitani I, Miyauchi A, Sugino K, et al. Prognostic factors and treatment outcomes for anaplastic thyroid carcinoma: ATC Research Consortium of Japan cohort study of 677 patients. World J Surg 2012;36(6):1247–54.
9. Iniguez Ariza NM, Ryder M, Morris JC, et al. EXTRA-Thyroidal anaplastic thyroid cancer: a single institution experience, in 87th Annual Meeting of the American Thyroid Association. Victoria, British Columbia, Canada, October 18–22, 2007.
10. Kebebew E, Greenspan FS, Clark OH, et al. Anaplastic thyroid carcinoma. Treatment outcome and prognostic factors. Cancer 2005;103(7):1330–5.
11. Talbott I, Wakely PE Jr. Undifferentiated (anaplastic) thyroid carcinoma: practical immunohistochemistry and cytologic look-alikes. Semin Diagn Pathol 2015;32(4): 305–10.
12. Bastman JJ, Serracino HS, Zhu Y, et al. Tumor-infiltrating T Cells and the PD-1 checkpoint pathway in advanced differentiated and anaplastic thyroid cancer. J Clin Endocrinol Metab 2016;101(7):2863–73.
13. Ryder M, Ghossein RA, Ricarte-Filho JC, et al. Increased density of tumor-associated macrophages is associated with decreased survival in advanced thyroid cancer. Endocr Relat Cancer 2008;15(4):1069–74.
14. Chintakuntlawar AV, Rumilla KM, Smith CY, et al. Expression of PD-1 and PD-L1 in anaplastic thyroid cancer patients treated with multimodal therapy: results from a Retrospective Study. J Clin Endocrinol Metab 2017;102(6):1943–50.
15. Ha EJ, Baek JH, Lee JH, et al. Core needle biopsy could reduce diagnostic surgery in patients with anaplastic thyroid cancer or thyroid lymphoma. Eur Radiol 2016;26(4):1031–6.

16. Landa I, Ibrahimpasic T, Boucai L, et al. Genomic and transcriptomic hallmarks of poorly differentiated and anaplastic thyroid cancers. J Clin Invest 2016;126(3): 1052–66.

17. Kunstman JW, Juhlin CC, Goh G, et al. Characterization of the mutational landscape of anaplastic thyroid cancer via whole-exome sequencing. Hum Mol Genet 2015;24(8):2318–29.

18. Bonhomme B, Godbert Y, Perot G, et al. Molecular pathology of anaplastic thyroid carcinomas: a retrospective study of 144 cases. Thyroid 2017;27(5):682–92.

19. Pozdeyev N, Gay LM, Sokol ES, et al. Genetic analysis of 779 advanced differentiated and anaplastic thyroid cancers. Clin Cancer Res 2018;24(13):3059–68.

20. Tiedje V, Ting S, Herold T, et al. NGS based identification of mutational hotspots for targeted therapy in anaplastic thyroid carcinoma. Oncotarget 2017;8(26): 42613–20.

21. Shi X, Liu R, Qu S, et al. Association of TERT promoter mutation 1,295,228 C>T with BRAF V600E mutation, older patient age, and distant metastasis in anaplastic thyroid cancer. J Clin Endocrinol Metab 2015;100(4):E632–7.

22. Liu Z, Hou P, Ji M, et al. Highly prevalent genetic alterations in receptor tyrosine kinases and phosphatidylinositol 3-kinase/akt and mitogen-activated protein kinase pathways in anaplastic and follicular thyroid cancers. J Clin Endocrinol Metab 2008;93(8):3106–16.

23. Bible KC, Smallridge RC, Morris JC, et al. Development of a multidisciplinary, multicampus subspecialty practice in endocrine cancers. J Oncol Pract 2012; 8(3 Suppl):e1s–5s.

24. Liu R, Zhang T, Zhu G, et al. Regulation of mutant TERT by BRAF V600E/MAP kinase pathway through FOS/GABP in human cancer. Nat Commun 2018;9(1):579.

25. Isham CR, Bossou AR, Negron V, et al. Pazopanib enhances paclitaxel-induced mitotic catastrophe in anaplastic thyroid cancer. Sci Transl Med 2013;5(166): 166ra3.

26. Marlow LA, von Roemeling CA, Cooper SJ, et al. Foxo3a drives proliferation in anaplastic thyroid carcinoma through transcriptional regulation of cyclin A1: a paradigm shift that impacts current therapeutic strategies. J Cell Sci 2012; 125(Pt 18):4253–63.

27. Parascandolo A, Laukkanen MO, De Rosa N, et al. A dual mechanism of activation of the Sonic Hedgehog pathway in anaplastic thyroid cancer: crosstalk with RAS-BRAF-MEK pathway and ligand secretion by tumor stroma. Oncotarget 2018;9(4):4496–510.

28. Williamson AJ, Doscas ME, Ye J, et al. The sonic hedgehog signaling pathway stimulates anaplastic thyroid cancer cell motility and invasiveness by activating Akt and c-Met. Oncotarget 2016;7(9):10472–85.

29. Hou P, Ji M, Xing M. Association of PTEN gene methylation with genetic alterations in the phosphatidylinositol 3-kinase/AKT signaling pathway in thyroid tumors. Cancer 2008;113(9):2440–7

30. Zhang L, Zhang Y, Mehta A, et al. Dual inhibition of HDAC and EGFR signaling with CUDC-101 induces potent suppression of tumor growth and metastasis in anaplastic thyroid cancer. Oncotarget 2015;6(11):9073–85.

31. Boufraqech M, Nilubol N, Zhang L, et al. miR30a inhibits LOX expression and anaplastic thyroid cancer progression. Cancer Res 2015;75(2):367–77.

32. Xiong Y, Zhang L, Kebebew E. MiR-20a is upregulated in anaplastic thyroid cancer and targets LIMK1. PLoS One 2014;9(5):e96103.

33. Byeon HK, Na HJ, Yang YJ, et al. Acquired resistance to BRAF inhibition induces epithelial-to-mesenchymal transition in BRAF (V600E) mutant thyroid cancer by c-Met-mediated AKT activation. Oncotarget 2017;8(1):596–609.

34. Ryder M, Gild M, Hohl TM, et al. Genetic and pharmacological targeting of CSF-1/CSF-1R inhibits tumor-associated macrophages and impairs BRAF-induced thyroid cancer progression. PLoS One 2013;8(1):e54302.

35. Brauner E, Gunda V, Vanden Borre P, et al. Combining BRAF inhibitor and anti PD-L1 antibody dramatically improves tumor regression and anti tumor immunity in an immunocompetent murine model of anaplastic thyroid cancer. Oncotarget 2016;7(13):17194–211.

36. French JD, Bible K, Spitzweg C, et al. Leveraging the immune system to treat advanced thyroid cancers. Lancet Diabetes Endocrinol 2017;5(6):469–81.

37. French JD. Revisiting immune-based therapies for aggressive follicular cell-derived thyroid cancers. Thyroid 2013;23(5):529–42.

38. Bogsrud TV, Karantanis D, Nathan MA, et al. 18F-FDG PET in the management of patients with anaplastic thyroid carcinoma. Thyroid 2008;18(7):713–9.

39. Smallridge RC, Ain KB, Asa SL, et al. American Thyroid Association guidelines for management of patients with anaplastic thyroid cancer. Thyroid 2012;22(11):1104–39.

40. Poisson T, Deandreis D, Leboulleux S, et al. 18F-fluorodeoxyglucose positron emission tomography and computed tomography in anaplastic thyroid cancer. Eur J Nucl Med Mol Imaging 2010;37(12):2277–85.

41. Amin MB, Edge SB, Greene FL, et al, editors. AJCC Cancer Staging Manual. 8th edition. New York: Springer; 2017.

42. Cabanillas ME, Williams MD, Gunn GB, et al. Facilitating anaplastic thyroid cancer specialized treatment: a model for improving access to multidisciplinary care for patients with anaplastic thyroid cancer. Head Neck 2017;39(7):1291–5.

43. Tallroth E, Wallin G, Lundell G, et al. Multimodality treatment in anaplastic giant cell thyroid carcinoma. Cancer 1987;60(7):1428–31.

44. Besic N, Auersperg M, Us-Krasovec M, et al. Effect of primary treatment on survival in anaplastic thyroid carcinoma. Eur J Surg Oncol 2001;27(3):260–4.

45. Wallgren A, Norin T. Combined chemotherapy and radiation therapy in spindle and giant cell carcinoma of the thyroid gland. Report of a case. Acta Radiol Ther Phys Biol 1973;12(1):17–20.

46. Werner B, Abele J, Alveryd A, et al. Multimodal therapy in anaplastic giant cell thyroid carcinoma. World J Surg 1984;8(1):64–70.

47. Tennvall J, Lundell G, Wahlberg P, et al. Anaplastic thyroid carcinoma: three protocols combining doxorubicin, hyperfractionated radiotherapy and surgery. Br J Cancer 2002;86(12):1848–53.

48. Schlumberger M, Parmentier C. Phase II evaluation of mitoxantrone in advanced non anaplastic thyroid cancer. Bull Cancer 1989;76(4):403–6.

49. Foote RL, Molina JR, Kasperbauer JL, et al. Enhanced survival in locoregionally confined anaplastic thyroid carcinoma: a single-institution experience using aggressive multimodal therapy. Thyroid 2011;21(1):25–30.

50. Prasongsook N, Kumar A, Chintakuntlawar AV, et al. Survival in response to multimodal therapy in anaplastic thyroid cancer. J Clin Endocrinol Metab 2017;102(12):4506–14.

51. Tennvall J, Andersson T, Aspegren K, et al. Undifferentiated giant and spindle cell carcinoma of the thyroid. Report on two combined treatment modalities. Acta Radiol Oncol Radiat Phys Biol 1979;18(5):408–16.

52. Kim JH, Leeper RD. Treatment of locally advanced thyroid carcinoma with combination doxorubicin and radiation therapy. Cancer 1987;60(10):2372–5.
53. Tennvall J, Lundell G, Hallquist A, et al. Combined doxorubicin, hyperfractionated radiotherapy, and surgery in anaplastic thyroid carcinoma. Report on two protocols. The Swedish Anaplastic Thyroid Cancer Group. Cancer 1994;74(4): 1348–54.
54. Schlumberger M, Parmentier C, Delisle MJ, et al. Combination therapy for anaplastic giant cell thyroid carcinoma. Cancer 1991;67(3):564–6.
55. Ain KB, Egorin MJ, DeSimone PA. Treatment of anaplastic thyroid carcinoma with paclitaxel: phase 2 trial using ninety-six-hour infusion. Collaborative Anaplastic Thyroid Cancer Health Intervention Trials (CATCHIT) Group. Thyroid 2000; 10(7):587–94.
56. Onoda N, Sugitani I, Higashiyama T, et al. Concept and design of a nationwide prospective feasibility/efficacy/safety study of weekly paclitaxel for patients with pathologically confirmed anaplastic thyroid cancer (ATCCJ-PTX-P2). BMC Cancer 2015;15:475.
57. Dandekar P, Harmer C, Barbachano Y, et al. Hyperfractionated Accelerated Radiotherapy (HART) for anaplastic thyroid carcinoma: toxicity and survival analysis. Int J Radiat Oncol Biol Phys 2009;74(2):518–21.
58. Mitchell G, Huddart R, Harmer C. Phase II evaluation of high dose accelerated radiotherapy for anaplastic thyroid carcinoma. Radiother Oncol 1999;50(1):33–8.
59. Swaak-Kragten AT, de Wilt JH, Schmitz PI, et al. Multimodality treatment for anaplastic thyroid carcinoma–treatment outcome in 75 patients. Radiother Oncol 2009;92(1):100–4.
60. Pierie JP, Muzikansky A, Gaz RD, et al. The effect of surgery and radiotherapy on outcome of anaplastic thyroid carcinoma. Ann Surg Oncol 2002;9(1):57–64.
61. Bhatia A, Rao A, Ang KK, et al. Anaplastic thyroid cancer: clinical outcomes with conformal radiotherapy. Head Neck 2010;32(7):829–36.
62. Venkatesh YS, Ordonez NG, Schultz PN, et al. Anaplastic carcinoma of the thyroid. A clinicopathologic study of 121 cases. Cancer 1990;66(2):321–30.
63. Chen J, Tward JD, Shrieve DC, et al. Surgery and radiotherapy improves survival in patients with anaplastic thyroid carcinoma: analysis of the surveillance, epidemiology, and end results 1983-2002. Am J Clin Oncol 2008;31(5):460–4.
64. Hu S, Helman SN, Hanly E, et al. The role of surgery in anaplastic thyroid cancer: a systematic review. Am J Otolaryngol 2017;38(3):337–50.
65. Haigh PI, Ituarte PH, Wu HS, et al. Completely resected anaplastic thyroid carcinoma combined with adjuvant chemotherapy and irradiation is associated with prolonged survival. Cancer 2001;91(12):2335–42.
66. Shaha AR, Ferlito A, Owen RP, et al. Airway issues in anaplastic thyroid carcinoma. Eur Arch Otorhinolaryngol 2013;270(10):2579–83.
67. Cabanillas ME, Ferrarotto R, Garden AS, et al. Neoadjuvant BRAF- and immune-directed therapy for anaplastic thyroid carcinoma. Thyroid 2018;28(7):945–51.
68. Shimaoka K, Schoenfeld DA, DeWys WD, et al. A randomized trial of doxorubicin versus doxorubicin plus cisplatin in patients with advanced thyroid carcinoma. Cancer 1985;56(9):2155–60.
69. Subbiah V, Kreitman RJ, Wainberg ZA, et al. Dabrafenib and trametinib treatment in patients with locally advanced or metastatic BRAF V600-mutant anaplastic thyroid cancer. J Clin Oncol 2018;36(1):7–13.
70. Takahashi S, K N, Yamazaki T, et al. Phase II study of lenvatinib in patients with differentiated, medullary, and anaplastic thyroid cancer: final analysis results. in 2016 ASCO Annual Meeting. Chicago, IL, 2016: J Clin Oncol.

71. Bible KC, Suman VJ, Menefee ME, et al. A multiinstitutional phase 2 trial of pazopanib monotherapy in advanced anaplastic thyroid cancer. J Clin Endocrinol Metab 2012;97(9):3179–84.
72. Casterline PF, Jaques DA, Blom H, et al. Anaplastic giant and spindle-cell carcinoma of the thyroid: a different therapeutic approach. Cancer 1980;45(7): 1689–92.
73. Kollipara R, Schneider B, Radovich M, et al. Exceptional response with immunotherapy in a patient with anaplastic thyroid cancer. Oncologist 2017;22(10): 1149–51.
74. Wirth LJ, Eigendorff E, Capdevila J, et al. Phase I/II study of spartalizumab (PDR001), an anti-PD1 mAb, in patients with anaplastic thyroid cancer. J Clin Oncol 2018;36(15 Suppl):6024.
75. Smallridge RC, Copland JA, Brose MS, et al. Efatutazone, an oral PPAR-gamma agonist, in combination with paclitaxel in anaplastic thyroid cancer: results of a multicenter phase 1 trial. J Clin Endocrinol Metab 2013;98(6):2392–400.

Management of Medullary Thyroid Cancer

David Viola, MD, Rossella Elisei, MD*

KEYWORDS

• Medullary thyroid cancer • Calcitonin • CEA • *RET* • MEN

KEY POINTS

• Medullary thyroid cancer (MTC) is a rare thyroid tumor but with a high prevalence of advanced cases at diagnosis.
• MTC can be sporadic or familial, in 75% and 25% of cases, respectively: genetic screening of the REarranged during Transfection (*RET*) oncogene can distinguish the 2 forms.
• Calcitonin is the specific serum marker of MTC and its doubling time is one of the most important prognostic factors: the shorter the worst.
• New targeted therapies are currently available that are able to block or reduce tumoral growth.

INTRODUCTION

Medullary thyroid cancer (MTC) is the third most common thyroid malignancy. It originates from the parafollicular or calcitonin-producing C cells and maintains the features of these cells.[1,2]

The exact incidence of MTC is unknown but its prevalence is approximately 3% to 5% of all thyroid malignancies and is estimated to be present in 0.4% to 1.4% of subjects with thyroid nodules. The incidence peak of MTC is between the fourth and fifth decades but with a wide range of age at presentation. No difference of prevalence between female and male subjects has been reported.[3] MTC can be sporadic or familial, in 75% and 25% of cases, respectively, and when familial it can be associated with other endocrine diseases, such as pheocromocytoma (PHEO) and parathyroid adenoma/hyperplasia causing hyperparathyroidism (HPTH).[4]

No environmental risk factors or ethnical predominance have been identified, although its pathogenesis has been recognized in the activation of the REarranged

Disclosure Statement. R. Elisei served as a consultant for Eisai, Sanofi Genzyme, Sobi (Exelixis), Ipsen, and Loxo. D. Viola served as a consultant for Sanofi Genzyme and Sobi (Exelixis).
Endocrine Unit, Department of Clinical and Experimental Medicine, University of Pisa, Via Paradisa 2, Pisa 56124, Italy
* Corresponding author.
E-mail address: rossella.elisei@med.unipi.it

during Transfection (*RET*) oncogene.[5,6] Germline mutations of *RET* are present in approximately 98% of hereditary cases whereas somatic *RET* mutation are reported in approximately 50% of sporadic cases. Of the latter group, approximately 20% of cases show a RAt Sarcoma (*RAS*) oncogene somatic mutation and 20% to 30% of cases are still orphan of any driver oncogene mutation.[7] The *RET* genetic screening can distinguish the familial from the sporadic form.

The prognosis of MTC is unfavorable, with a 10-year survival rate of MTC patients of approximately 50%. Both the cure and survival rates of these patients are positively affected by an early diagnosis and precocious surgical treatment.[8,9]

CLINICAL PRESENTATION

Most commonly, MTC is diagnosed in a subject with a thyroid nodule, either single or in the context of a multinodular goiter, without any other specific symptom. In a few cases, however, untreatable diarrhea and/or flushing (**Fig. 1**) is present and associated with advanced metastatic disease. Familial history must be carefully investigated because it can be positive for the presence of other cases of MTC, thus suggesting a familial/hereditary case. The same hypothesis should be done if a patient has also a PHEO or a HPTH.

The hereditary syndromes present with MTC (100%) but involve multiple endocrine and non-endocrine organs and can be distinguished in (1) multiple endocrine neoplasia type 2A (MEN 2A), in which PHEO (50%) and HPTH (25%) can be present; (2) multiple endocrine neoplasia type 2B (MEN 2B), in which MTC is associated with PHEO (50%); and (3) familial MTC (FMTC), which is the most frequent and characterized by the presence of isolated MTC. A distinctive feature of MEN 2A is cutaneous lichen amyloidosis (CLA) (15%–20%) (**Fig. 2**) whereas cutaneous/mucosal neuromas (100%), megacolon (100%), and marfanoid habitus (100%) are peculiar to MEN 2B (**Fig. 3**).[10]

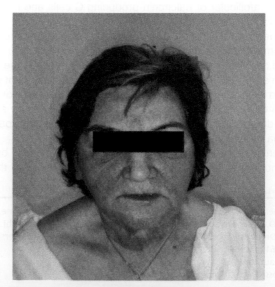

Fig. 1. Typical flushing syndrome in a patient with elevated serum levels of calcitonin: the patient becomes markedly red in the face at various intervals of time. The phenomenon is more frequent in advanced and metastatic cases.

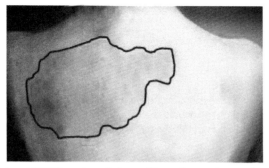

Fig. 2. Typical CLA in a MEN 2A patient: itchy and hyperkeratotic papules that are brownish-red in color are located in the interscapular region. The lesion is due to the extracellular deposition of amyloid proteins in that particular region of the body. It is present preferentially in patients with a Cys 634 *RET* mutation.

The clinical course of MTC varies considerably in the three syndromes, being very aggressive and almost invariably unfavorable in MEN 2B, indolent in a majority of patients with FMTC, and with an intermediate degree of aggressiveness in MEN 2A patients. For this reason, the clinical abnormalities, described previously, that are

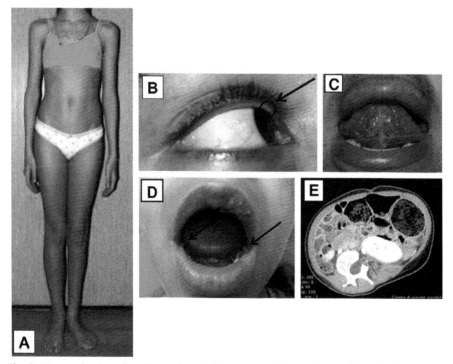

Fig. 3. Non-endocrine alterations almost always present in patients affected with MEN 2B syndrome: (*A*) marfanoid habitus characterized by long arms and long legs with respect to the trunk; (*B*) a neuroma of the conjunctiva is indicated by the arrow; (*C*) bumpy lips and neuromas of the tongue; (*D*) bilateral mucosal neuromas of the mouth as indicated by the 2 arrows; and (*E*) CT of the abdomen showing a megacolon due to an abnormal dilation of the colon secondary to the ganglioneuromatosis typical of the MEN 2B syndrome.

peculiar to MEN 2, should be early recognized to perform an early diagnosis and an early treatment.

DIAGNOSIS
Sporadic Form

As discussed previously, the most common presentation of sporadic cases is thyroid nodular disease. In this case, physical examination, neck ultrasound (US), and US-guided fine-needle aspiration cytology are among the most important diagnostic tools for MTC.

A cytologic smear of an MTC is characterized by isolated, oval to round, large polygonal or spindled cells. Although the cytologic pattern is generally typical, there are several series that show a high percentage of failure in making a presurgical diagnosis.[11–13]

At variance, elevated basal levels of serum calcitonin, especially when greater than 100 pg/mL,[14] are diagnostic of MTC. Routine measurement of serum calcitonin in nodular thyroid diseases allows the preoperative diagnosis of unsuspected sporadic MTC.[15–18] Calcitonin screening allows the precocious diagnosis of MTC, usually when the tumor is still at its early stages, thus favoring successful surgical treatment and patient cure. Patients diagnosed by serum calcitonin screening were demonstrated to have significantly better prognosis than those diagnosed by cytology or at histology.[17] There are several other conditions, however, in which basal levels of serum calcitonin may be elevated.[19–25] Differential diagnosis can be performed by calcium stimulation test.[26] Although in patients with MTC and elevated basal levels of calcitonin, calcium stimulation determines a 5-fold to 10-fold increase of serum levels of calcitonin, in other diseases, the calcitonin increase is limited or absent.

An additional tool for the diagnosis of MTC, especially when serum calcitonin is elevated but less than 100 pg/mL, is the measurement of calcitonin in the washout fluid of the needle used for the puncture of a suspected thyroid nodule.[27] This approach is of particular diagnostic importance to ascertain the nature of suspicious neck lymph nodes detected at neck US to plan the most appropriate surgical treatment.

Although calcitonin is the most reliable tumor marker due to its high sensitivity and specificity, there are other peptides that may be released by the malignant transformed C cell. Serum carcinoembryonic antigen (CEA) is usually elevated in advanced cases when distant metastases are present.[28] Recently, high levels of serum carbohydrate antigen 19.9 have been demonstrated to identify a subset of MTC patients with a worse prognosis and a higher risk of mortality in the short term. As in many other neuroendocrine tumors, serum chromogranin, somatostatin, gastrin-releasing peptide, vasoactive intestinal peptide, neuron-specific enolase, and other neuroendocrine substances may be abnormally produced but none of them is useful for diagnosis.[28] Moreover, some MTC-secreted peptides may result in significant clinical manifestations: vasoactive intestinal peptide, serotonin, and prostaglandins may all contribute to flushing and diarrhea whereas ACTH may cause ectopic Cushing syndrome in approximately 1% of MTC cases.[29]

RET genetic analysis should always be performed when the diagnosis of MTC has been established because it allows defining the sporadic or hereditary nature of MTC.[30] The presence of the mutation in an apparently sporadic case or in a family member of hereditary forms is of fundamental importance to guide future diagnostic and therapeutic strategies. Different types of RET gene mutations account for different biological behavior and may guide the future examinations that should be performed. A complete and updated database of all reported RET germline mutations and their clinical behavior are available online (http://www.arup.utah.edu/database/MEN2/MEN2_welcome.php).

Hereditary Form

The hereditary nature of the MTC may be suspected on the basis of a positive family history or for the presence of other endocrine (ie, PHEO and/or HPTH) or non-endocrine disorders (ie, mucosal or cutaneous neuromas, marfanoid habitus, megacolon for MEN 2B [see **Fig. 3**], and CLA [see **Fig. 2**] for MEN 2A). However, 7% to 15% of apparently sporadic MTC are found to be hereditary cases.[30–32]

Usually PHEO diagnosis follows the development and diagnosis of MTC, and the mean age at presentation is 30 to 40 years. An elevated 24-hour urinary excretion of metanephrines is the most sensitive and specific test to diagnose PHEO that is often asymptomatic. Once PHEO is suspected, an abdomen US for the localization of the adrenal mass should be performed but in some cases a computerized tomography (CT) scan and/or an MRI may be necessary.[28] The screening for PHEO should begin according to the type of *RET* mutation because the disease was diagnosed as early as 8 years, 12 years, and 19 years of age in subjects with more or less aggressive *RET* mutations.[28]

Parathyroid glands may also be involved but only in MEN 2A. Both adenomas and hyperplasia may be associated with an increase of the parathyroid hormone secretion, resulting in hypercalcemia and hypercalciuria.[33] In contrast with MEN 1 patients, HPTH is mild and often asymptomatic. The mean age of HPTH diagnosis in MEN 2A is approximately 30 years and almost all experts agree that the screening for HPTH should begin not earlier than 11 years and 16 years in patients with more aggressive or less aggressive *RET* mutations, respectively. In some families with MEN 2A Hirschsprung disease can be associated with MTC and the other endocrine neoplasias. This association is peculiar because the pathogenesis of Hirschsprung disease is due to a loss-of-function mutation of *RET* gene whereas the mutations related to the MEN 2 syndromes are caused by gain-of-function mutations.[34] There are only 4 *RET* codons (**Fig. 4**) that give origin to mutations with gain-of-function and loss-of-function and for this reason they are called Janus mutations.[34]

Once the index case has been identified has a hereditary case, all first-degree relatives should be analyzed for the possibility of carrying the same *RET* germline mutation. The genetic screening allows distinguishing the gene carriers, who are at risk to develop the syndrome, from those who do not carry the mutation and do not need to perform any specific follow-up and can be reassured. At variance, gene carriers should be immediately submitted to a clinical and biochemical evaluation to establish if one disease of the syndrome is already present. For gene carriers who have not yet developed any diseases belonging to the MEN 2 syndrome, a strict follow-up is suggested. Many germline *RET* mutations have been recognized and are clearly associated with specific phenotypes.[35] According to the different *RET* mutations and their associated phenotypes, the American Thyroid Association (ATA) has distinguished the *RET* mutations into 3 levels of risk to develop MTC: highest (ATA-HST), high (ATA-H), and moderate (ATA-MOD) (see **Fig. 4**). This classification, together with the serum levels of serum calcitonin,[36] is relevant to better plan screening and treatment strategies.[28]

THERAPY AND FOLLOW-UP
Initial Treatment

An early diagnosis and complete surgical treatment are the bases for the definitive cure of MTC patients. Total/near total thyroidectomy is considered standard treatment

RET receptor			CODON	EXON	ATA risk	HPTH	PHEO	CLA	HD	MH/MG/MN/BL
EXTRACELLULAR DOMAIN	CD		533	8	MOD	-	+	A	A	A
			609	10	MOD	+	+/++	A	P	A
			611	10	MOD	+	+/++	A	P	A
			618	10	MOD	+	+/++	A	P	A
			620	10	MOD	+	+/++	A	P	A
			630	11	MOD	+	+/++	A	A	A
			631	11	MOD	-	+++	A	A	A
			634	11	H	++	+++	P	A	A
TRANSMEMBRANE DOMAIN	TM	{	666	11	MOD	-	+	A	A	A
INTRACELLULAR DOMAIN	TK	{	768	13	MOD	-	-	A	A	A
			790	13	MOD	-	+	A	A	A
			804	14	MOD	+	+	P	A	A
			883	15	H	-	+++	A	A	A
			891	15	MOD	+	+	A	A	A
			912	16	MOD	-	-	A	A	A
			918	16	HST	-	+++	A	A	P

Fig. 4. Genotype-phenotype correlation and level of risk (according to the ATA classification) to develop the endocrine neoplasia and the other non-endocrine diseases associated with MTC. +, 10%; ++, 20%–30%; +++, 50%; A, absent; BL, bumpy lips; CD, cysteine-rich domain; H, high risk; HD, Hirschsprung disease; HST, highest risk; MG, megacolon; MH, marfanoid habitus; MN, mucosal neuromas; MOD, moderate risk (ATA 2015 guidelines) to develop; P, present; TK, tyrosine kinase domain.

in both sporadic and hereditary MTC. The need for total thyroidectomy is supported by the presence of multicentric and bilateral disease in a majority of hereditary and in approximately 6% of sporadic MTCs.[37] An additional reason in favor of total thyroidectomy is that 7% to 15% of apparently sporadic cases are hereditary forms with multicentric/bilateral disease associated with C-cell hyperplasia.[30–32]

Due to the high prevalence of central compartment lymph node metastases (50%–75%), many clinicians suggest performing central compartment lymph node dissection (CCLND) with total thyroidectomy as initial treatment. Considering that this prevalence is the same whether the primary tumor is less than 1 cm or greater than 4 cm, prophylactic CCLND should be performed independently of the primary tumor size and the presurgical evidence of lymph node involvement.

More recent evidences suggest using preoperative calcitonin values to determine the extent of lymph node dissection. It seems that there is virtually no risk of lymph node metastases when preoperative calcitonin level is less than 20 pg/mL (normal reference range <10 pg/mL).[38] In these cases, the prophylactic CCLND, that is affected by a high risk of surgical complications, particularly of permanent hypoparathyroidism, might be avoided. At variance, calcitonin values higher than 20 pg/mL, 50 pg/mL, 200 pg/mL, and 500 pg/mL seem associated with the presence of lymph node metastases in the ipsilateral central and ipsilateral lateral neck, in the contralateral central neck, in the contralateral lateral neck, and in the upper mediastinum, respectively.[38] It is demonstrated, however, that the highest values of serum calcitonin are the expression of metastatic disease, and the prophylactic CCLND would probably not change the course of the disease. In these cases, the surgery extension could be limited to the lymph nodes compartments that have been demonstrated involved by the disease at neck US.

The age at thyroidectomy is a well-known risk factor for morbidity and mortality, particularly in infants. In this regard, a greater concern is represented by young *RET* gene carriers who, if rendered hypoparathyroid, would be exposed to the need of calcium and vitamin D supplementation for the rest of their lives. According to the ATA guidelines, total thyroidectomy should be performed in the first year/first months of life in MEN 2B (ATA-HST), before 5 years of age in MEN 2A (ATA-H), and when calcitonin levels become elevated or in childhood if the parents do not wish to embark on a lengthy period of evaluation in MEN 2A (ATA-MOD).[28] Considering the great heterogeneity, however, in the age of onset among different families and within the same family and recent evidences that patient cure could be achieved by tailoring the surgical treatment in different subjects according to basal and stimulated calcitonin levels, an individualized approach is proposed. This is mainly because also experienced surgeons have great difficulty localizing the parathyroid glands in young children and infants. Moreover, some pediatricians have some concerns regarding the potential detrimental effects of insufficient thyroid hormone replacement that can impair brain development and normal growth. Thus, prophylactic thyroidectomy associated with CCLND within the first year of life should be reserved for MEN 2B children. Moreover, because the CCLND in children, as well as in adults, is the major cause of hypoparathyroidism, the ATA guidelines suggest that children with MEN 2 who have been decided to be submitted to total thyroidectomy can avoid prophylactic CCLND when calcitonin values are less than 40 pg/mL and there is no US evidence of lymph node metastases.[28,36,39]

Regardless of age and presenting symptoms, all hereditary MTC patients and apparently sporadic cases not yet definitively ascertained as true sporadic must be investigated for the presence of PHEO and HPTH. PHEO, if present, must be treated before MTC and patients need to be adequately prepared to avoid hypertensive crisis that could be life threatening. The diagnosis of HPTH is not less important because the delay in diagnosis could lead to further surgical treatment in the same region exposing the patient to a higher rate of surgical complications.

Hormone replacement therapy with L-thyroxine (LT4) should be started immediately after thyroidectomy. At variance with differentiated thyroid cancer parafollicular C cells and MTC are not dependent on thyrotropin; thus, there is no need to treat patients with "LT4 suppressive" therapy. Substitutive LT4 treatment aiming to keep thyrotropin values within the normal range is adequate.

In cases of aggressive local disease, the initial surgical treatment can be incomplete. In these cases, external beam radiotherapy (EBRT) can be considered but its real therapeutic role is still controversial because of the absence of prospective randomized trials comparing EBRT to observation. From a recent Surveillance, Epidemiology, and End Results program analysis, it seems clear that there is no survival benefit in patients with MTC and positive lymph nodes.[40] For this reason, the benefit of an EBRT treatment should be compared with the risks of exposing patients to the acute and chronic toxicity of this treatment. Moreover, the surgeons and clinicians should accurately consider the possibility that the patients could be candidates for reoperation in the neck because the procedure is more difficult and associated with significant complications if EBRT has been previously performed.

Follow-up and Diagnosis of Persistent/Recurrent Disease

Three months after the initial treatment, a control, including physical examination, neck US, and measurement of serum thyrotropin, basal calcitonin, and CEA, should be performed. Due to the prolonged half-lives, if performed too early, measurement of serum calcitonin and CEA may be misleading, especially if high serum values were present before surgery. If basal calcitonin is undetectable, the patient can be considered in clinical remission with a low risk of recurrence (10%).[41] If a calcium stimulation test for calcitonin is also negative, the risk of recurrence drops to 3%.[42] Measurement of CEA is not necessary in cases of undetectable levels of serum calcitonin.

Subjects who are still having low but detectable calcitonin values (<150 pg/mL) after initial surgery can present distant metastatic disease but in a majority of cases persistent/recurrent disease is confined to neck lymph nodes. These patients can be followed every 6 months to 12 months with physical examination, neck US, and measurement of serum basal calcitonin and CEA. Detectable serum calcitonin levels are compatible with long-term survival during which calcitonin may remain stable over time or slowly increase. In this case, frequent and repeated imaging studies (eg, CT, PET, and bone scan) are unnecessary and harmful.[28]

In cases of postoperative basal calcitonin values higher than 150 pg/mL or in those in which calcitonin increase substantially over time, patients should be evaluated with imaging studies. In particular, patients with calcitonin higher than 5000 pg/mL present distant metastatic disease in more than 50%, and sites of metastases can be detected in almost all cases in which calcitonin is higher than 20,000 pg/mL.[43] The most sensitive imaging studies to detect MTC in different sites are US for the neck, CT for the chest, MRI for the liver, and MRI and bone scintigraphy for the skeleton.[44] In some cases, other imaging techniques, such as PET with different tracers (fluorodeoxyglucose F 18 [^{18}FDG], dihydroxyphenylalanine F 18 [^{18}F-DOPA], dotatate gallium Ga 68 [^{68}Ga-DOTATATE], and so forth) may be useful. To avoid repeated and unnecessary imaging studies in patients who are usually long survivors, after initial staging, except in rare cases, CT scans should be performed no more than annually and according to the serum calcitonin trend of increase.

Both serum calcitonin and CEA levels doubling times (DTs) are good predictors of survival, in particular the former,[45] and can also predict disease progression, as demonstrated by the evidence that when calcitonin and CEA DTs were concordant and less than 25 months, progressive disease (PD) was observed in almost all cases (94%), whereas when calcitonin and CEA DTs were discordant and less than 25 months, PD was still present but in a lower number of cases (56%).[46] The DTs of calcitonin and CEA can be easily calculated on the ATA Web site and is useful in choosing the most appropriate time to submit a patient to a new CT scan (www.thyroid.org/thyroid-physicians-professionals/calculators/thyroid-cancer-carcinoma).

Other Treatments for Persistent/Recurrent Disease

A second surgical treatment with a curative intent is generally not recommended, in fact, only one-third of MTC patients has been demonstrated to have postoperative basal and stimulated serum calcitonin in the normal range and more rarely calcitonin is undetectable.[47,48] In the clinical management of patients with MTC, the identification of those who might benefit from this treatment is of great importance; however, no clinical trials randomized to observation alone or reoperation are available. Repeat neck surgery should be suggested for rapidly growing lymph node metastases at risk of infiltration of vital neck structures, symptomatic lesions, or ulceration that is unlikely in MTC. Capsular invasion and more than 10 lymph node metastases in the primary surgical specimens are significant predictors of poor response to reoperation.[49,50] Neck lymph node metastases after adequate initial diagnosis and treatment are present mostly in metastatic patients and can be followed by neck US in a majority of cases.

Similarly to lymph node recurrence, surgical treatment of distant metastatic lesions is not indicated except for those that could compromise vital structures and/or be life threatening. Liver metastases may be amenable to surgical treatment in some cases.

This procedure may be useful in large, single, increasing in size liver metastases, particularly if associated with symptoms, such as diarrhea or pain. As an alternative, local treatments, such as radiofrequency ablation, thermablation chemoembolization, and transarterial radioembolization,[28] can be appropriate and less invasive. These local approaches could be always considered also for lung or bone metastases, because, if feasible, they can be useful to delay systemic therapy.

External beam radiotherapy (EBRT) can be used only occasionally for the treatment of lung metastases and be reserved for rare symptomatic cases (cough, dyspnea, difficulty in swallowing, and so forth). The main reason is that EBRT of lungs carries a high risk of radiation fibrosis and respiratory failure that can become the real risk of death for these patients. In cases of painful bone metastases present, EBRT may be useful to provide relief. A monthly intravenous infusion of zoledronic acid or a monthly subcutaneous administration of denosumab possibly reduces the skeletal-related adverse events (AEs) and should be performed especially when bone lesions are multiple. Alternative approaches to prevent/delay fractures may be radiofrequency ablation, vertebroplasty, or kyphoplasty.

Brain metastases may also be treated with EBRT or stereotaxic radiosurgery to obtain local control, prolong survival, and improve quality of life. Surgical resection for asymptomatic brain metastases is almost always not indicated because it exposes patients with rapidly progressive systemic disease to useless risks.

When metastatic lesions are multiple and localized in different organs, systemic therapy should be considered if disease progression is documented. Classical cytotoxic chemotherapy for advanced metastatic MTC has shown limited response rates (15%–20%) and short duration.[28] Treatment with several radiolabeled molecules has been widely explored. A promising approach documenting complete remission or partial remission seems to come from the treatment of MTC patients with radiolabeled (yttrium 90 or lutetium 177) peptides targeting somatostatin receptors. Furthermore, better designed studies evaluating more patients are needed to establish its therapeutic efficacy.

Since 2005, a new interest for targeted therapy in MTC has been growing.[51] The rationale for this interest was represented by the presence of RET mutation in virtually all familial cases and in a majority of advanced sporadic cases.[52] In addition to RET, other important targets (ie, vascular endothelial growth factor receptor [VEGFR], epidermal growth factor receptor [EGFR], hepatocyte growth factor receptor [MET], and so forth) were demonstrated to be overexpressed in this tumor and represented the molecular basis of treating this disease with tyrosine kinase inhibitors (TKIs). The most important drugs and targets investigated in MTC are summarized in **Table 1**.

One of the first drugs investigated on MTC was motesanib.[53] In a phase II trial, the lack of a placebo arm and strict inclusion criteria led to the enrollment of many patients with stable disease and poor results in terms of efficacy. For these reasons the drug never reached the market. In the following years, other phase II clinical trials with axitinib, pazopanib, and lenvatinib have been performed. All of them showed interesting results[54–56] but these drugs were never evaluated in a phase III study. At variance, the efficacy of vandetanib has been investigated in MTC with a prospective, randomized, double-blind phase III trial that showed good results in terms of efficacy and tolerability compared with placebo (ZETA trial).[57] The improvement of symptoms and a significant prolongation of the progression-free survival (PFS) in patients treated with vandetanib compared with those treated with placebo have been considered relevant. For this reason, in 2011 and 2013, vandetanib was approved for the treatment of symptomatic and progressive MTC by the Food and Drug Administration and the European Medicines Agency, respectively.

Table 1
Results of clinical trials with targeted drugs in patients with medullary thyroid cancer

Drug	Target	Phase	Patients (n)	Partial Response (%)	Stable Disease ≥6 mo (%)	Median Progression-Free Survival (mo)	Median Overall Survival (mo)	References
Axitinib	VEGFR1, VEGFR3, PDGFR, cKIT	II	13	23.1	NE	9.4	18.9	Capdevila et al,[54] 2017
Cabozantinib	VEGFR2, cKIT, RET, MET	III	330	28	NE	11.2	26.6	Elisei et al,[58] 2013
Lenvatinib	VEGFR1, VEGFR3, RET, FGFR, cKIT, PDGFR	I	59	36	67	9	16.6	Schlumberger et al,[56] 2016
Motesanib	VEGFR1, VEGFR3, PDGFR, cKIT, RET	II	91	2	48	12	NE	Schlumberger et al,[53] 2009
Pazopanib	VEGFR1, VEGFR3, cKIT, PDGFR	II	35	14.3	>70%	9.4	19.9	Bible et al,[55] 2014
Vandetanib	VEGFR2, RET, FGFR, cKIT, EGFR	III	331	45	87	NE	NE	Wells et al,[57] 2012

Abbreviations: EGFR, epidermal growth factor receptor; FGFR, fibroblast growth factor receptor; KIT, v-kit Hardy-Zuckerman 4 feline sarcoma viral oncogene; MET, hepatocyte growth factor [HGF] receptor; NE, not estimated; PDGFR, platelet-derived growth factor receptor; *RET*, REarranged during Transfection receptor; VEGFR-1,-2,-3, vascular endothelial growth factor receptor.

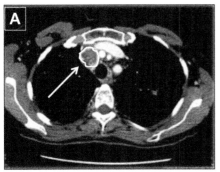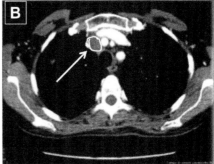

Fig. 5. Metastatic hilar lymph node of the lung detected at the CT scan (*A*) before and (*B*) 3 months after the initiation of TKI treatment (*white arrows*): a significant reduction of the lesion size and a change of its CT aspect, due to the devascularization of the lesion, can be observed.

Cabozantinib is the second Food and Drug Administration–approved and the European Medicines Agency–approved drug for the treatment of advanced and progressive MTC. The approval arrived in 2012 in the United States and in 2014 in Europe after the very good results of a randomized phase III study in which 330 patients with advanced and progressive MTC were randomized either to cabozantinb (140 mg) or placebo (EXAM trial).[58] The prolongation of the PFS of patients treated with cabozantinib with respect to those treated with placebo showed a significant difference, not only in patients who were naïve from other TKI but also in those who were previously treated with other TKI. These results clearly indicated that cabozantinib can be successfully used either as first-line or second-line treatment.

Despite these good results in PFS, both cabozantinib and vandetanib seem unable to prolong overall survival (OS) in MTC patients even if in the subgroup of M918T *RET*–mutated patients those treated with cabozantinib were demonstrated to have a higher OS than those treated with placebo (44.3 months vs 18.9 months).[59] Despite that they are cytostatic and not cytotoxic, however, a significant objective response of the target lesions have been observed after few weeks/months of treatment (**Fig. 5**).

Both drugs have several AEs that represent the major limit of these therapies (**Table 2**). One of the reasons for which TKI systemic therapy is delayed until disease progression according to Response Evaluation Criteria In Solid Tumors is that AEs can severely affect the quality of life of these patients. Several AEs can be managed by introducing other drugs, such as for hypertension or diarrhea, but others, such as QT prolongation, fatigue, or weight loss, require daily dose reduction.[60] The different design of the 2 phase III trials (EXAM and ZETA) do not allow a direct comparison of the 2 drugs. For this reason, when a systemic therapy is needed, the choice between these drugs should be made by carefully considering patient comorbidities, potential toxicities, need of a more or less rapid response, and history of previous treatments. In this regard, it is relevant to say that several reports demonstrated that vandetanib can reverse or control ectopic Cushing syndrome that can be present in advanced MTC and associated with a poor prognosis. All this evidence and these considerations indicate that the management of these patients should be done by an experienced team, including at least endocrinologists, oncologists, cardiologists, dermatologists, and radiologists.

Most of these AEs are due the multitarget activity of these drugs and mainly to the anti-VEGFR activity. For this reason, other new promising drugs (ie, LOXO-292 and BLU-667), directed against *RET*, are under investigation in phase I/II studies.[61,62]

Table 2
Adverse events reported in at least 10% of patients treated with vandetanib (ZETA trial)[56] or cabozantinib (EXAM trial)[57]

Adverse Events, Any Degree	Vandetanib, % of Patients with This Adverse Event	Adverse Events, Any Degree	Cabozantinib, % of Patients with This Adverse Event
Diarrhea	56	Diarrhea	63
Rash	45	Palmar-plantar erythrodysesthesia	50
Nausea	33	Decreased weight	48
Hypertension	32	Decreased appetite	46
Fatigue	24	Nausea	43
Headache	26	Fatigue	41
Decreased appetite	21	Dysgeusia	34
Acne	20	Hair color changes	34
Dry skin	15	Hypertension	33
Dermatitis	15	Stomatitis	29
Asthenia	14	Constipation	27
Vomiting	14	Hemorrhage	25
Abdominal pain	14	Vomiting	24
QT prolongation	14	Mucosal inflammation	23
Insomnia	13	Asthenia	21
Nasopharyngitis	11	Dysphonia	20
Cough	10	Rash/dry skin	19
Decreased weight	10	Headache/oropharyngeal pain	18
		Abdominal pain	17
		Alopecia	16
		Pain and back pain	15
		Dyspnea/oral pain/dry mouth	13
		Cough/muscle spams	12
		Dyspepsia	11
		Erythema/glossodynia	10

SUMMARY

MTC is a rare thyroid tumor but with a high prevalence of advanced cases at diagnosis. Its definitive cure can be obtained only if, at the time of diagnosis, the tumor is still intrathyroid. MTC can be sporadic or familial in 75% and 25% of cases, respectively. The genetic screening of *RET* oncogene can distinguish the two forms. Once an index case of a family is recognized, all first-degree relatives should undergo the *RET* genetic screening. The early identification of gene carriers allows their early thyroidectomy and their definitive cure. Calcitonin is the specific serum marker of MTC and its DT is one of the most important prognostic factors both for survival and progression of the disease. The CEA, although not specific, is also important in the follow-up of MTC patients, related to the tumoral burden. Moreover, its DT must be taken into consideration in the follow-up of MTC patients. Approximately 30% of MTC patients arrive at first observation when already metastatic. These cases are likely to enter into progression. After considering the possibility of using local treatments, especially if the growing lesion is unique and appropriately located, a systemic therapy should be considered with one of the two new approved targeted drugs, vandetanib or cabozantinib. An accurate evaluation of the case must be performed by a multidisciplinary team to choose the drug and to follow-up the patient.

ACKNOWLEDGMENTS

This manuscript was supported by the Associazione Italiana per la Ricerca sul Cancro (AIRC), Investigator Grant 21790.

REFERENCES

1. Hazard JB, Hawk WA, Crile G. Medullary (solid) carcinoma of the thyroid—a clinicopathologic entity. J Clin Endocrinol Metab 1959. https://doi.org/10.1210/jcem-19-1-152.
2. Melvin KE, Tashjian AH Jr. The syndrome of excessive thyrocalcitonin produced by medullary carcinoma of the thyroid. Proc Natl Acad Sci U S A 1968. https://doi.org/10.1073/pnas.59.4.1216.
3. Bergholm U, Adami HO, Telenius-Berg M, et al. Incidence of sporadic and familial medullary thyroid carcinoma in Sweden 1959 through 1981: A nationwide study in 126 patients. Acta Oncol (Madr) 1990. https://doi.org/10.3109/02841869009089985.
4. Keiser HR, Beaven MA, Doppman J, et al. Sipple's syndrome: medullary thyroid carcinoma, pheochromocytoma, and parathyroid disease. Studies in a large family. NIH conference. Ann Intern Med 1973. https://doi.org/10.7326/0003-4819-78-4-561.
5. Donis-keller H, Dou S, Chi D, et al. Mutations in the RET proto-oncogene are associated with MEN 2a and FMTC. Hum Mol Genet 1993. https://doi.org/10.1093/hmg/2.7.851.
6. Mulligan LM, Kwok JBJ, Healey CS, et al. Germ-line mutations of the RET proto-oncogene in multiple endocrine neoplasia type 2A. Nature 1993. https://doi.org/10.1038/363458a0.
7. Ciampi R, Mian C, Fugazzola L, et al. Evidence of a low prevalence of RAS mutations in a large medullary thyroid cancer series. Thyroid 2013. https://doi.org/10.1089/thy.2012.0207.
8. GHARIB H, McCONAHEY WM, TIEGS RD, et al. Medullary thyroid carcinoma: clinicopathologic features and long-term follow-up of 65 patients treated during 1946 through 1970. Mayo Clin Proc 1992. https://doi.org/10.1016/S0025-6196(12)60923-9.
9. Kebebew E, Ituarte PHG, Siperstein AE, et al. Medullary thyroid carcinoma: Clinical characteristics, treatment, prognostic factors, and a comparison of staging systems. Cancer 2000;88(5):1139–48.
10. Romei C, Pardi E, Cetani F, et al. Genetic and clinical features of multiple endocrine neoplasia types 1 and 2. J Oncol 2012. https://doi.org/10.1155/2012/705036.
11. Trimboli P, Treglia G, Guidobaldi L, et al. Detection rate of FNA cytology in medullary thyroid carcinoma: a meta-analysis. Clin Endocrinol (Oxf) 2015. https://doi.org/10.1111/cen.12563.
12. Chang TC, Wu SL, Hsiao YL. Medullary thyroid carcinoma: Pitfalls in diagnosis by fine needle aspiration cytology and relationship of cytomorphology to RET proto-oncogene mutations. Acta Cytol 2005. https://doi.org/10.1159/000326191.

13. Papaparaskeva K, Nagel H, Droese M. Cytologic diagnosis of medullary carcinoma of the thyroid gland. Diagn Cytopathol 2000;22(6):351–8.

14. Costante G, Filetti S. Early diagnosis of medullary thyroid carcinoma: is systematic calcitonin screening appropriate in patients with nodular thyroid disease? Oncologist 2011. https://doi.org/10.1634/theoncologist.2010-0344.

15. Pacini F, Fontanelli M, Fugazzola L, et al. Routine measurement of serum calcitonin in nodular thyroid diseases allows the preoperative diagnosis of unsuspected sporadic medullary thyroid carcinoma. J Clin Endocrinol Metab 1994. https://doi.org/10.1210/jcem.78.4.8157706.

16. Niccoli P, Wion-Barbot N, Caron P, et al. Interest of routine measurement of serum calcitonin: Study in a large series of thyroidectomized patients. J Clin Endocrinol Metab 1997. https://doi.org/10.1210/jcem.82.2.3737.

17. Elisei R, Bottici V, Luchetti F, et al. Impact of routine measurement of serum calcitonin on the diagnosis and outcome of medullary thyroid cancer: experience in 10,864 patients with nodular thyroid disorders. J Clin Endocrinol Metab 2004. https://doi.org/10.1210/jc.2003-030550.

18. Vierhapper H, Raber W, Bieglmayer C, et al. Routine measurement of plasma calcitonin in nodular thyroid diseases. J Clin Endocrinol Metab 1997. https://doi.org/10.1210/jcem.82.5.3949.

19. Borchhardt KA, Hörl WH, Sunder-Plassmann G. Reversibility of "secondary hypercalcitoninemia" after kidney transplantation. Am J Transplant 2005. https://doi.org/10.1111/j.1600-6143.2005.00908.x.

20. Bevilacqua M, Dominguez LJ, Righini V, et al. Dissimilar PTH, gastrin, and calcitonin responses to oral calcium and peptones in hypocalciuric hypercalcemia, primary hyperparathyroidism, and normal subjects: a useful tool for differential diagnosis. J Bone Miner Res 2006. https://doi.org/10.1359/JBMR.051210.

21. Schuetz M, Duan H, Wahl K, et al. T lymphocyte cytokine production patterns in Hashimoto patients with elevated calcitonin levels and their relationship to tumor initiation. Anticancer Res 2006;26(6B):4591–6.

22. Pratz KW, Ma C, Aubry MC, et al. Large cell carcinoma with calcitonin and vasoactive intestinal polypeptide-associated Verner-Morrison syndrome. Mayo Clin Proc 2005. https://doi.org/10.1016/s0025-6196(11)62968-6.

23. Shi X, Liu R, Basolo F, et al. Differential clinicopathological risk and prognosis of major papillary thyroid cancer variants. J Clin Endocrinol Metab 2016;101(1). https://doi.org/10.1210/jc.2015-2917.

24. Sim SJ, Glassman AB, Ro JY, et al. Serum calcitonin in small cell carcinoma of the prostate. Ann Clin Lab Sci 1996;26(6):487–95.

25. Machens A, Haedecke J, Holzhausen HJ, et al. Differential diagnosis of calcitonin-secreting neuroendocrine carcinoma of the foregut by pentagastrin stimulation. Langenbecks Arch Surg 2000. https://doi.org/10.1007/s004230000169.

26. Mian C, Perrino M, Colombo C, et al. Refining calcium test for the diagnosis of medullary thyroid cancer: cutoffs, procedures, and safety. J Clin Endocrinol Metab 2014;99(5):1656–64.

27. Boi F, Maurelli I, Pinna G, et al. Calcitonin measurement in wash-out fluid from fine needle aspiration of neck masses in patients with primary and metastatic medullary thyroid carcinoma. J Clin Endocrinol Metab 2007. https://doi.org/10.1210/jc.2007-0326.

28. Wells SA, Asa SL, Dralle H, et al. Revised American thyroid association guidelines for the management of medullary thyroid carcinoma. Thyroid 2015. https://doi.org/10.1089/thy.2014.0335.

29. Barbosa SL-S, Rodien P, Leboulleux S, et al. Ectopic adrenocorticotropic hormone-syndrome in medullary carcinoma of the thyroid: a retrospective analysis and review of the literature. Thyroid 2005. https://doi.org/10.1089/thy.2005.15.618.

30. Romei C, Cosci B, Renzini G, et al. RET genetic screening of sporadic medullary thyroid cancer (MTC) allows the preclinical diagnosis of unsuspected gene carriers and the identification of a relevant percentage of hidden familial MTC (FMTC). Clin Endocrinol (Oxf) 2011;74(2). https://doi.org/10.1111/j.1365-2265.2010.03900.x.

31. Elisei R, Romei C, Cosci B, et al. Brief report: RET genetic screening in patients with medullary thyroid cancer and their relatives: experience with 807 individuals at one center. J Clin Endocrinol Metab 2007. https://doi.org/10.1210/jc.2007-1005.

32. Kihara M, Miyauchi A, Yoshioka K, et al. Germline RET mutation carriers in Japanese patients with apparently sporadic medullary thyroid carcinoma: a single institution experience. Auris Nasus Larynx 2016. https://doi.org/10.1016/j.anl.2015.12.016.

33. Bilezikian JP, Bandeira L, Khan A, et al. Hyperparathyroidism. Lancet 2018. https://doi.org/10.1016/S0140-6736(17)31430-7.

34. Moore S, Zaahl M. The Hirschsprung's–multiple endocrine neoplasia connection. Clinics (Sao Paulo) 2012. https://doi.org/10.6061/clinics/2012(Sup01)12.

35. Romei C, Ciampi R, Elisei R. A comprehensive overview of the role of the RET proto-oncogene in thyroid carcinoma. Nat Rev Endocrinol 2016. https://doi.org/10.1038/nrendo.2016.11.

36. Elisei R, Romei C, Renzini G, et al. The timing of total thyroidectomy in RET gene mutation carriers could be personalized and safely planned on the basis of serum calcitonin: 18 Years experience at one single center. J Clin Endocrinol Metab 2012. https://doi.org/10.1210/jc.2011-2046.

37. Essig GF, Porter K, Schneider D, et al. Multifocality in sporadic medullary thyroid carcinoma: an international multicenter study. Thyroid 2016. https://doi.org/10.1089/thy.2016.0255.

38. Machens A, Dralle H. Biomarker-based risk stratification for previously untreated medullary thyroid cancer. J Clin Endocrinol Metab 2010. https://doi.org/10.1210/jc.2009-2368.

39. Rohmer V, Vidal-Trecan G, Bourdelot A, et al. Prognostic factors of disease-free survival after thyroidectomy in 170 young patients with a RET germline mutation: a multicenter study of the Groupe Français d'Etude des Tumeurs Endocrines. J Clin Endocrinol Metab 2011. https://doi.org/10.1210/jc.2010-1234.

40. Martinez SR, Beal SH, Chen A, et al. Adjuvant external beam radiation for medullary thyroid carcinoma. J Surg Oncol 2010. https://doi.org/10.1002/jso.21557.

41. Pellegriti G, Leboulleux S, Baudin E, et al. Long-term outcome of medullary thyroid carcinoma in patients with normal postoperative medical imaging. Br J Cancer 2003. https://doi.org/10.1038/sj.bjc.6600930.

42. Franc S, Niccoli-Sire P, Cohen R, et al. Complete surgical lymph node resection does not prevent authentic recurrences of medullary thyroid carcinoma. Clin Endocrinol (Oxf) 2001. https://doi.org/10.1046/j.1365-2265.2001.01339.x.

43. Machens A, Schneyer U, Holzhausen HJ, et al. Prospects of remission in medullary thyroid carcinoma according to basal calcitonin level. J Clin Endocrinol Metab 2005. https://doi.org/10.1210/jc.2004-1836.

44. Giraudet AL, Vanel D, Leboulleux S, et al. Imaging medullary thyroid carcinoma with persistent elevated calcitonin levels. J Clin Endocrinol Metab 2007. https://doi.org/10.1210/jc.2007-1211.

45. Barbet J, Campion L, Kraeber-Bodéré F, et al. Prognostic impact of serum calcitonin and carcinoembryonic antigen doubling-times in patients with medullary thyroid carcinoma. J Clin Endocrinol Metab 2005. https://doi.org/10.1210/jc.2005-0044.

46. Giraudet AL, Al Ghulzan A, Aupérin A, et al. Progression of medullary thyroid carcinoma: Assessment with calcitonin and carcinoembryonic antigen doubling times. Eur J Endocrinol 2008. https://doi.org/10.1530/EJE-07-0667.

47. Tisell LE, Hansson G, Jansson S, et al. Reoperation in the treatment of asymptomatic metastasizing medullary thyroid carcinoma. Surgery 1986;99(1):60–6.

48. Fialkowski E, DeBenedetti M, Moley J. Long-term outcome of reoperations for medullary thyroid carcinoma. World J Surg 2008. https://doi.org/10.1007/s00268-007-9317-7.

49. Scollo C, Baudin E, Travagli JP, et al. Rationale for central and bilateral lymph node dissection in sporadic and hereditary medullary thyroid cancer. J Clin Endocrinol Metab 2003. https://doi.org/10.1210/jc.2002-021713.

50. Miccoli P, Minuto MN, Ugolini C, et al. Clinically unpredictable prognostic factors in the outcome of medullary thyroid cancer. Endocr Relat Cancer 2007. https://doi.org/10.1677/ERC-07-0128.

51. Viola D, Valerio L, Molinaro E, et al. Treatment of advanced thyroid cancer with targeted therapies: ten years of experience. Endocr Relat Cancer 2016;23(4):R185–205.

52. Romei C, Casella F, Tacito A, et al. New insights in the molecular signature of advanced medullary thyroid cancer: evidence of a bad outcome of cases with double RET mutations. J Med Genet 2016;53(11). https://doi.org/10.1136/jmedgenet-2016-103833.

53. Schlumberger MJ, Elisei R, Bastholt L, et al. Phase II study of safety and efficacy of motesanib in patients with progressive or symptomatic, advanced or metastatic medullary thyroid cancer. J Clin Oncol 2009. https://doi.org/10.1200/JCO.2008.18.7815.

54. Capdevila J, Trigo JM, Aller J, et al. Axitinib treatment in advanced RAI-resistant differentiated thyroid cancer (DTC) and refractory medullary thyroid cancer (MTC). Eur J Endocrinol 2017. https://doi.org/10.1530/EJE-17-0243.

55. Bible KC, Suman VJ, Molina JR, et al. A multicenter phase 2 trial of pazopanib in metastatic and progressive medullary thyroid carcinoma: MC057H. J Clin Endocrinol Metab 2014. https://doi.org/10.1210/jc.2013-3713.

56. Schlumberger M, Jarzab B, Cabanillas ME, et al. A phase II trial of the multitargeted tyrosine kinase inhibitor lenvatinib (E7080) in advanced medullary thyroid cancer. Clin Cancer Res 2016. https://doi.org/10.1158/1078-0432.CCR-15-1127.

57. Wells SA, Robinson BG, Gagel RF, et al. Vandetanib in patients with locally advanced or metastatic medullary thyroid cancer: a randomized, double-blind phase III trial. J Clin Oncol 2012. https://doi.org/10.1200/jco.2011.35.5040.

58. Elisei R, Schlumberger MJ, Müller SP, et al. Cabozantinib in progressive medullary thyroid cancer. J Clin Oncol 2013. https://doi.org/10.1200/JCO.2012.48.4659.

59. Schlumberger M, Elisei R, Müller S, et al. Overall survival analysis of EXAM, a phase III trial of cabozantinib in patients with radiographically progressive medullary thyroid carcinoma. Ann Oncol 2017. https://doi.org/10.1093/annonc/mdx479.

60. Matrone A, Valerio L, Pieruzzi L, et al. Protein kinase inhibitors for the treatment of advanced and progressive radiorefractory thyroid tumors: From the clinical trials to the real life. Best Pract Res Clin Endocrinol Metab 2017;31(3). https://doi.org/10.1016/j.beem.2017.06.001.

61. Subbiah V, Velcheti V, Tuch BB, et al. Selective RET kinase inhibition for patients with RET-altered cancers. Ann Oncol 2018. https://doi.org/10.1093/annonc/mdy137.

62. Subbiah V, Gainor JF, Rahal R, et al. Precision targeted therapy with BLU-667 for RET-driven cancers. Cancer Discov 2018. https://doi.org/10.1158/2159-8290.CD-18-0338.

Printed and bound by CPI Group (UK) Ltd, Croydon, CR0 4YY

08/05/2025

01864723-0009